# Philosophy and Medicine

Volume 137

The Philosophy and Medicine series is dedicated to publishing monographs and collections of essays that make important contributions to scholarship in bioethics and the philosophy of medicine. The series addresses the full scope of issues in bioethics and philosophy of medicine, from euthanasia to justice and solidarity in health care, and from the concept of disease to the phenomenology of illness. The Philosophy and Medicine series places the scholarship of bioethics within studies of basic problems in the epistemology, ethics, and metaphysics of medicine. The series seeks to publish the best of philosophical work from around the world and from all philosophical traditions directed to health care and the biomedical sciences. Since its appearance in 1975, the series has created an intellectual and scholarly focal point that frames the field of the philosophy of medicine and bioethics. From its inception, the series has recognized the breadth of philosophical concerns made salient by the biomedical sciences and the health care professions. With over one hundred and twenty-five volumes in print, no other series offers as substantial and significant a resource for philosophical scholarship regarding issues raised by medicine and the biomedical sciences.

More information about this series at http://www.springer.com/series/6414

Afifi al-Akiti • Aasim I. Padela
Editors

# Islam and Biomedicine

Springer

*Editors*
Afifi al-Akiti
Oxford Centre for Islamic Studies
Oxford, UK

Aasim I. Padela
Department of Emergency Medicine &
Institute for Health and Equity
Medical College of Wisconsin
Milwaukee, WI, USA

ISSN 0376-7418 ISSN 2215-0080 (electronic)
Philosophy and Medicine
ISBN 978-3-030-53800-2 ISBN 978-3-030-53801-9 (eBook)
https://doi.org/10.1007/978-3-030-53801-9



This Springer imprint is published by the registered company Springer Nature Switzerland AG
The registered company address is: Gewerbestrasse 11, 6330 Cham, Switzerland

# Preface

Although many deserve to be appreciated and acknowledged, not least of all those who contributed to our conversations throughout the journey, I wish to thank especially my project partner, Dr Aasim I. Padela, who has heroically been ever so patient with me in giving birth to this volume. It is arguably providential that the two partners – a theologian and a scientist, one originating from the world of *naql*, the other coming from the world of *ʿaql* – should meet and start this journey, and then complement each other, thus exemplifying what we do indeed believe, the true complementarity between both *Islam* and *Biomedicine*. We were indeed fortunate to have had the support from our patron, the Templeton Religion Trust, for our original joint-project entitled, 'Conversations on Islam and the Human Sciences.'[1] Special appreciation therefore is reserved for Michael Murray, at the John Templeton Foundation, who supported this project from conception through implementation and served as a critical interlocutor for the chapter authors, and W. Christopher Stewart who trusted our team to carry out the project under the auspices of the Templeton Religion Trust. I should also mention Professors Abdulaziz Sachedina and Omar Qureshi who also served as key interlocutors. Professor Sachedina doubled as a Keynote Speaker at the special dinner event billed as 'Trivia with the *ʿUlamāʾ*' (when there is nothing trivial about sitting with the *ʿulamāʾ* actually!), staged on the sidelines of the two-day Multidisciplinary Symposium and Workshop on Islam and Biomedicine at the University of Chicago in September 2018. That Symposium was indeed the return match from the weekly Seminar Series on 'Islam and Biomedicine' I had convened a year earlier at the Oxford Centre for Islamic Studies in Michaelmas Term 2017. For this, I would like to thank the Director of the Centre, Dr Farhan Nizami, CBE, who supported and allowed the Centre to host the project from the get-go.

Oxford, UK　　　　Afifi al-Akiti

[1] The project website is at: https://www.medicineandislam.org/conversations-on-islam-and-the-human-sciences

I echo Dato' Dr Afifi's sentiments in thanking our sponsors, chapter authors, and interlocutors. I am truly indebted to him for agreeing to embark on this project journey with me. We could not have produced this volume without his steadfastness in the face of obstacles, his trust in our abilities, and his scholarly insights. I also would like to thank Dr Don Fette Barrett at Arizona State University for his editorial assistance. Much gratitude goes to Drs Rosie Duivenbode and Shaheen Nageeb who supported the project in many ways and arranged our retreat and symposium at the University of Chicago. I also thank the volunteers, participants, and supporters for allowing that weekend to be one of much learning and camaraderie. I also acknowledge the hospitality of Dr Farhan Nizami and the Fellows at the Oxford Centre for Islamic Studies for hosting me and my family in Michaelmas Term 2017 so that Dr Afifi and I could work on this and other projects. Last but not least, all praise and gratitude are due to Allāh for arranging our affairs to make this all possible, may He make this work one of benefit to its readers.

Milwaukee, WI, USA Aasim I. Padela

# Contents

# Chapter 1
# Taking On the Ghazālian Challenge of Integrating Religion and Science in Islam and Biomedicine

**Afifi al-Akiti and Aasim I. Padela**

## 1.1 Introduction

Advances in the sciences, particularly in the biomedical and life sciences, have created a knowledge gap that leaves various Muslim lay persons feeling bewildered even as Muslim scientists and religious scholars (*ulamā*ʾ) labour to integrate religious teachings with new scientific knowledge. For example, breakthroughs in artificial intelligence technology force Muslim theologians to consider anew traditional ideas of sentience and the nature of the soul. Advanced predictive epidemiologic modelling techniques, such as those used to forecast COVID-19 disease spread and mortality, spur Muslim legists to reconsider classical views on the obligation of establishing congregational Friday prayer. And the human-animal chimeras used to grow organs in the lab pose multiple questions to Muslim scholars about the nature of a 'human' organ, as well as the ethical limits of biomedical research and healthcare enterprises. These topics are but the tip of the iceberg as biomedical development pushes new frontiers on a daily basis, and accordingly pushes religious scholars to bridge scientific discoveries and religious understandings.

This book, *Islam and Biomedicine*, engages this exciting problem-space by initiating conversations at the intersection of the Islamic intellectual tradition, specifically its theological, legal, and metaphysical frameworks, as well as the diverse

A. al-Akiti (✉)
Oxford Centre for Islamic Studies, Oxford, UK
e-mail: afifi.al-akiti@worc.ox.ac.uk

A. I. Padela
Department of Emergency Medicine & Institute for Health and Equity, Medical College of Wisconsin, Milwaukee, WI, USA
e-mail: apadela@mcw.edu



A. al-Akiti, A. I. Padela (eds.), *Islam and Biomedicine*, Philosophy and Medicine 137, https://doi.org/10.1007/978-3-030-53801-9_1

disciplines of biomedicine.[1] More specifically, our original project, supported generously by the Templeton Religion Trust, brought scholars from diverse backgrounds together in order to engage with the critical question of integration: how might scientific knowledge inform, and work with, the various Muslim theologies[2] on the nature of being and life.

Biomedical advancements herald new insights on the fundamental questions about the nature of human beings, the natural world, and the experiences of life. This new knowledge, coupled with the latest technological breakthroughs, increasingly enables humans, in their diverse societies, to shape the world according to their own vision. Consequently, while humankind grapples with the new possibilities brought about by biomedicine, religious understandings of life and death, as well as the notion of the human person itself, are debated and, at times, reconfigured. Certainly, the Islamic tradition is not immune to the vicissitudes and vagaries produced by modern biomedical science. Its teachings and frameworks are also reviewed, (re) developed, and at times, revised. Such engagement between Islam and biomedicine deserves focused study, and the chapters in this book seeds such research.

To be sure, although conversations have long taken place between the two traditions,[3] our colloquy here is unique in that it gathers together scholars whose academic and/or professional lives are devoted, in one way or another, to the intersection of Islam and biomedicine. As will be noted in greater detail shortly, this volume contains chapters authored by intellectual historians whose expertise is on medieval 'Islamic' medicine, Muslim physicians who conduct research on the healthcare and ethical challenges faced by Muslim patients, and Muslim theologians who focus on describing how science and theology come together within the intellectual tradition. Over the course of two years, this diverse group convened to exchange ideas, sharpen analyses, and discover how and where integration may be accomplished. This volume captures some of those rich conversations to reveal core challenges facing scholars working to integrate Islam and biomedicine. Perceived and, sometimes, actual conflicts emerge as a result of the competing ontological visions, different epistemic frameworks, and diverse theologies of life and living presented and upheld by these two bodies of knowledge. Such differences must be bridged in order for some form of integration to occur.

[1] The term 'biomedicine' refers to the multiple bodies of knowledge related to the biomedical enterprise within society, including the biological sciences, healthcare delivery, health policy, biolaw, and others.

[2] We use the term 'theology' here in its broadest sense to refer to the articulation of a worldview based on understandings and interpretations of the revealed texts of Islam. We acknowledge that there can be no singular Islamic/Muslim theology because theological exposition is undertaken in light of a particular hermeneutic and accompanying epistemological framework. It is also conducted within a particular context, and often in response to critical interlocutors, thus leading to multiple Muslim/Islamic theologies. At the same time, there is similarity and coherence among Muslim/Islamic theologies arising from their common focus on revealed texts and shared creeds.

[3] See, for example: Sachedina (2011), Pormann (2011), Sajoo (2008). For similar engagement in the Christian tradition: Austriaco (2011), Clark (2000); in the Jewish tradition: Rosner (2006); in the Buddhist tradition, see Unger and Ikeda (2016); and in the Hindu tradition: Crawford (2006).

This volume, therefore, presents part of the ongoing story of Muslim engagement with, and responses to, developments in biomedical science. Our hope is that these conversations will stimulate more robust interpretations of Islam, as well as of science, by Muslim theologians and jurists as they address issues of biosocial and biomedical concern. And conversely, a better appreciation among clinicians and scientists of the richness of understanding and of values that Islamic scholars bring to the dialogue as they draw upon scriptural disciplines. To put it another way, by bringing together theologians, clinicians, and intellectual historians, this volume seeks to draw sustained attention to the intersection of Islam and biomedicine and provide a foundation for dedicated research at the junction of these bodies of knowledge for many years to come.

## 1.2 The Ghazālian Challenge

This project was inspired by the historic theological engagement of one of Islam's most celebrated religious scholars, al-Ghazālī (d. 505/1111),[4] with the scientific tradition of his medieval world. Afifi al-Akiti has previously characterized Ghazālī's sustained attention to the challenge of integrating Islamic theology and science as one of 'the good, the bad, and the ugly.'[5] This crude Hollywood description, indeed, does express the results of a Muslim theologian's systematic engagement with any body of scientific knowledge. Al-Ghazālī suggests Muslim *ʿulamāʾ* have to urgently, positively, and engage fully with nature and the deliverables of science, because at times their skepticism of science may arise out of a hostile and unsympathetic reading of science, which in turn may have begun from doubts and uncertainty produced by unfamiliar or 'alien' scientific methods and data. Such misreadings lead to misadventures and generate much confusion. Of course, instead of engaging with the Greek-inspired Aristotelian science from Ghazālī's own time, we are contending with the contemporary biomedical sciences. And alongside changes in the nature and enterprise of today's science, the Islamic religious sciences have also developed and advanced from Ghazālī's time. This colloquy, therefore, is the first of many steps required on the challenging stairway that leads to a fruitful integration of contemporary biomedical knowledge with the faith and practice of Islam – a journey that both the *ʿulamāʾ* and the scientists need to embark upon together as enjoined by the great al-Ghazālī.

Today, unlike at the time of al-Ghazālī, the question of the nature and sources of *fides et ratio* or *naql wa-ʿaql* – one of revealed knowledge, the other of rational knowledge – is well-understood and their complementarity agreed upon by many,

[4] Where possible, the death years of pre-modern persons are given throughout this book; and where relevant, the *Anno Hegirae* (AH) year precedes the Common Era (CE) or *Anno Domini* (AD) year. When uncertain, converted *Hijrī* dates have been made approximate to the earliest possible year.

[5] Al-Akiti (2009).

though disputed by some.[6] The basic sources of the Islamic religion are primarily from revelation, while scientific knowledge *per se* is based on reason and rationality. Yet, many thinkers throughout the ages have sought a rapprochement between these two seemingly opposite epistemological sources. The Ghazālīan challenge, so to speak, for both the theologian and the scientist, is to harmonize. His own biography reflects an amazing intellectual journey undertaken by one of Islam's most gifted critical thinkers, and it also confirms al-Ghazālī as a man of deep spirituality and religious belief. Truly, his intellectual prowess and his faith equipped him to become one of the world's great harmonizers. In his works we see a dependence on God is still there: he is explicit in stating that all true knowledge, indeed whatever is, comes from Him, and all knowledge leads back to Him. In our volume as well, we see this suprarational spirit of al-Ghazālī throughout the strategies for integration proposed by the scholars who participated in this project. *Yet*, there was also an admirable and innovative spirit of rational inquiry in al-Ghazālī's writings, where blind faith in God was challenged and partially delimited, but never trivialized. He confidently declares that there is no true bifurcation between religion and science, but rather a complementarity exists between them. Al-Ghazālī expresses this paradox best for us, when he describes revealed knowledge (*sharʿ* = *naql*)[7] as 'an intellect (*ʿaql*) from outside of this world' and scientific knowledge (*ʿaql*) as 'a scripture (*sharʿ*) from within ourselves.'[8] Likewise, the spirit of our project on *Islam and Biomedicine* – in the face of the polarizing challenges posed by *naql* and *ʿaql*, especially at the outset of the long scholarly journey that our volume anticipates – presupposes a genuine complementarity between these knowledges.

## 1.3 The Chapters

As noted above, this volume has the modest aim of shedding light on a set of problems at the the intersection of two vast bodies of knowledge, the Islamic tradition and the biomedical sciences. Each of the authors, themselves situated at different junctions between these fields, brings to bear different analytic tools to describe, and at times propose solutions to, the thorny challenges of splicing together knowledge coming from the two fields. Some authors address theoretical challenges while others focus on more practical ones, and some deal with questions of epistemology while others tackle problems in law. Far from being disconnected, however, each chapter tackles the challenge of bridging the two fields at a slightly different register. In so doing the volume, as a whole, seeds future theoretical and applied research on Islam and biomedicine. In what follows we map out the journey the reader will undertake in

---

[6] See especially: Brooke and Numbers (2011), Morvillo (2010), Brooke (2014).

[7] The terms *sharʿ* (lit., path) and *naql* (lit., transmission) can be treated as synonyms and used interchangeably in Arabic to mean 'revelation' and 'scripture.' Although in this case al-Ghazālī employed the former, we prefer to use the latter here as it appears in consonance with *ʿaql*.

[8] Al-Ghazālī (1927), p. 60, ll. 7–8 (*bayān* 8): *fa-l-sharʿu ʿaqlun min khārijin wa-l-ʿaqlu sharʿun min dākhilin*.

this multidisciplinary volume by situating each author's contribution within the discourse.

Our journey begins with the first part of this book, *From Greek Sources to Islamic Conceptions of Health and Biomedicine*, containing four chapters which delve into biomedical epistemes, concepts, and frameworks in Islamic history and the tradition more broadly.

In Chap. 2, 'Medical Epistemology in Arabic Discourse: From Greek Sources to the Arabic Commentary Tradition,' Peter Pormann, a prominent historian of medicine and philosophy in the classical period, focuses on contentions regarding medical epistemology as they are discussed in the medieval Arabic exegetical corpus. In doing so he traces the science's Hellenic roots and describes the flowering of home-grown medical theoreticians as well as practitioners within the medieval Muslim world. When it comes to bridging Islam and biomedicine, his chapter informs us that the engagement between these two fields in the history of the Islamic civilization was fruitful and can even help guide discussions today.

Pormann handily walks us through the engagement with the Greek tradition on the part of three medical authors who all penned commentaries on the Hippocratic *Aphorisms*, namely Abū Bakr al-Rāzī (d. *ca.* 313/925), ʿAbd al-Laṭīf al-Baghdādī (d. 629/1231), and al-Kilānī (*fl. ca.* 750s/1350s). The *Canon of Medicine* (*al-Qānūn fī al-ṭibb*) by Avicenna (d. 428/1037) and one of the commentaries on it by Ibn al-Nafīs (d. 687/1288) also come under scrutiny. Pormann dissects both theoretical discussions about the nature of medical knowledge, and practical ones about the efficaciousness of drugs. He demonstrates that, far from merely receiving and preserving the body of Greek medical knowledge, the medieval Arabic commentaries on the *Aphorisms* were sites of germination. These medical writers – though not necessarily all Muslims – went beyond their Greek sources, be it by using a control group in a medical experiment, and defining conditions for the testing of drugs, or by qualifying medicine as 'knowledge of probabilities' and offering reflections on the physicians' inabilities to always get things right. This set of medieval conversations, involving mostly scholars from the *ʿaqlī* tradition embracing scientists and physicians, became a platform for intense debates about epistemology and the reality of disease and cure, and in turn set up the practices of biomedical research and patient care we take for granted today.

Debates about medical epistemology necessarily include discussions about health and disease. To this end, motivated in part by the Prophet's experience of illness, classical Islamic religious writings offer various definitions for health, disease, and healing. Indeed, religious scholars, the *ʿulamāʾ*, paid (and continue to pay) significant attention to these concepts because of the need to determine the moral status of seeking medical treatment and advise pious Muslims about how and why they need to care for their bodies. Moreover, Islamic bioethical advice needs to account for both ontological notions of God's control over health and healing, as well as theological and biomedical accounts of the human healer's role in moving individuals from states of illness to states of well-being.

The next chapter in the volume assists us in thinking about how to align such theological and biomedical views in constructing health. Chapter 3, 'The Piety of Health: The Making of Health in Islamic Religious Narratives,' deals directly with the challenges of conceptualizing 'health' from an Islamic lens. Ahmed Ragab, an intellectual historian of Islam who has also undergone medical training, investigates the concept as a medical, theological, and socio-cultural category. In doing so, he asks, firstly, whether health is a divine blessing, and analyses the behaviours and attitudes expected from healthy, pious believers. Secondly, he considers health as a natural, but fragile physical state that requires active maintenance and preservation. Finally, he considers health as the antithesis of illness, and explores debates found in the theological texts around the legality (and/or desirability) of seeking medical treatment, and the attendant pietistic debates around being patient and relying on God (*tawakkul*).

Ragab skilfully demonstrates the pietistic tension brought about by the *naqlī* tradition like the famous *ḥadīth*, 'God has not created an illness without also creating a cure for it.'[9] He shows that the role of sickness in the pietistic cosmology posed important questions about the appropriateness of seeking cure and whether it was better for Muslims to withstand illness and not seek help. Resolving these tensions within Islamic ethics and law turns on the conceptualization of health, and may demand that we resist definitions of health and healing which draw solely upon the biomedical sciences.

Taking off from Ragab's preliminaries on cosmology and integration, Chap. 4, 'The Concept of a Human Microcosm: Exploring Possibilities for a Synthesis of Traditional and Modern Biomedicine,' tackles these higher-up issues more directly. Osman Bakar, an eminent Muslim philosopher whose work revolves around scientific thought in the tradition, introduces us to the notion of the 'human microcosm' in Islamic philosophy. This idea, as understood from within the intellectual tradition, is important to natural theology as well as more applied branches of knowledge like medicine. Following many famous Muslim theologians and philosophers before him, Bakar identifies the three most important constituent parts of the human microcosm as the body (*jism*), the soul (*nafs*), and the spirit (*rūḥ*). In the past, attempts were made to harmonize the theological and the scientific approaches to the formulation and understanding of the interrelationships linking these three microcosmic entities. While the two approaches were held to be complementary to each other, in this chapter, he tries to formulate the biological dimension of these microcosmic interrelationships and its implications for the theory and practice of medicine. In his view, the human microcosm must be viewed as bearing a certain 'relationship of correspondence' with its macrocosmic counterpart, and this correspondence when considered at a biological level can inform medical theory and practice in the contemporary era. His work makes tentative arguments and offers entry-points for synthesizing medical understandings and philosophical ones. In the end, Bakar argues that the 'atomistic' and mechanistic approach to the treatment of the human body in present-day biomedical science sharply contrasts with the holistic and qualitative approach that a traditional Islamic biomedicine did/would stand for. While these two 'biomedicines' have their respective merits and virtues, he encourages an epistemological synthesis and outlines what, tentatively, such a synthesis would entail.

[9] This *ḥadīth* has many different versions and narrators, one example is in al-Bukhārī (1422/2001), 7:122 (*ḥadīth* no. 5678).

The concluding chapter of this section is Adi Setia Md. Dom's discussion on 'Islamic Ethics in Engagement with Life, Health, and Medicine.' This chapter takes a critical analytic approach and lays bare the many salient aspects of modern medicine that may pose challenges to Islamic conceptions of life, health, and general well-being. He explores these issues first at the metaphysical and theoretical level – through first principles, theories, and methodology – and thereafter at the practical level of ethics and law. Any integration between the concepts, theories, and applications of 'Islam' and 'biomedicine' demands that the critiques he levels be taken seriously. Following in Ghazālian footsteps, Adi Setia systematically engages with the 'good, the bad, and the ugly' of biomedical science. He does this by drawing upon pertinent insights from the rich history of the analytical engagement of Muslim theologians and philosophers with the received Hellenistic medical and scientific tradition. He then levels a wide-ranging critique and rethinking of the premises, methods, practices, and ethics of contemporary biomedicine. Here Adi Setia observes the rising problem of the 'divergence between technics and ethics.'[10] He argues that this has become acute, for instance in the current era of -omics research and machine learning with its tendency to downplay the reality that ethics should concern human agency. He further contends that the biomechanical model of medicine tends to marry biological to technological determinism, and maintains that it is both unintellectual and unethical to allow this double determinism to subvert traditional Islamic understandings of human nature, namely that mankind is a free moral agent capable of choice (*ikhtiyār*), in fact 'to choose for the better,' and hence invested with responsibility and accountability for the consequences of his or her actions. Adi Setia continues by arguing that if ethics is to be taken seriously it has to be taken *structurally* as a proactive point of departure, and applied consistently throughout the 'value chain' of any medical procedures and techniques, including the whole process of decision-making involved in their design, fabrication, and deployment in research to their actual therapeutical deployment, from upstream to midstream to downstream. Otherwise ethics runs the risk of becoming a mere afterthought, an *ad hoc*, overly reactive appendage to an essentially amoral biomedical enterprise in which the technical systemically overrides the ethical by *subsuming* it.

The second part of the book, *The Meaning of Life and Death*, consists of five chapters. It begins with the primordial question, 'When Does a Human Foetus Become Human?' Chapter 6 is authored by Hamza Yusuf, one of the most influential Muslim theologians in the West. Yusuf is helped in his analysis by his dual training as a theologian and a nurse, and weaves together metaphysical and legal discussions within the Islamic tradition with biomedical and sociological controversies about abortion and infanticide. He investigates the idea of the soul and the definition of life by skilfully navigating the scriptural and theological texts of Islam and comparing such received understandings with how biomedical scientists today define the concept of life, particularly as it relates to practices of contraception and abortion.

Hamza Yusuf argues that the traditional 'ensoulment' (*nafkh al-rūḥ*) date of 120 days – the minimum threshold by which the majority of classical Sunnī Muslim

[10] Adi Setia, 116 (Chap. 5, below).

jurists, especially Shāfiʿīs and Ḥanafīs, qualifiedly permitted abortion – was based on a misunderstanding of the biomedical knowledge underpinning it. This point is debated in the literature, for example, in a co-authored work, Aasim I. Padela notes that classical Ḥanafī jurists were well aware that the human form took shape much earlier than 120 days post-conception. Some preferred to interpret the Prophetic tradition declaring ensoulment at 120 days as a metaphysical occurrence while others viewed the ḥadīth to also have a physical manifestation. As a result two different views regarding the relative prohibition of abortion arose.[11] Nonetheless, Hamza Yusuf argues for a downward revision of that period to within 40 days based on the biomedical fact that both the nervous and circulatory systems begin to function at that time. We thus see the chapter propose an integration of sorts between the Islamic and the biomedical where biomedical data inform ethico-legal judgements and interpretation of metaphysical realities, albeit in a limited way. In making this call to reconsider Islamic legal rulings regarding abortion, Hamza Yusuf is making common cause not only with al-Ghazālī, but also with the medieval scholar often regarded as his nemesis, Ibn Taymiyya (d. 728/1328). On this controversial biomedical issue, both Muslim theologians were ardently against abortion as a practice. This chapter thus offers an interesting real-life example of how understanding the *ʿaqlī* tradition might lead to a revision in the understanding of the *naqlī* texts.

In Chap. 7, 'Where the Two Oceans Meet: The Theology of Islam and the Philosophy of Psychiatric Medicine in Exploring the Human Self,' Asim Yusuf, a psychiatrist and an Imam serving the British Muslim community, and Afifi al-Akiti, a Muslim theologian and the principal editor of the present volume, expand our understanding of mental health and its dysfunction by working with the Islamic tradition and the biomedical one in parallel. The question of mental health is core to Asim Yusuf's identity as a psychiatrist and a religious counselor, and the chapter advances to a practical discussion by first working through the lens of philosophy of medicine and philosophy of religion, describing where they overlap and interface with each other. The authors state that any theory of mental well-being that does not tackle the fundamental theological ideas of the mind and its functions cannot claim to be thoroughgoing. They thus investigate the various theories of the nature of the human being, evaluating medical, scriptural, theological, philosophical, and even mystical formulations of these ideas. Thereafter, they examine how notions of function and dysfunction of the mind become explicable in relation to Islamic understandings of the origin of humankind and its ultimate purpose, and thus the meaning of human life – in terms of their usefulness for achieving a 'holistic, bio-psycho-socio-spiritual model' of mental well-being and illness.

At the root of it, the chapter seeks to interrogate, via the notion of a mental illness, the bedrock assumptions upon which medicine and psychiatry are founded. Respectively, these are: 'what is life/health?' and 'what is self/mind?' The authors explore the limitations of a purely naturalistic or mechanistic approach to these questions, and examine what a religious metaphysical perspective might add. In unpacking the meanings of life and health, they touch upon holistic and reductionist

[11] Stodolsky and Padela (2021), 127–136.

approaches (the biopsychosocial and medical models respectively), before exploring naturalistic and Islamic theological perspectives on the nature and purpose of life – the preservation and quality of which is the final goal of seeking health. They ultimately proffer a unique consideration, that life and health are *desiderata* because they are necessary preconditions to experience God and 'Ultimate Reality.' Turning to the idea of the 'self,' they examine two approaches to modern psychiatry (the minimalist and strong medical models), as well as the closely allied field of cognitive neuroscience, in terms of their exploration of the nature of selfhood: what it is, how it arises, and why is it there. Again, this chapter seeks to demonstrate the inadequacies of a purely reductive, naturalistic approach. The authors then proceed to consider the strengths and drawbacks of three classical Islamic approaches to the idea of the soul and its relationship with the body, before providing an integrative account of the unitary self. They incorporate scripture and classical theological frameworks with contemporary scientific understandings to suggest that the human entity is equipped with consciousness, sentience, physical faculties, and a higher intellect in order to experience fully and respond to Ultimate Reality – which constitute the purpose and goal of human existence. Having drawn Islamic and biomedical models together the authors argue that it is possible to attempt a non-contradictory and satisfactory answer to the descriptive, explanatory, and functional questions of consciousness. Although the scientific approach finds accounting for the nature of the self to be problematic, it is largely silent on its purpose; meanwhile the religious approach is largely silent or out-of-date on the mechanics of mind-body interactivity. The 'sciences' must work together to fill in the gaps and thereby enhance or even advance our collective understanding. As they sharply put the *ʿaql-naql* conundrum: 'It is at the mingling of the waters of science and religion, then, that the answer may be found, provided one abandons an *a priori* commitment to metaphysical naturalism.'[12]

Chapter 8, 'Muslim Values and End-of-Life Healthcare Decision-making: Values, Norms and Ontologies in Conflict?', is written by Mehrunisha Suleman, a bioethicist with training in both clinical medicine and in Islamic theology. In this chapter, she notes that receiving religiously sensitive end-of-life healthcare is increasingly important to British Muslims because the population is both increasing in religiosity and advancing in age. Through a qualitative study of the experiences, practices, and moral deliberations of patients, clinicians, and chaplains, she examines how religious values and notions interact with biomedical paradigms in end-of-life healthcare delivery. The challenge at this intersection of Islam with biomedicine is that Muslim beliefs and practices in relation to death and dying emerge from a deep commitment to a metaphysical reality that is independent of empirical knowledge. Yet, within biomedicine, empirical studies such as randomized-control trials and meta-analyses establish healthcare values and best practices.

Suleman's thematic analysis of over 70 interviews reveals deep friction over the integration of biomedical knowledge with the theological understandings of death and dying. Families and clinicians struggle with understanding each other's worldviews and values, and in making decisions that balance theology with science.

---

[12] Asim Yusuf and Afifi al-Akiti, 175 (Chap. 7, below).

Notably, patients, chaplains, and physicians alike rely on multiple sources to make prudential decisions about end-of-life care (scientific biomedicine being only one source), and they face anxiety and frustration when the different sources come into conflict. Despite this, her study reveals active synchronicity between Islam and biomedicine in decision-making in end-of-life care. This is embodied by Muslim chaplains who are literate in the two traditions and can bridge perceived divides between clinicians and families. This dual expertise enables the appropriate translation of values, beliefs, and practices of faith alongside an evaluation of scientific data in joint deliberations over clinical goals. Her piece emphasizes the growing need for such experts who can navigate both spheres of knowledge, i.e., understanding and practice, in hospital and community settings.

Rafaqat Rashid, a practising physician who is also a Muslim theologian, authors the final chapter in this section. Entitled 'The Intersection between Science and Sunnī Theological and Legal Discourse in Defining Medical Death,' Chap. 9 explores the relationship between the body, the soul, and the mind, through the writings of various Muslim theologians in history. This exploration aims at defining the death of the individual from within the religious tradition. Next Rafaqat Rashid analyses the various ways in which death is defined and/or diagnosed in biomedicine to see where the tradition of Islam may support such medical notions. The chapter also discusses controversies, both biomedical and religious, over notions of 'brain death'[13] and the meaning of consciousness in order to map out the difficult terrain more fully. In the end he offers a pragmatic solution that accepts biomedical notions but also coheres with some theological notions of death. Thus he calls for the notion of *physiological* death to guide Muslim patients, physicians, and jurists, when participating in end-of-life healthcare decision-making.

The final and third part of the book, *Interfacing Biomedical Knowledge and Islamic Theology*, consists of four chapters. It begins with a chapter that addresses discursive methods and how analyses of the deliverables and truth claims of science should take place. Written by Omar Qureshi, an academic with advanced training in education and Islamic theology presently serving as Provost for a Muslim liberal arts college, alongside the editors of this volume, Afifi al-Akiti and Aasim I. Padela, Chap. 10 is titled 'Islam and Science: Reorienting the Discourse.'

While our project sought to address how the religious and biomedical sciences might be integrated, this chapter concedes that one approach might be to side-line specific products, and accompanying truth claims, of one type of knowledge with respect to the other. Indeed, discourses abound regarding the relationship between religion and science, where researchers and scholars, in peer-reviewed publications, lectures, and even on social media, debate the conflict or compatibility between these two bodies of knowledge. In recent years these debates have entered the Islamic world, and Muslim scientists and the *ʿulamāʾ* assess how Western philosophical and Christian perspectives on the debate compare with Islamic

[13] For an overview of some of these controversies: Padela, Arozullah, and Moosa (2013): 132–139; and Padela and Basser (2012): 433.

understandings of science and religion. Qureshi, al-Akiti, and Padela contend that at present, many of these discussions appear broad and superficial, invoking thin conceptions of Islam and science. This has resulted in piecemeal solutions for boundary negotiation between the claims of religion and of modern science. As scholarly work at the intersection of Islam and biomedicine increases, a deeper engagement is needed, in which substantive conceptions of both religious tradition and contemporary science are brought together to facilitate a meaningful, fruitful dialogue between the two.

They note that the truth claims of science and of religion are both developed through particular self-contained sets of assumptions and suppositions about knowledge and reality. So they propose that on the Islamic side, the dialogue with science (and hence biomedicine) should be based on the scholastic methods and results established by one of the schools of theology and law in the Islamic tradition. Engaging modern science from within a particular Islamic school will allow fundamental metaphysical and doctrinal commitments to be put into the foreground, and they contend that this will facilitate negotiations about how empirical findings and posited knowledge about nature can be accommodated in light of established theological frameworks and authority structures of the Islamic tradition.

This part of the book continues with 'Science in the Framework of Islamic Legal Epistemology: An Exploratory Essay,' by Kamaluddin Ahmed, an academically and seminary-trained Muslim theologian. Chapter 11 reflects upon the understandings of life and humanity as received from modern biomedicine and from the Islamic tradition. This chapter intersects with, and offers slightly different vantage-points upon, moral and analytic questions addressed by the preceding chapters authored by Hamza Yusuf, Asim Yusuf, Afifi al-Akiti, and Rafaqat Rashid.

Kamaluddin Ahmed's core concern is the metaphysical and existential question of what constitutes human life. He traces how this question was traditionally approached by the Muslim *ʿulamā*, through verses in the Qur'an and Prophetic reports that talk about the developmental stages in human embryology. Yet, in biomedicine, the question is addressed with different data sources; genetic analyses affirm that the fertilized zygote is a unique creature and can be used to predict aspects of its functioning and behaviour. The main thrust of the chapter is to utilize the sciences of Islamic law and legal epistemology (*fiqh* and *uṣūl al-fiqh*) to offer strategies for reconciling disparities between how modern biomedicine and the Islamic tradition resolve this question and related matters. Indeed, the perceived tensions arise from the separation of revealed and/or *naqlī* knowledge and non-revealed and/or *ʿaqlī* knowledge.

Kamaluddin Ahmed recounts how the early Muslim *ʿulamāʾ* were not only aware of these separate domains, but that they pragmatically assessed how non-revelatory sources of knowledge might complement revealed knowledge. Here he suggests that Muslim jurists have always ascribed value to knowledge that comes from non-revelatory sources. Such knowledge has even informed their understanding and application of Islamic law (*fiqh*). His resolution thus comes from the epistemic values ascribed to customary practices, *ʿurf,* and to rational empiricism, *ʿaql.* Ahmed argues that the notion of *ʿurf* – which usually refers to prevailing customs and practices of society that constitute *social* reality – can be used to evaluate, and at times incorporate, certain scientific claims. Similarly, empirical claims can be graded by jurists as *ʿaql* and thus be used to generate better understandings of the world and derive more nuanced legal rulings. Thus natural and social scientific data and understandings find entry-points into the Islamic tradition. In other words, when scientific truth claims are plotted on the same scale of probabilities (*ẓann*) and certainties (*qaṭʿ*) that Muslim jurists use to classify sources of knowledge such as rational empiricism (*ʿaql)* and customary practices (*ʿurf*), some *empirical* and *social* realities may be integrated within the tradition without any resultant confrontation or contradiction with scriptural revelation and prophecy.

While reproductive technology has overcome intractable infertility conditions, genetic technology has opened a major new chapter in the history of medicine. Despite impressive achievements, however, these technologies raise serious concerns over their potential impact on both existing and prospective family members. Muslim responses to these concerns reveal a sober realization that these technologies pose significant challenges to various aspects of Muslim theology. That is the central thrust of the penultimate chapter, Chap. 12, 'Interface between Islamic Law and Science: Ethico-Legal Construction of Science in Light of Islamic Bioethical Discourses on Genetic and Reproductive Technologies,' contributed by Ayman Shabana, an al-Azhar and UCLA-trained Islamic legal scholar.

Like Kamaluddin Ahmed, Shabana examines how biomedical data can be integrated within the traditional frameworks of Islamic law to resolve tensions between the two bodies of knowledge. Shabana draws upon the deliberations of prominent jurists and juridical councils to investigate several important questions at the intersection of Islam and biomedicine including: To what extent does science, as an alternative body of positive knowledge that does not recognize religious or metaphysical assumptions, play a role in Islamic bioethical discourses? And to what extent does science aid or challenge the normative authority of the Islamic legal tradition? Ultimately, Shabana demonstrates that preeminent jurists and juridical councils are open to biomedical understandings, yet they are also wary of the ethical values that underpin the biomedical enterprise. They see themselves as addressing the needs of Muslims struggling with questions about personal health and health policy, but also as 'ethical gate-keepers' trying to separate the wheat from the chaff when it comes to accepting biomedical science and technology coming from the 'West.' Shabana's description of the discursive and reasoning exercises suggest that the medical *fiqh* academies do not follow the school-based approach proposed by Qureshi, al-Akiti, and Padela. The analysis also suggests that the uptake of biomedical science and technology is fraught with some measure of inconsistency as some biomedical applications are embraced, while others are rejected without convincing yardsticks. Moreover, as Aasim I. Padela has demonstrated, the embrace of assisted reproductive technologies by juridical councils in order to solve infertility necessitates a biomedicalization of childlessness into disease and an acceptance, more or less, of biomedical (read: genetic) definitions of parenthood. Yet, in order to maintain an ethical gate-keeping function, this embrace of biomedicine cannot be a full one; the Qur'an does not recognize childlessness as a disease to be remedied, and Islamic law recognizes lineal bonds on the basis of social rearing or marital ties in addition to genetic ones.[14] Shabana's chapter thus calls for greater research into how juridical councils incorporate the various biomedical sciences into their legal deliberation, and for identifying the pros and cons of various methods of integrating the two bodies of knowledge in Islamic bioethical deliberation.

The final chapter of the book, Chap. 13, 'Integrating Science and Scripture to Produce Moral Knowledge: Assessing *Maṣlaḥa* and *Ḍarūra* in Islamic Bioethics,' is authored by Aasim I. Padela. A physician-bioethicist with advanced training in Islamic moral theology, Padela's chapter intersects with Shabana's in that it relates to producing moral knowledge within the field of Islamic bioethics. It also relates to Kamaluddin Ahmed's chapter by addressing how natural and social scientific realities may inform Islamic ethico-legal constructs.

We know that as scientific knowledge advances and societies grow ever more complex, religious traditions struggle to provide a moral compass for humanity. Often, Muslim theologians and jurists encounter difficulties in bridging the separate worlds of *ʿaql* and *naql*, scripture and science, religion and reason, and traditional and modern epistemic frameworks. Drawing upon the epistemological ideas of Thomas F. Torrance (d. 2009) about the relational structure and constructivist nature of knowledge, as well as borrowing from various Islamic theories of knowledge and law, Padela describes a conceptual framework and process model for generating 'new' moral knowledge. Principally, he argues that the notions of *maṣlaḥa* (human interest/societal benefit) and *ḍarūra* (dire necessity) relate to social realities, and thus jurists who apply these concepts to address contemporary biomedical questions must tie scriptural insights and social scientific understandings together. Only by integrating these knowledges can the essential moral goal of Islam 'to forestall harms and procure benefits' (*dar' al-mafāsid wa-jalb al-maṣāliḥ*) be actualized. To illustrate the utility of this model, Padela turns to the case of organ donation. In his case study, he demarcates specific biomedical and social scientific data needed in order to delineate, properly, Islamic perspectives on the moral status of donation as well as address pressing policy issues surrounding organ donation and transplantation.

It is fitting indeed that we have adjourned, but not ended, this journey into the Islam and biomedicine discourse with a biomedical scientist's reflections on integrating science and scripture – just as we opened the book with a theologian's thoughts on framing the challenge of integration as 'Ghazālian' in nature.

## References

al-Akiti, Afifi. 2009. 'The Good, the Bad, and the Ugly of *Falsafa*: Al-Ghazālī's *Maḍnūn*, *Tahāfut*, and *Maqāṣid*, with Particular Attention to Their *Falsafī* Treatments of God's Knowledge of Temporal Events. In *Avicenna and His Legacy: A Golden Age of Science and Philosophy*,

[14] See: Padela, Klima and Duivenbode (2020): 17–37.

ed. Y. Tzvi Langermann. Cultural Encounters in Late Antiquity and the Middle Ages, no. 8. Turnhout: Brepols.

Austriaco, Nicanor Pier Giorgio. 2011. *Biomedicine and Beatitude: An Introduction to Catholic Bioethics*. Washington, DC: The Catholic University of America Press.

Brooke, John Hedley. 2014. *Science and Religion: Some Historical Perspectives*. Cambridge: Cambridge University Press.

Brooke, John Hedley, and Ronald L. Numbers, eds. 2011. *Science and Religion around the World*. Oxford: Oxford University Press.

al-Bukhārī. 1422/2001. *Ṣaḥīḥ al-Imām al-Bukhārī al-musammá al-Jāmiʿ al-musnad al-ṣaḥīḥ al-mukhtaṣar min umūr Rasūl Allāh wa-sunanihi wa-ayyāmih*, ed. Muḥammad Zuhayr ibn Nāṣir al-Nāṣir (the Sulṭāniyya edition). 9 vols. Beirut: Dār Ṭawq al-Najāh.

Clark, Stephen R. L. 2000. *Biology and Christian Ethics*. Cambridge: Cambridge University Press.

Crawford, S. Cromwell. 2006. *Hindu Bioethics for the Twenty-first Century*. Albany, NY: SUNY Press.

al-Ghazālī. 1927. *Maʿārij al-quds fī madārij maʿrifat al-nafs*, ed. Muḥyī al-Dīn Ṣabrī al-Kurdī. Cairo: Maṭbaʿat al-Saʿāda.

Morvillo, Nancy. 2010. *Science and Religion: Understanding the Issues*. Malden, MA: Wiley-Blackwell.

Padela, Aasim I., and Taha A. Basser. 2012. 'Brain Death: The Challenges of Translating Medical Science into Islamic Bioethical Discourse.' *Medicine and Law* 31 (3): 433–450.

Padela, Aasim I., Ahsan Arozullah, and Ebrahim Moosa. 2013. 'Brain Death in Islamic Ethico-Legal Deliberation: Challenges for Applied Islamic Bioethics.' *Bioethics* 27 (3): 132–139.

Padela, Aasim I., Katherine Klima, and Rosie Duivenbode. 2020. 'Producing Parenthood: Islamic Bioethical Perspectives and Normative Implications.' *The New Bioethics* 26 (1): 17–37.

Pormann, Peter E., ed. 2011. *Islamic Medical and Scientific Tradition*. Critical Concepts in Islamic Studies, 4 vols. London: Routledge.

Rosner, Fred. 2006. *Contemporary Biomedical Ethical Issues and Jewish Law*. Hoboken, NJ: Ktav Publishing.

Sachedina, Abdulaziz. 2011. *Islamic Biomedical Ethics: Principles and Application*. Oxford: Oxford University Press.

Sajoo, Amyn B. 2008. *Muslim Ethics: Emerging Vistas*. London: IB Tauris.

Stodolsky, Muhammed V., and Aasim I. Padela. 2021. 'Abortion in Hanafī Law.' In *Global Positions and Practices, Religious and Legal Perspectives*, ed. Alireza Bagheri. Cham: Springer.

Unger, Felix, and Daisaku Ikeda. 2016. *The Humanist Principle: On Compassion and Tolerance*. London: IB Tauris.

**Dato' Dr Afifi al-Akiti** is the Kuwait Fellow in Islamic Studies at the Oxford Centre for Islamic Studies, and teaches in the Faculty of Theology, University of Oxford. He is a Fellow of Worcester College, Oxford. Dato' Afifi is trained as a theologian in both the Islamic and Western traditions. His areas of expertise are Islamic theology, law, and science. He has worked on several BBC documentaries, including the award-winning *Science and Islam* (2009). Since 2010, Dato' Dr Afifi has been listed in *The Muslim 500: The World's 500 Most Influential Muslims*.

**Dr Aasim I. Padela** is a clinician, health researcher, and bioethicist at the Medical College of Wisconsin. He utilizes methodologies from health services research, religious studies, and comparative ethics to examine the encounter of Islam with contemporary biomedicine through the lives of Muslim patients and clinicians, and in the writings of Islamic scholars. His scholarship develops intellectual frameworks through which Islamic theology (both moral and scholastic) can engage with contemporary natural and social scientific data.

# Part I
# From Greek Sources to Islamic Conceptions of Health and Biomedicine

# Chapter 2
# Medical Epistemology in Arabic Discourse: From Greek Sources to the Arabic Commentary Tradition

**Peter E. Pormann**

*Medical practice has been evidence-based since antiquity. What has changed is our understanding of what constitutes evidence*

(Edwards 2004: 1657).

## 2.1 Introduction

Philosophy is sometimes (if erroneously) described as a series of footnotes to Plato (d. *ca.* 347 BC). Likewise, one could argue (erroneously, I hasten to say) that modern medical theory and practice constitutes a series of footnotes to Hippocrates; after all, the main topics of medicine such as physiology, aetiology, deontology, nosology, therapeutics, surgery, and gynaecology all figure in the *Hippocratic Corpus*.[1] And yet modern medical theory and practice both are totally different from that of antiquity, the Middle Ages, and the Renaissance, when the model of humoral pathology dominated, namely the idea that health consists of a balance of the four humours, black bile, yellow bile, blood, and phlegm. There is one area of ancient medicine, however, that still grapples with the same problems as modern medicine: epistemology. Can we know the inner workings of the body? How do we find new treatments? And how can we ascertain whether a given drug works?

It is for this reason that I have chosen to contribute an essay on this topic, especially since so many interesting things were happening in the field of medical epistemology in the medieval Islamic world. Physicians there innovated in many areas

[1] For a recent overview of both Hippocrates and the *Hippocratic Corpus*, see Pormann (2018b).

P. E. Pormann (✉)
University of Manchester, Manchester, UK
e-mail: peter.pormann@manchester.ac.uk



A. al-Akiti, A. I. Padela (eds.), *Islam and Biomedicine*, Philosophy and Medicine 137, https://doi.org/10.1007/978-3-030-53801-9_2

and did not just receive and preserve the heritage of the Greeks.[2] And yet it is important to comprehend the Greek antecedents in order to understand the later Arabic debates. For this reason, I shall first review the main strands of medical epistemology in Antiquity, and look at how Greek ideas were adopted and adapted through translation into Arabic. Throughout this chapter, one focus will be commentary discourse. Commentaries are often seen as derivative and their authors as lacking critical thinking, but the examples here will show that nothing could be further from the truth. For instance, the first Hippocratic Aphorism ('Life is short, the Art long, …') led to interesting debates about medical epistemology.

The arguably most innovative medieval clinician, Abū Bakr al-Rāzī (d. *ca.* 313/925), for instance, produced arguments about testing therapies against the backdrop of another influential Hippocratic work, the *Epidemics*, and we shall look at the question whether he developed the notion of group thinking and the use of control groups. Next comes the discussion by Avicenna (d. 428/1037) of what conditions need to be met in order for drug tests to be valid. His *Canon of Medicine* attracted an enormous amount of exegetical activity, and we shall consider how one commentator, Ibn al-Nafīs (d. 687/1288), interpreted Avicenna. A sharp critic of Avicenna was ʿAbd al-Laṭīf al-Baghdādī (d. 629/1231), who talks about medicine as 'knowledge of probabilities (*maʿrifa aktharīyya*)' and reflects on uncertainties in medical practice. Finally, we shall discuss another commentary on the *Aphorisms* by al-Kilānī (*fl. ca.* 750s/1350s), who offers a fascinating take on the concept of qualified experience, an idea first developed by Galen of Pergamum (d. 216). It is to these Greek antecedents that we shall now turn.

## 2.2 Greek Background

Debates about medical epistemology go back to the beginning of Greek medical literature, and notably the *Hippocratic Corpus*.[3] This *Corpus* consists of a group of texts from the fifth century BC to the first and second centuries AD which are all attributed to Hippocrates. Although there can be no doubt that a famous physician called Hippocrates lived some time in the second half of the fifth century BC, scholars now are sceptical whether we will ever know for certain which works in the *Corpus* were written by the historical Hippocrates.[4] The most important and sophisticated work in terms of epistemology is *On Ancient Medicine*.[5] Although several modern scholars regard it as potentially reflecting Hippocrates' views, it was, nevertheless, not translated into Arabic and had no impact on the Arabic medical tradition. The reason for this is that Galen of Pergamum regarded this work as spurious, and therefore the Arabic translators did not bother with it.

---

[2] See Pormann (2018a).

[3] Craik (2015).

[4] Van der Eijk (2016), 15–47.

[5] Hippocrates (2005).

Epistemology does, however, also feature in other works of the *Hippocratic Corpus*. Arguably the most famous example is *Aphorisms* 1.1, which runs as follows:

> ὁ βίος βραχὺς, ἡ δὲ τέχνη μακρὴ, ὁ δὲ καιρὸς ὀξὺς, ἡ δὲ πεῖρα σφαλερὴ, ἡ δὲ κρίσις χαλεπή. δεῖ δὲ οὐ μόνον ἑωυτὸν παρέχειν τὰ δέοντα ποιεῦντα, ἀλλὰ καὶ τὸν νοσέοντα, καὶ τοὺς παρεόντας, καὶ τὰ ἔξωθεν.
>
> العمر قصير والصناعة طويلة والوقت ضيّق والتجربة خطر والقضاء عسر. وقد ينبغي أن لك لا تقتصر على توخّي فعل ما ينبغي دون أن يكون ما يفعله المريض ومن يحضره كذلك والأشياء التي من خارج.
>
> Life is short, and the Art long; the crisis fleeting; experiment perilous; and decision difficult. The physician must not only be prepared to do what is right himself, but also to make the patient, the attendants, and externals cooperate.

This first aphorism encompasses two parts: one that makes five statements related to the art of medicine; and another that provides an ethical injunction not just to the doctor, but also the patient and the entourage. Although both parts had an enormous influence, let us look at the first part in particular here, and notably the statement that 'experience is perilous, and decision difficult (*al-tajribatu khaṭarun wa-l-qaḍāʾu ʿaṣirun*).' It raises the question of how experience relates to medical judgment, and also whether there are other sources of medical knowledge.

The most important Greek commentator, Galen of Pergamum, also penned a number of highly influential works in this area, the most famous being his *On the Sects for Beginners* (Gk. Περὶ αἱρέσεων τοῖς εἰσαγομένοις; Ar. *Fī firaq al-ṭibb*).[6] In it, he distinguished three 'sects' or 'medical schools': the 'rationalists' (Gk. οἱ λογικοί; Ar. *aṣḥāb al-qiyās*); the 'empiricists' (Gk. οἱ ἐμπειρικοί, Ar. *aṣḥāb al-tajriba*); and the so-called 'methodists' (Gk. οἱ μεθοδικοί; Ar. *aṣḥāb al-ḥiyal*), not to be confused with the Christian church founded by John Wesley (d. 1791). For these methodists, Galen had only scorn, and we need not concern ourselves with them here.

But the first two sects represent important epistemological positions.[7] The rationalists argued that one had to use reason to understand the inner workings of the body, and therefore also favoured dissection. Only when one understands the causal relations between the patient and the disease, can one develop the right therapy. The empiricists adopted a sceptical position, saying that the human body is too complex for us to understand its various functions; they therefore also rejected dissection. Our knowledge is limited to experience: our own experience (called *autopsía*) and that of others (*historía*, in the sense of 'narrative'); a third element is the transfer from one similar thing to another (*metábasis toû homoíou eis tò hómoion*): if an ointment, for instance, works on the skin of the hand, it might also work on the skin of the foot; or if lemon helps against a cold, so might lime, a similar substance.

Galen illustrates the difference between the rationalists and the empiricists with an example, namely what to do in case of being bitten by a rabid dog. Both sects advocate to cleanse the wound and keep it open, yet for different reasons. The empiricists say that they have observed repeatedly that when one cleanses the wound and

---

6 Galen (1985), 3–20.

7 Frede (1990), 225–50.

applies the appropriate remedies, rabies does not occur; this is therefore the correct treatment. The rationalists argue that rabies is provoked by a poison (Gk. *iós*; Ar. *samm*) that enters the body through the wound. Therefore, one has to prevent it from reaching the body by cleansing the wound and applying the appropriate remedies.

Galen himself did not adhere to any of the three sects, but rather developed the idea of 'qualified experience' (*peîra dihōrisménē*).[8] It is necessary for experience to be qualified or ruled by a number of conditions in order to be valid. In his *On Critical Days*, Galen specified three conditions ('*sharāʾiṭ*' in the Arabic translation) for experience about crisis to be valid:

1. not all patients are suitable, but only those about whom there is no doubt;
2. the patient must know exactly when the crisis comes about;
3. in the case of prolonged crises, one must be able to establish on which day exactly the crisis began.

It is this combination of experience and reason that became the mainstay of medical epistemology in the late antique Greek and the subsequent Arabic traditions.

## 2.3 Graeco-Arabic Translations and the Formation of a New Technical Language

How did these ideas about medical epistemology reach the Arabic tradition? The main translator of medical texts was Ḥunayn ibn Isḥāq (d. *ca.* 260/873) and his workshop or 'school,' including his son Isḥāq and his nephew Ḥubaysh. Drawing on an earlier layer of translations produced during the eighth century, Ḥunayn created a technical and highly sophisticated medical language capable to expressing the most subtle nuances.[9]

Ḥunayn and his team rendered most of Galen's work into Arabic, and in the wake of Galen's commentaries on Hippocratic works, also a significant number of treatises contained in the *Hippocratic Corpus*. Certain of these translated works enjoyed particular popularity, such as the *Hippocratic Aphorisms* and Galen's *On the Sects for Beginners*. They had already been core curriculum in the amphitheatres of Alexandria and became influential medical textbooks in Arabic translation in Baghdad and beyond as well.

In the area of epistemology, core concepts were translated from Greek into Arabic. Take the semantic field of 'testing' as an example. Greek expressions such as *exetázein* ('to test'), *tḕn exétasin poieîsthai* (lit. 'to carry out a test'), and *analambánein eis tḕn básanon* (lit. 'to put to the test') are rendered through Arabic words from the root *m-ḥ-n* such as '*miḥna*' (test) and '*imtaḥana*' (to test). Likewise, experience (Gk. *peîra*, *empeiría*) and reason (*lógos*) are translated as *tajriba* and *qiyās*,

[8] Van der Eijk (1997), 35–57; reproduced in van der Eijk (2005), 279–98.

[9] Pormann (2011b): 493–515; and Pormann (2012), 143–62.

respectively. The latter has a very specific meaning in the context of Islamic jurisprudence (*fiqh*), namely that of 'analogy,' but in the context of medical epistemology, it simply refers to reason and rational thought as opposed to experience.

We can take Galen's commentary on the *Aphorisms* as an example. It is a massive work, divided into seven books, in which Galen first quotes the aphorism in question – this is the lemma – and then explains it. Ḥunayn gives an account of how he translated the works of Galen in a famous Epistle (*Risāla*); the entry on the commentary on the *Book of Aphorisms* runs as follows:[10]

> He [*sc.* Galen] composed this work in seven books [*maqālāt*]. Ayyūb [al-Ruhāwī, d. after 216/832] had translated it badly [*sc.* into Syriac]. Jibrīl ibn Bukhtīshūʿ wanted to improve it, but he only corrupted it further. Then I collated the Greek with it, and corrected it in a way that amounted to retranslating it. Then I added the lemmas of Hippocrates' text [*faṣṣ kalām Buqrāṭ*] in their own right.
>
> Aḥmad ibn Muḥammad, known as Ibn al-Mudabbir, had asked me to translate it for him [into Arabic]. I translated one book of it into Arabic. Then he asked me not to begin with the translation of another book before he had read the one that I had translated. Yet, the man was too busy, and therefore, the translation was interrupted. When Muḥammad ibn Mūsā saw this book, he asked me to complete [the translation] of the [whole] work. Therefore I translated it completely [into Arabic].

This description consists of two main parts. Ḥunayn first speaks of his use of Greek manuscripts and earlier Syriac translations, and how he produced a new Syriac version on the basis of them. He then turns to the Arabic translation, which was completed in stages.

This Arabic translation spawned a huge commentary tradition in its own right.[11] The list of at least partially extant commentaries in Arabic is long. The earlier works include Pseudo-Palladius' *Commentary*;[12] and fragments by Abū Bakr al-Rāzī. From the eleventh century we have works by Abū Sahl Saʿīd ibn ʿAbd al-ʿAzīz al-Nīlī (d. 419/1029), ʿAlī ibn Riḍwān (d. 460/1068), and Ibn Abī Ṣādiq (d. after 460/1068), who became known as the 'second Hippocrates (*Buqrāṭ al-thānī*),' and whose commentaries were the most popular. Two commentators hailed from Muslim Spain, Ibn Bājja (Lat. Avempace; d. 533/1138), who only worked on the first aphorism (1.1); and the Jewish scholar Mūsā ibn ʿUbayd Allāh al-Qurṭubī (Maimonides, d. 1204). Others from the central lands of Islam include al-Sinjārī (*fl.* 7th/12th cent.); ʿAbd al-Laṭīf al-Baghdādī; Najm al-Dīn Aḥmad ibn al-Minfākh (d. *ca.* 655/1258); and Ibn al-Nafīs, who wrote at least three different versions of his commentary. By far the longest commentary is by Ibn al-Quff (d. 684/1286), a Christian author from Syria. Later exegesis was provided by ʿAbd Allāh ibn ʿAbd al-ʿAzīz ibn Mūsā al-Sīwāsī (early 8th/14th cent.); Ibn Qāsim al-Kilānī (*fl.* 740–756/1340–1356); Ibrāhīm al-Kīshī and ʿAbd al-Raḥīm al-Ṭabīb; and al-Manāwī (d. 893/1488).

---

[10] Ḥunayn ibn Isḥāq (2016), 94–7.

[11] Pormann and Karimullah (2017): 1–52; see also, Pormann and Joosse (2012), 211–249.

[12] It was previously thought to be an Arabic translation by Yaḥyā ibn al-Biṭrīq (d. *ca.* 200/815) (late 2nd/8th cent.) of a Greek original; but this assumption has been proved to be wrong by Pormann et al. (2017), *pace* Manfred Ullmann (2002) and Biesterfeldt (2007).

These commentators came from different religious backgrounds, be it Christian, Jewish or Muslim, and different localities, and yet partook in a scientific dialogue across cultures and creeds. We shall return to one relatively unknown commentator's debate of the first aphorism below. For now suffice it to say that early Hippocratic observations about medical epistemology impacted Islamic medicine mainly through the commentary tradition. One of these commentators was the arguably greatest medieval clinician, Abū Bakr al-Rāzī.

## 2.4 Abū Bakr al-Rāzī (d. *ca.* 313/925), *Comprehensive Book*

Like Galen, Abū Bakr al-Rāzī adhered to the idea that experience on its own is dangerous. For instance, in his *Epistle to One of His Students*, he inveighs against the idea 'that one can hit on [the right treatment] by experience [*tajriba*] without any reference to [scientific] knowledge [*ʿilm*]' and he quotes the Hippocratic first aphorism in support of his dismissal of unqualified experience.[13] This underscores the importance of the *Aphorisms* for al-Rāzī's thought. Yet it is in the context of the Hippocratic *Epidemics* that he made what appears to be his most remarkable contribution to medical epistemology: the use of a control group in a medical experiment.

Let us very briefly go over the evidence for this use of a control group. It occurs in al-Rāzī's *Comprehensive Book* (*al-Kitāb al-Ḥāwī*), a massive collection of notes arranged thematically and posthumously published by his students. These note files contain quotations from a variety of sources, many Greek (in Arabic translation), and they are interspersed with al-Rāzī's personal remarks. It was Albert Z. Iskandar, then a graduate student at Oxford in the 1950s, who discovered this example and first published it in a seminal article in the Lebanese Journal *Al-Mashriq* in 1962.[14] The context for the quotation is the following: al-Rāzī discussed the topic of burning fevers (*ḥummā muḥriqa*), including *phrenîtis* or 'brain fever,' called *sirsām* in Arabic. He quoted from the *Questions on the 'Epidemics,'* an abridgment by Ḥunayn ibn Isḥāq of Galen's *Commentary on Hippocrates' 'Epidemics.'* Then al-Rāzī added his own observation, introduced by '*lī* (mine),' in which he listed the main symptoms of brain fever – including heaviness, continuous pain in the head and neck, yawning accompanied by severe insomnia, and extreme exhaustion – and then continued:[15]

> So when you see these symptoms, resort to bloodletting. For I once saved one group [of patients (*jamāʿa*)] by it [bloodletting], whilst I intentionally left another group (*jamāʿa*), so as to remove the doubt from my opinion through this. Consequently all of these [latter] contracted brain fever.

---

[13] Pormann (2008), 95–118; reprinted in Pormann (2011a), 1:179–206, on p. 99–100 and 183–4.

[14] Iskandar (1962): 238–9; translated in Pormann (2011a), 1: 207–53; the passage is conveniently discussed by Tibi (2005).

[15] Al-Rāzī, *al-Kitāb al-Ḥāwī fī al-ṭibb* (1955–75), 15:122, ll. 1–3.

Although we do not recognize today the therapeutic effect of bloodletting in case of meningitis and similar conditions, the use of a control group here seems quite extraordinary. From the context, it is clear that al-Rāzī divided the patients into two groups here intentionally (*mutaʿammidan*). The language of the passage suggests that this is not a thought experiment, but one where he confronts what he read in the literature with his own experience, or, as he put it 'according to what I have seen by way of experience and what I have read in this book (*ʿalā mā raʾaytu bi-l-tajribati wa-mā raʾaytu fī hādhā l-kitābi*).'

This use of a control group and the occurrence of the word 'group (*jamāʿa*)' twice might suggest that al-Rāzī adhered to group or population thinking. In fact, in a previous article in the James Lind Library, republished by the *Journal of the Royal Society of Medicine*, I argued that al-Rāzī referred to patient 'groups' (Arabic '*jamāʿa*') in two further examples; and discussed large patient cohorts (e.g., 'two thousand').[16] We therefore have to ask whether these references to groups are underpinned by a concept of patient groups, an awareness that large cohorts of patients and some statistical methods are needed to determine whether treatments are effective; or whether these are general expressions without any special significance. If the former were the case, that would certainly fly in the face of the scholarly consensus that population thinking with its patient groups in which treatment outcomes are carefully counted emerges in the modern period.[17] A recent investigation of the occurrence of the word 'group' in the *New England Journal of Medicine*, for instance, shows that its use increases dramatically from the beginning of the twentieth century, peaks in the mid-1970s and then declines somewhat but is still frequently encountered, as a hitherto unpublished investigation shows.[18]

In order to shed additional light on the question of how al-Rāzī used the word '*jamāʿa* (group),' I have systematically searched an electronic file of his *Comprehensive Book*. The file, shared on the website Al-Shāmila, is based on the reprint of this work by the Beirut publisher Dār al-Kutub al-ʿIlmīya in 2000.[19] The file (as well as the printed edition) contains numerous misprints and mistakes, and, as such, introduces a certain margin of error to my enquiry.[20] Yet, as the examples below demonstrate, it is a powerful tool for assessing the usage of '*jamāʿa*' within this limited corpus.

The first result from this search is that the famous passage quoted above is the only one to use '*jamāʿa*' twice in the whole of the *Comprehensive Book*, comprising some 1.1 m words and 23 volumes in the printed edition. The other occurrences of the word '*jamāʿa*' can usefully be divided into two kinds: (1) general usage and (2) specific references to groups of patients. Let us begin by reviewing the first. Here,

[16] Pormann (2013): 370–72.

[17] Morabia (2014).

[18] Through personal communication with David Armstrong of King's College London.

[19] The website is at http://shamela.ws/index.php/book/10704

[20] On the quality of the various editions of al-Rāzī, see Oliver Kahl (2015), xi-xiv, who argues that the Hyderabad edition remains the most reliable, despite its own shortcomings.

moreover, I would like to begin with a quotation from a Greek source, Galen's book *On the Method of Healing*. Al-Rāzī quotes a passage extolling the virtues of honey water (water mixed with honey, called *melíkraton* in Greek and *mā' al-ʿasal* in Arabic) in case of fever where the patient is weak. Galen enjoins to 'use honey water alone during the first three days, massaging *in turn* (τῷ μελικράτῳ μόνῳ χρῆσθαι κατὰ τὰς τρεῖς τὰς πρώτας ἡμέρας, *ἐκ διαδοχῆς* τρίβοντα)' (my emphasis).[21] In al-Rāzī, this becomes 'use honey water alone for three days, whilst they are constantly given a massage by a group [of people] taking turns (*wa-yudlakūna dalikan dā'iman tatadāwaluhū jamāʿatun*).'[22] So the Greek expression 'in turn (*ek diadochês*)' is rendered periphrastically, but the word *jamāʿa* has no terminological meaning here. This is not surprising, as we know from the Graeco-Arabic translation literature that *jamāʿa* can translate a whole range of words meaning 'large group of people' such as *óchlos*.[23]

Likewise, we have five other examples of this kind where '*jamāʿa*' refers to a group of other people, such as:

- 'a group [of people] counted among the ophthalmologists (*jamāʿat al-maʿdūdīn bayn al-kaḥḥālīn*)';[24]
- 'the group said in the *Compilation on the Eye* (*al-jamāʿatu qālat fī l-Kitābi l-Majmūʿi fī l-ʿayni*)';[25]
- 'a group [of people] who have tested colocynth root (*jamāʿatun jarrabū aṣla l-ḥanẓali*)';[26]
- 'a group of physicians (*jamāʿa min al-aṭibbā'*)';[27]
- 'one of modern authors said (and a group agreed with this), (*wa-qāla baʿḍu l-muḥdathīna wa-jtamaʿa ʿalā dhālika jamāʿatun*).'[28]

This shows that the word '*jamāʿa*' could certainly be used for a 'large number of people' without any technical or terminological meaning.

Let us now turn to the examples where '*jamāʿa*' refers to a group of patients. I have previously published two such examples.[29] In one, al-Rāzī advocates the use of a sternutatory (*saʿūṭ*) against epilepsy, saying that 'a group [of patients] were cured by it (*qad bari'a ʿalayhi jamāʿatun*).'[30] In the other, al-Rāzī recommends bloodlet-

[21] Greek text (10.823 K), and translation taken from Galen (2011), 242–5.

[22] Al-Rāzī, *al-Kitāb al-Ḥāwī*, 14:3, l. 15–14:4, l. 2; 14:3, l. 15–14:4, l. 2. I was able to identify this quotation thanks to Weisser (1997).

[23] Ullmann (2002).

[24] Al-Rāzī (1955–75), 2:20, ll. 12–13.

[25] Ibid., 2:109, l. 9.

[26] Ibid., 19:290, l. 12.

[27] Ibid., 23(1):304, l. 6.

[28] Ibid., 20:123, l. 15.

[29] Pormann (2013): 370–71.

[30] Al-Rāzī (1955–75), 1:142, l. 2.

ting in the corner of the eye in case of inveterate pannus (*sabal qadīm*), trachoma (*jarab*), and red 'ulcerative blepharitis' (*al-sulāq al-aḥmar*); he then reports that 'In front of me, a group (*jamāʿa*) was phlebotomized who were suffering from pannus. It [the pannus] receded and they were able to rest.' In both these previously published examples, there is no suggestion of a control group and it would appear that al-Rāzī could have easily referred to a 'sizeable number of patients' when using the word '*jamāʿa*.' The same can be said for the first three of the four new examples: in each case, a 'group of patients' was cured. Only in the last is the outcome possibly negative. Let us discuss them in turn.

The first new example comes from the section in the *Comprehensive Book* dealing with warm swellings (*waram ḥārr*) in the stomach. It runs as follows:[31]

على ما رأيت في العلل المرارية في المعدة: الإيارج في طبيخ الأفسنتين لا نظيرَ له. ونقيع الصبر سقيته جماعة ممعودين فبرؤا عليه. أفسنتين عشرة دراهم، دارصيني خمسة دراهم، عود البلسان ثلاثة، سنبل ثلاثة، ورق ورد درهمان، عود درهم، مصطكى درهمان. يطبخ وينقع الصبر فيه. يسقى في كل يوم أوقية.

My opinion about bilious diseases affecting the stomach is that the 'holy remedy' in epithyme decoction has no equal. I have given aloe mucilage to drink to a group [of patients] suffering from stomach disorders (*jamāʿat mamʿūdīn*), and they were cured by it. [This is how to administer it. Take] epithyme, ten dirham; cinnamon, ten dirham; balsam wood, three; nard, three; rose leaves, two disham; aloeswood, one dirham; mastix, two dirham. Cook, macerate the aloe in it, and give to drink each day, one ounce.

Here, the gist appears to be that in al-Rāzī's opinion *iyāraj*, a kind of compound drug going back to Greek *hierá* the 'holy (remedy),' is best for bilious diseases, but that he also treated a number of patients successfully with aloe mucilage.[32]

The second example concerns limbs that are paralysed because they are too cold. The treatment should consist of strongly warming remedies, containing, for instance, 'sulphur not touched by fire and pellitory (*ʿāqirqarḥā*).' Al-Rāzī continues:[33]

وقد داويت بهذا الطريق جماعة فبرؤوا.

I have treated a group [of patients] in this way, and they were cured (*wa-qad dāwaytu … jamāʿatan fa-bariʾū*).

In a third quotation, al-Rāzī states:[34]

فأما القروح الحادثة في قصبة الرئة في الغشاء الداخل خاصة إذا كانت قريبا من الحنجرة أو في الحنجرة نفسها، فقد يمكن أن تبرأ. وقد أصابه ذلك فبرأ. داوينا نحن جماعة ممن

In case of ulcers occurring in the windpipe on the inside of the membrane, especially when they are close to the larynx or in the larynx itself, a cure may be effected. We, ourselves,

[31] Ibid., 5:87, ll. 13–17.

[32] At first, one might think that *wa-naqīʿu/a/i l-ṣabiri* ought to be vocalized *wa-naqīʿi l-ṣabiri* with the *wa-* taken as *wāw-rubba* in the sense of 'many an aloe mucilage have I given to drink …,' but *wāw-rubba* normally is followed by an indetermined noun in the genitive. Therefore, we probably just have to read *wa-naqīʿu* and take this as *casus pendens*.

[33] Al-Rāzī (1955–75), 6:272, l. 1.

[34] Ibid., 13:99, ll. 10–12.

treated a group of [patients] affected by this, and they were cured (*wa-qad dāwaynā naḥnu jamāʿatan mimman aṣābahū dhālika fa-bariʾa*).

In both these examples, nearly the same form of words is used; al-Rāzī merely records the success of a certain treatment that he has just described.

The fourth example, however, is different. In the context of discussing smallpox (*judarī*), a subject on which al-Rāzī had wrote a separate and rightly famous monograph, he says the following:[35]

ورأيت جماعة خرج بهم جدري حار عظيم وأصابهم كلهم وجع الساق في آخر أمرهم.

I have seen a group [of patients] in which a severe warm [type of] smallpox erupted. All were affected by a pain in the leg at the end.

After this remark follows another one introduced by 'mine (*lī*),' that is not directly related to this one. Therefore, it is difficult to say whether the expression 'at the end (*fī ākhari amrihim*)' suggests a negative outcome, as seems plausible, or whether this is just another symptom before the disease runs its course without killing the patient. Be that as it may, all four examples here do not offer us any indication that al-Rāzī meant more than 'a large number of patients' when employing the term *jamāʿa*.

Moreover, previously, I have presented some examples of al-Rāzī's using crude statistics when talking about patients, taken from his work *Doubts about Galen*. One example includes a small number of patients: 'Three were cured whilst one was affected by dropsy more quickly than those who were not treated, but by a lighter variety'; another example involves large numbers: 'For there were approximately three hundred out of two thousand patients whose state developed in a contrary fashion.'[36] But these two remarks, too, appear to be *ad hoc* and only suggest a very rough counting of clinical outcomes.

Therefore, we are left with a rather negative conclusion. The one famous example of al-Rāzī's using a control group does not appear to have any similar cases in the whole of his *Comprehensive Book*. Likewise, the very few cases of al-Rāzī's using numbers when describing the outcome of treatments should not be used to extrapolate general practice; they, too, are rather rare, with no examples from the *Comprehensive Book*. We should therefore resist the temptation to read the present into the past: although al-Rāzī uses the word 'group (*jamāʿa*)' in connection with patients, and although there are some cases of his quantifying clinical outcomes, these instances, when taken together, do not suggest that al-Rāzī adhered to population thinking or used sophisticated statistical methods. His use of a control group remains an intriguing, but singular example.

Before we turn to the most influential medieval medical author, Avicenna, and his ideas about the use of experience, it is necessary to dispel an oft related rumour, namely that al-Rāzī tested drugs on animals; or that physicians in the Arabo-Islamic tradition generally tested drugs on animals before giving them to humans.

---

[35] Ibid., 17:25, ll. 7–8.

[36] Pormann (2013): 371.

It is a case of a rumour growing as it is transmitted (*fama crescit eundo*). It started with the 1959 Oxford DPhil thesis of the Egyptian medical historian Albert Z. Iskandar, who found the following report in al-Rāzī's *Book for al-Manṣūr* (*al-Kitāb al-Manṣūrī*):[37]

> I do not think that pure mercury causes much damage. When one drinks it, however, it does cause a lot of pain in the stomach and the bowels. It is secreted in its [original] form, especially if the patient moves. I, myself, have administered it to an ape in my possession. I observed exactly the symptoms which I have just mentioned.

Therefore, al-Rāzī in fact tested the poisonous effects of mercury on an ape, and not a drug. In other words, this is not a drug test at all, but rather one to establish how poisonous mercury is. Yet, this was reported as 'animal testing' and misunderstood to refer to animal drug testing. But I do not know of a single example where medieval physicians tested drugs on animals. Avicenna even warned specifically against animal drug testing, as we shall see next.

## 2.5 Avicenna (d. 428/1037), *Canon of Medicine*

Avicenna is, as already mentioned, the most influential medical writer of the medieval period, and possibly of all times—perhaps with the exception of Galen of Pergamum.[38] He penned a large number of medical treatises ranging from topics such as cardiac drugs, bloodletting, anatomical topics and druglore, including some didactic poems on medicine in general, sexual hygiene and the preservation of health. Yet, his greatest and most influential work is the *Canon of Medicine (al-Qānūn fī al-ṭibb)*, a medical encyclopaedia in five books, dealing with the 'Generalities' (*kulliyyāt*, Book 1); 'simple drugs' (Book 2); 'topical diseases' (diseases affecting a specific part of the body, from tip to toe; Book 3); 'other diseases' (Book 4); and 'compound drugs' (Book 5). This *Canon* attracted an incredible amount of exegetical attention, with dozens of commentaries, supercommentaries (that is, commentaries of commentaries), abridgments and commentaries of abridgments; I shall return to one interesting example from the commentary tradition below.

This substantial output in the area of medicine could seem surprising for a thinker like Avicenna. For he himself classed medicine as a derivative natural science (*ḥikma ṭabīʿiyya farʿiyya*) on the same level as astrology, dream interpretation, and the production of talismans and amulets – all subjects for which Avicenna had very little time. He also claimed that he had mastered medicine at a young age, as it was not complicated. For him, philosophy was of far greater importance. Yet, his *Canon*

---

[37] Iskandar (1959), 1:306, 2:107; the passage can also be found in the modern edition of the text: al-Rāzī (1987), 368.

[38] See Pormann (2013).

overlaps in certain areas with his philosophical writings, for instance when he talks about the functional anatomy of the brain.

Like Galen and al-Rāzī, Avicenna appears to adhere to the notion of qualified experience. At the beginning of the second book, he has a chapter on 'How to ascertain the faculties of the mixtures of drugs through experience,' and specifies seven conditions for the use of experience.[39] These conditions are:

1. 'it should be free from any acquired quality';
2. 'the experience should be conducted on a simple illness (*ʿilla mufrada*)';
3. it should be tested on a drug and its opposite as well;
4. the strength in the drug should correspond to the strength in the illness;
5. the time that the drug requires to take effect should not be too long;
6. the effect should be constant and occur in most cases (*ʿalā l-akthari*);
7. the human body should be used for testing (*an takūna l-tajribatu ʿalā badani l-insāni*), and not that of animals.

Let us look more closely at the seventh condition:[40]

والسابع: أن تكون التجربة على بدن الإنسان فإنه إن جرب على غير بدن الإنسان جاز أن يتخلّف من وجهين: أحدهما: أنه قد يجوز أن يكون الدواء بالقياس إلى بدن الإنسان حاراً وبالقياس إلى بدن الأسد والفرس بارداً إذا كان الدواء أسخن من الإنسان وأبرد من الأسد والفرس ويشبه فيما أظن أن يكون الراوند شديد البرد بالقياس إلى الفرس وهو بالقياس إلى الإنسان حار. والثاني أنه قد يجوز أن يكون له بالقياس إلى أحد البدنين خاصية ليست بالقياس إلى البدن الثاني مثل البيش فإن له بالقياس إلى بدن الإنسان خاصية السمية وليست له بالقياس إلى بدن الزرازير.

> The seventh [condition] is that experiments should be carried out on the human body. If the experiment is carried out on the bodies of [other animals] it is possible that it might fail for two reasons. First, the medicine might be warm in relation to the human body, yet cold in relation to the body of a lion or a horse, if the drug is hotter than the human being and colder than the lion and the horse. I believe that it may be possible that rhubarb is extremely cold in relation to a horse, but warm in relation to a human being. Second, it is possible that the drug has a specific quality in relation to one body, but not the other. For instance, aconite (*bīsh*) has a specifically poisonous quality in relation to the human body which it does not have in relation to the body of starlings (*zarāzīr*).

In other words, Avicenna contemplates the possibility of testing drugs on animals, but rejects it, because it may act differently on animals than it would on humans. This difference could be twofold: it may affect the so-called primary qualities of drugs, such as hot and cold, and dry and moist. Or it may have specific qualities in the cases of humans, but not animals: aconite can be poisonous for human beings, but not birds.

Since Avicenna argues against animal drug testing, does this not suggest that it must have been practised, for why would he otherwise reject it? The answer to this question is no. As Avicenna explains at the beginning of the *Canon*, he deals with the theory of practice in this book, not actual practice. And the arguments proffered here certainly have something theoretical about them. This can also be seen in the rich commentary tradition on the *Canon*, out of which we are going to discuss a prominent example next.

---

[39] See Nasser, Tibi and Savage-Smith (2009): 78–80.

[40] Translation from Nasser, Tibi and Savage-Smith (2009) (with modifications).

## 2.6 Ibn al-Nafīs (d. 687/1288), *Commentary on the 'Canon'*

Ibn al-Nafīs wrote a lemmatic commentary on the *Canon* which survives in its entirety in a manuscript in the library of the Wellcome Trust. The continuity of the epistemological debates can nicely be illustrated by looking at how he comments on Avicenna's seventh condition for the testing of drugs, quoted and discussed above. Ibn al-Nafīs begins by quoting the beginning of the passage on which he is going to comment; this quotation is the lemma, but he only gives it in abbreviated form and expects the reader to have the whole passage in question from the *Canon* in mind. After the lemma and a brief summary of Avicenna's argument, Ibn al-Nafīs makes three main points: (1) he comments on a drug called '*bīsh*' (aconite) and equates it with hemlock, which he says is called *euphórbion* in Greek; in reality, Greek *kṓneion* means 'hemlock,' whereas *euphórbion* is spurge; (2) he gives a possible objection to Avicenna's argument, and (3) then refutes this objection. This is the passage:[41]

« الشرط السابع أن تكون التجربة على بدن الإنسان »

وقد ذكر الشيخ علة ذلك، وهي أنه يجوز أن يكون غير الإنسان مخالفا للإنسان في انفعاله عن ذلك الدواء من جهتين: أحدهما أن غير الإنسان مخالف لإنسان في مزاجه، فقد يكون دواء واحد بالنسبة إلى ذلك الحيوان حارا أو باردا، ولا يكون كذلك بالنسبة إلى الإنسان ؛ وثانيهما أنه قد يكون لبدن ذلك الحيوان خاصية في الانفعال عن ذلك الدواء، وليست تلك الخاصية للإنسان. وقد مثل الشيخ على ذلك بالبيش المفسد للإنسان دون الزرازير. ويشبه أن يكون بدل البيش الشوكران. وسبب هنا الغلط أن البيش يسمى باليونانية فربيون، وفربيون يترجم بالبيش، ويترجم بالشوكران ولهنا قال بعضهم إن الشوكران ضرب من البيش

ولقائل أن يقول «إن غير الإنسان كما جاز أن يخالف الإنسان بهذين الوجهين اللذين ذكرتم، فكذلك يجوز أن يكون بدن الإنسان الذي يجرب عليه الدواء مخالفا لأبدان باقي الناس بهذين الوجهين أيضا. وحينئذ لا يكون للتجربة دلالة على قوى الأدوية. وليس لكم أن تقولوا إنّا إنما نثق بالتجربة بعد استعمال الأدوية على أبدان كثيرة. وظاهر أن تلك الأبدان لا تكون كلها مخالفة لباقي أبدان الناس، لأنا نقول ‹هب أن هذا يصح، فالبدن الواحد الذي يريد أن تستعمل فيه الدواء عرفت قوته بالستعماله في تلك الأبدان، أليس أنه يجوز أن يكون مخالفا لها ؟ وحينئذ لا يكون لنا ثقة بنفع ذلك الدواء فيه، فلا يكون للتجربة فائدة».

والجواب أن هذا الاعتراض غير مختص بدلالة التجربة إذ الأدوية التي يعرف حكمها بالقياس حالها أيضا كذلك ونحن عند استعمال الأدوية على كل بدن لا نكون جازمين بنفعها وإنما نتبع في ذلك الظن الغالب. فإن ظاهر الحال <أن> يشابه حال هذا البدن لأبدان باقي الناس وما يتفق من مخالفة بعض الأبدان لبعض فإنما هو على خلاف الظاهر.

[Avicenna:] 'The seventh [condition] is that experiments should be carried out on the human body.'

The master mentioned the cause for this, namely that it is possible for a non-human to be differently affected by a given drug in two ways. First, a non-human differs from a human being in mixture, so that one drug may be warm or cold in relation to an animal, but not a

[41] MS Wellcome Or. 51, fol. 195a, ll. 20–29.

> human being. Second, the body of the animal may have a special quality in the way it is affected by the drug, whereas the human being does not have it. The master gave the example of aconite (*bīsh*), which has a devastating effect on humans, but not starlings (*zarāzīr*). One should probably [read] hemlock [*shawkarān*] instead of aconite. This mistake occurred because aconite [*bīsh*] is called spurge [*furbiyūn*, from εὐφόρβιον] in Greek, 'spurge [*furbiyūn*, from εὐφόρβιον]' being the translation of 'aconite [*bīsh*]' and of hemlock [*shawkarān*]. Therefore, some people say that hemlock is a kind of aconite.
>
> One may object that just like non-humans may differ from humans in these two ways which you have mentioned, so the human body on which the drug is tested may differ from the bodies of other humans in these two ways as well. In this case, the experiment [*tajriba*] would not provide an indication about the faculties of drugs. Therefore you cannot just say that we can trust experience only after having used a drug on many bodies. For it is clear that these bodies are not all different from all the other human bodies. We could say: 'Let us assume that this is right: you know the power of one body on which you want to use the drug by using it on those [other] bodies. Could it [the body] then not be different from them? That would mean that we cannot have trust that this drug will be useful for it [the body], and therefore, experience has no benefit.
>
> One may retort that this objection is not specific to the probative value (*dalāla*) of the experience. For the case is similar for drugs on which one knows how to decide through reason. When we use drugs on any body, we do not know for certain whether they will be beneficial. In this regard, we only follow a prevailing opinion [*al-ẓann al-ghālib*]. For the case is clear: the case of this body is similar to the other human bodies. The fact that some bodies happen to differ from others is the opposite of the clear [case].

The discussion of *bīsh* illustrates the difficulty with identifying foreign *materia medica*, a topic on which a lot of ink has been spilled. More interesting in our context is the epistemological debate. At the heart of this debate is the (theoretical) question whether testing treatments on animals is a viable process – a question with which we still struggle today. Avicenna states that animal bodies differ from human bodies. But human bodies also differ from other human bodies. Therefore, any drug testing, any use of medical experience is futile. Ibn al-Nafīs refutes this objection by saying that the same could also be said about knowledge of drugs through reason (as opposed to experience). Ibn al-Nafīs' implication appears to be that this is patently not the case, and therefore this objection neither applies to knowledge about drugs through reason nor through experience.

## 2.7 ʿAbd al-Laṭīf al-Baghdādī (d. 629/1231)

Let us now turn to a physician who was highly critical of the *Canon* and in particular of his contemporaries' habit of focussing merely on the first book, the *Generalities* to the exclusion of studying ancient medical authorities such as Hippocrates and Galen. This physician is ʿAbd al-Laṭīf al-Baghdādī, who hailed from Baghdad but spent most of his career in Syria and Egypt.[42] Among medical historians he is famous for criticising certain anatomical notions of Galen, such as the idea that the jawbone consists of two parts joined near the chin; on the basis of a large number of skeletons seen during an epidemic in Egypt, ʿAbd al-Laṭīf argued (correctly) that the jawbone is one.[43]

ʿAbd al-Laṭīf was also a very original thinker in the area of medical epistemology. For instance, his *Book of the Two Pieces of Advice* (*Kitāb al-Nasīḥatayn*) is directed against contemporaneous physicians and philosophers, respectively. In his attack against the physicians, he refers to Galen's three sects – the rationalists, the empiricists and the methodists – and praises the latter over the former, saying:[44]

> He [Galen] complained about the methodist sect and the empiricist sect. Even though they all generally fall short and are deficient, they have useful rules and principles, which it is best to acquire and learn, especially those of the empiricists. […] Our contemporaries do not belong to any of the three sects which he [Galen] defined in his book *On the Sects* [*for Beginners*], but rather rely on luck and chance [*al-bakht wa-l-ittifāq*] like a blind man shooting [an arrow] without knowing in which direction the target is. The sects of the methodists and empiricists know the direction of the target, but shoot [the arrow] without first examining its [the target's] specific position. The rationalists know the direction and examine the position of the target, directing their arrow there in the most perfect and correct fashion. The empiricists examine certain aspects of the target, such as its shadow, so that they deserve to hit the mark. The people of our time, however, do not examine the target, nor its direction, and one is therefore surprised not by their making a mistake, but by their getting things right, whereas one is surprised by the mistake of the rationalists, and their not getting things right. For the latter get things mostly right – and essentially right at that [*wa-bi-l-dhāti*], whilst making mistakes only rarely – and accidentally [*bi-l-ʿaraḍi*]. But these freeloaders rarely get things right, and only accidentally, whilst mostly making mistakes, and essentially at that.

We can immediately see that ʿAbd al-Laṭīf no longer adheres to Galen's idea of qualified experience. For him as a true Aristotelian, there is a clear hierarchy of knowledge, and theoretical knowledge is superior to empirical one, as his arrow shooting simile shows. Empiricists have some idea of where to shoot, but only rationalists hit the target consistently. 'They get things … essentially right,' that is to say, their success is not accidental, in both senses of the word: it is not by happenstance or chance, nor is it a non-essential feature of their craft.

ʿAbd al-Laṭīf also uses the simile of archery to describe the inherently uncertain nature of medical practice as opposed to medical theory, saying:[45]

> When the conditions of the medical art are fully adhered to, then it never makes a mistake. The intelligent physician only errs occasionally, but gets things right a hundred times, as Galen said. Moreover, his mistake will be neither decisive nor great nor far from what is

[42] Joosse and Pormann (2010).

[43] Fancy (2018), 46–7.

[44] Translation from Joosse and Pormann (2010), 9–10.

[45] Translation from Joosse and Pormann (2008), 426.

correct. One can compare him to an expert in archery who mostly hits the mark, and when he misses, then it [i.e., his arrow] will not be far off, but it will rather land near [the target]. But in the event of the arrow falling entirely in the opposite direction, then [this is like] a physician committing an error.

In other words, theoretical medicine which respects all the rules of the art can be always correct, but practical medicine, even by the best physician, must sometimes make mistakes. ʿAbd al-Laṭīf then continues and compares this inability to be completely correct to the mathematical inability to determine irrational numbers such as *pi* or the square root of 10.[46]

This discussion about uncertainty in medicine is not accidental to ʿAbd al-Laṭīf's thinking. He wrote two commentaries on key Hippocratic works: on the *Aphorisms*, as we have already seen, but also on the *Prognostic*, a text concerned not just with prognosis, but also diagnosis. When commenting on the opening sentence of this text, ʿAbd al-Laṭīf offers the following reflection:[47]

The subject of medicine is the knowledge of probabilities [*wa-mawḍūʿu l-ṭibbi l-maʿrifatu l-ʾakthariyyatu*], especially in the case of acute diseases. Therefore, Hippocrates said in the *Aphorisms* [2.19]: 'To determine beforehand [the course] of acute diseases, whether it is death or health, is not entirely trustworthy [*laysa yakūnu ʿalā ghāyati l-thiqati*].' The probable [*al-aktharī*] has an element of happenstance [*ʿaraḍ*] which is more or less likely. For the necessary and the impossible are two extremes which do not have an element of happenstance [*ʿaraḍ*]. The possible is like something that is in the middle over a wide range. That which is close to the extreme of necessity is more probable, whereas that which is close to the extreme of impossible is less likely. Medicine investigates things which probably occur, although it also considers the less probable and that which is equally likely in a different way, although it is not here the place to explain it.

Before discussing this quotation further, it is useful to look at part of what ʿAbd al-Laṭīf has to say in his *Commentary on the Aphorisms*:[48]

فأبقراط يتقدم بالقضية في الأمراض المزمنة على غاية الثقة، وليس هو في جميع الأمراض الحادة من الثقة على تلك الحال، لكنه قد أقر بأنه يمكن أن يقع في بعضها خطأ كأنه ليس يصح الحكم على الأمراض الحادة في جميع الحالات بل قد يخطئ الطبيب الحاذق في الندرة وصوابه أكثر، وإنما يعرض له الخطأ لسرعة تغير المرض عن كيموس حاد، ولأن الكيموس ربما سال من عضو إلى آخر بغتة فوقع ما لم يكن في حسبان الطبيب.

In the case of chronic and long-lasting diseases, Hippocrates makes predictive judgments that are entirely trustworthy. He does not, however, possess this level of trust [or certainty, *thiqa*] in the case of all chronic diseases, but has established that in some of them, a mistake can be made. To put it differently, the judgment about acute diseases is not correct in all cases. Even an intelligent physician may rarely make mistakes, although he mostly gets things right. He only commits a mistake because the disease changes quickly owing to a sharp humour, and the humour may suddenly flow from one part of the body to another, so that something which the physician did not expect occurs.

---

[46] Ibid.

[47] Joosse and Pormann (2012), 280.

[48] Al-Baghdādī (2017), p. 21, l. 6–11: https://doi.org/10.3927/51688912

We therefore see that on the basis of a Hippocratic *Aphorism*, ʿAbd al-Laṭīf develops the idea that medicine deals with probabilities. In practice, even the best physician sometimes makes mistakes, but only rarely (*fī l-nadrati*). The definition of medicine as 'knowledge of probabilities' of course suggests something incredibly modern. But as in the case of Abū Bakr al-Rāzī, we should not impose our modern ideas onto the medieval text. ʿAbd al-Laṭīf is obviously not talking about population statistics or outcomes of various groups of patients which are then statistically analysed. He merely makes the (important) point that clinical outcomes are linked to chance, and that good medical practice is characterized by relative, not absolute, success.

## 2.8 Al-Kilānī (*fl. ca.* 750s/1350s)

Among the many Arabic commentaries on the *Aphorisms* we find a particularly interesting, if difficult example, namely that by al-Kilānī. We know very little about the author, and his commentary only survives in two manuscripts: an older one with significant water damage, and a younger one which is directly descended from the older one.[49] The text is often difficult to understand, because it seems lacunose or corrupt. And yet, even despite these difficulties, it certainly deserves our attention, as al-Kilānī often proffers interesting arguments and ideas. He is therefore an excellent example to study the commentaries on *Aphorism* 1.1 further, as he was unknown to Franz Rosenthal when he surveyed the *Aphorisms* commentary tradition through the lens of the first aphorism more than half a century ago.[50]

We have already seen that the first *Aphorism* contains the advice that 'experience is perilous and decision difficult (ἡ δὲ πεῖρα σφαλερὴ, ἡ δὲ κρίσις χαλεπή; *al-tajribatu khaṭarun wa-l-qaḍāʾu ʿaṣirun*).' Al-Kilānī offers the following explanation on this momentous phrase:[51]

> Hippocrates mentioned 'experience' before 'decision,' which is explained by the rationalists as meaning reason, although experience comes after reasoning in rank, in order to teach us that there is danger in experience that precedes reasoning. This is experience by the ignorant, and the test of something which begins without reasoning and does not stem from a principle or guideline. This is the [type of experience] which the wise Hippocrates means by saying 'experience is dangerous,' because a single disease varies according to whether the disease matter is plentiful or small, thick or thin, simple or compound, and similar accidental qualities associated with it. Thus the single disease becomes multiple in number and in the way it is experienced in as much as it is impossible to grasp all of them [*sc.* the accidents] by experience.

---

[49] Pormann and Karimullah (2017), 28.

[50] Rosenthal (1966).

[51] Translation from Pormann (2017), 22 (with modifications).

It is impossible for all of the specific conditions of natural and unnatural states to occur, for not all of these states are actualized in the bodies and the times over which a single person is able to gain mastery. Nor can a single individual learn the natures of bodies and all of their conditions, the nature of diseases and their extent, the faculties of drugs with which one treats them, the different drugs of greater and lesser strength, the reason why each drug is useful or harmful, and the climates in relation to each disease, without sound reasoning and the general guidelines which encompass all of the specifics of this art.

Some have said that the intended meaning of 'decision (*qaḍāʾ*)' is 'judgment (*ḥukm*).' In this case, its difficulty lies in judging the benefit and harm that follows from treating, for example, a severe headache with purging and bleeding, hot compresses, perfumes, and ointments.

Al-Kilānī's first point is this: in the hierarchy of knowledge, reason is higher than experience, and yet Hippocrates mentions experience first to warn against its use without reason. We therefore find here again the idea of qualified experience that underlies al-Kilānī's explanation. Al-Kilānī then makes the point that experience cannot be total and all encompassing. It is simply not possible for anyone to witness all possible permutations of health and disease: they are too manifold. Therefore, one needs 'sound reasoning (*al-aqyisa al-ṣaḥīḥa*).' Only the 'general guidelines (*al-qawānīn al-kulliyya*)' can encompass all the particulars of the art of medicine.

Al-Kilānī's commentary is thematically arranged, meaning that it does not follow the standard division into seven 'sections' (Greek *thēmata*), but group them around subject areas. The second *Aphorism* which al-Kilānī discusses is 2.19, mentioned earlier. He gives the following explanation[52]:

يعني التقدم بالقضية والمبادرة إلى الحكم في الأمراض الحادة بلا علامات السلامة وأمارات التلف بأن صاحبها يبرأ أو يتلف غير موثوق به...

فالمبادرة إلى الحكم قبل ظهور دليل وقياس يؤديان إليه في الأمراض الحادة ليس يكون على غاية الثقة، وذلك لأن لها علامات وأمارات يستدل بها على كيفية حال قوة الطبيعة أو قوة المرض، وغلبة إحداهما على الأخرى عند البحران فالتقدم بالحكم عند عِلّام العلامة بالبرء أو بالموت ليس يكون على غاية الثقة لأنه يكون رجماً بالغيب أو متابعة الظن إن الظن لا يغني عن الحق شيئاً.

واعلم أن المرض الحاد هو الذي مع سرعة انقضائه عظيم ويحدث من أخلاط حارة مع حمى كالحمرة والحصبة وفرانيطس، ومن أخلاط باردة بلا حمى كالسكتة والكزاز والصرع فإنّه قد يبرأ المريض من هذه الأمراض عند نهوض القوة المدبرة وغلبتها بلا دليل الغلبة فلا ينبغي أن يحكم على التلف وقد يهلك العليل بعد ظهور النضج وأيام الإنذار في أوان البحران عند خور القوة وضعفها.

[52] Al-Kilānī (2017), p. 6, ll. 4–6 and l. 10–17: https://doi.org/10.3927/51688739 (with modifications).

> He [*sc*. Hippocrates] means this: determining beforehand (*al-taqaddum bi-l-qaḍiyya*) and coming to a decision about acute diseases without signs of health or indications of death through which [one can ascertain] that the patient recovers or dies is not trustworthy. …
>
> Coming to a decision before the appearance of an indicator and reasoning, both of which lead to it [*sc*. the decision], in the case of acute diseases is not entirely trustworthy. For they have signs and indications through which one can deduce the state of the strength of nature, or the strength of the disease, or whether one of them [i.e., nature or disease] dominates the other during the crisis. Therefore, coming to a decision when a sign indicating recovery or death appears is not entirely trustworthy, because it amounts to guessing (*ragjm bi-l-ghayb*) and following a [mere] opinion (*ẓann*), for an opinion cannot do at all without truth.[53]
>
> Know that a chronic disease is powerful, as it runs its course quickly; it is brought about by warm humours accompanied by fever, as in the case of erysipelas, measles, and brain fever; [or it is brought about] by cold humours without fever as in the case of apoplexy, tetanus, and epilepsy. A patient may recover from these diseases when the governing faculty (*al-quwwa al-mudabbira*) reasserts itself. It gains dominance, however, without any indication for this dominance. Therefore, one should not make the judgement that [the patient] will die. The patient may die after the digestion appears [to be working normally]. During moments of crisis, one ought to be careful on days when the strength [of the body] recedes and becomes weak.

We therefore see that al-Kilānī first paraphrases the aphorism, but then provides his own interpretation. A clinical judgement in the case of certain acute diseases is simply guesswork. He cautions against quick judgements, as the signs can be deceptive, or simply absent. This epistemological scepticism could easily be reconciled with ʿAbd al-Laṭīf al-Baghdādī's position that even the best physician errs from time to time.

## 2.9 Conclusion

The examples above demonstrate the vibrancy of the Arabo-Islamic tradition and the interesting debates that took place about medical methodology and epistemology. In one extraordinary case, one physician used a control group to ascertain the medical efficacy of a treatment, in another, he tested the toxicity of mercury on an ape. Likewise, physicians refined the conditions under which drugs are tested and debated uncertainty in medical practice. Another physician even went so far as to talk of medicine as a 'knowledge of probabilities (*maʿrifa aktharīyya*).' All this sounds very modern, but we also have to resist the temptation to read the present into the past, or just to search in the past for what is now deemed correct or scientific.

What can we learn from these examples, and why do they matter? First of all, they show that in the medieval Islamic tradition, physicians from different backgrounds partook in a shared scientific discourse that transcended country and creed.

[53] I.e., requires verification to see whether it is true.

In these medical texts, confessions are largely irrelevant, and the points debated are those of science: Avicenna and ʿAbd al-Laṭīf al-Baghdādī can disagree about medical epistemology, and the latter criticized the former quite heavily, but this criticism is couched in terms of medical and scientific, and not religious discourse.

And yet this medical and scientific discourse also has implications for the religious sciences. For instance, the famous Ḥanbalite jurist, *ḥadīth* scholar and specialist in Prophetic medicine Ibn Qayyim al-Jawziyya (d. 751/1350) quoted a Hippocratic aphorism in his book *The Beloved's Gift on How to Treat Newborns* (*Tuḥfat al-mawdūd bi-aḥkām al-mawlūd*);[54] importantly, he does so in the manner as one would cite a Prophetic tradition. Likewise, Ibn al-Nafīs, who wrote at least three different versions of *Aphorisms* commentaries, was also a famous theologian, and his medical ideas are reflected in his understanding of human physiology and the nature of the soul as they appear in his theological works.[55] The medical ideas of the time represented the dominant paradigm according to which many Islamic theologians of the formative and classical period understood the human being. This, then, is yet another reason why it is so important to understand the medieval medical tradition: it is an important facet of Islamic theology and culture, which cannot be comprehended without it. But, most importantly, this medical tradition is of great intrinsic interest and therefore deserve further study in its own right.

## References

al-Baghdādī, ʿAbd al-Laṭīf. 2017. *al-Maqāla al-thāniya min sharḥ Fuṣūl Abuqrāṭ*, eds. Peter E. Pormann, Karim I. Karimullah, Nicola Carpentieri, Taro Mimura, Emilie Selove, Aileen Das, and Hammood Obaid. Manchester: University of Manchester. Available at https://doi.org/10.3927/51688912

Biesterfeldt, Hans Hinrich. 2007. 'Palladius on the Hippocratic Aphorisms.' In *The Libraries of the Neoplatonists*. Philosophia Antiqua, no. 107, ed. Cristina D'Ancona. Leiden: Brill.

Craik, Elizabeth M. 2015. *The Hippocratic Corpus: Content and Context*. London: Routledge.

Edwards, Martin. 2004. 'Historical Keywords: Trial.' *Lancet* 363 (9446): 1659.

Fancy, Nahyan. 2013. *Science and Religion in Mamluk Egypt: Ibn al-Nafīs, Pulmonary Transit and Bodily Resurrection*. New York, NY: Routledge.

———. 2018. 'Anatomy.' In *1001 Cures: Contributions in Medicine and Healthcare from Muslim Civilisation*, ed. Peter E. Pormann. Manchester: Foundation for Science Technology and Civilisation.

Frede, Michael. 1990. 'An Empiricist View of Knowledge: Memorism.' In *Epistemology*. Companions to Ancient Thought, no. 1, ed. Stephen Everson. Cambridge: Cambridge University Press.

Galen. 1985. *Three Treatises on the Nature of Science*, trans. R. Walzer and M. Frede. Indianapolis, IN: Hackett.

[54] Ibn Qayyim al-Jawziyya (1998), 191.

[55] Fancy (2013).

———. 2011. *Method of Medicine: Volume III, Books 10–14*, ed. and trans. Ian Johnston and G. H. R. Horsley. Loeb Classical Library, no. 518. Cambridge, MA: Harvard University Press.
Hippocrates. 2005. *On Ancient Medicine*, ed. and trans. Mark J. Schiefsky. Leiden: Brill.
Ḥunayn ibn Isḥāq. 2016. *On His Galen Translations*, ed. and trans. John C. Lamoreaux. Provo, UT: Brigham Young University Press.
Ibn Qayyim al-Jawziyya. 1998. *Tuḥfat al-mawdūd bi-aḥkām al-mawlūd*, ed. Bassām ʿAbd al-Wahhāb al-Jābī. Beirut: Dār al-Bashā'ir al-Islamiyya.
Iskandar, Albert Z. 1959. 'A Study of ar-Rāzī's Medical Writings, with Selected Texts and English Translations.' 2 vols. DPhil diss., University of Oxford.
———. 1962. '*al-Rāzī al-Ṭabīb al-Iklīnī: Nuṣūṣ min makhṭūṭāt lam yasbiq nashruhā* (Al-Rāzī, the Clinical Physician: Texts from Manuscripts not Previously Published).' *al-Mashriq* 56.
Joosse, N. Peter, and Peter E. Pormann. 2008. 'Archery, Mathematics, and Conceptualising Inaccuracies in Medicine in 13th Century Iraq and Syria.' *Journal of the Royal Society of Medicine* 101 (8): 425–427.
———. 2010. 'Decline and Decadence in Iraq and Syria after the Age of Avicenna: ʿAbd al-Laṭīf al-Baghdādī (1162–1231) between Myth and History.' *Bulletin of the History of Medicine* 84 (1): 1–29.
———. 2012. "ʿAbd al-Laṭīf al-Baġdādī's Commentary on Hippocrates' "*Prognostic*": A Preliminary Exploration.' In *Epidemics in Context: Greek Commentaries on Hippocrates in the Arabic Tradition*, ed. Peter E. Pormann. Scientia Graeco-Arabica, no. 8. Berlin: De Gruyter.
Kahl. Oliver. 2015. *The Sanskrit, Syriac and Persian Sources in the Comprehensive Book of Rhazes*. Islamic Philosophy, Theology and Science: Texts and Studies, no. 93. Leiden: Brill.
al-Kilānī, Ibn Qāsim. 2017. *Sharḥ Fuṣūl Abuqrāṭ*, eds. Peter E. Pormann, Karim I. Karimullah, Nicola Carpentieri, Taro Mimura, Emilie Selove, Aileen Das, and Hammood Obaid. Manchester: University of Manchester. Available at https://doi.org/10.3927/51688739
Kruk, Remke, and Gerhard Endress, eds. 1997. *The Ancient Tradition in Christian and Islamic Hellenism: Studies on the Transmission of Greek Philosophy and Sciences: Dedicated to H. J. Drossaart Lulofs on His Ninetieth Birthday*. CNWS, no. 50. Leiden: Research School CNWS.
Morabia, Alfredo. 2014. *Enigmas of Health and Disease: How Epidemiology Helps Unravel Scientific Mysteries*. New York, NY: Columbia University Press.
Nasser, Mona, Aida Tibi, and Emilie Savage-Smith. 2009. 'Ibn Sina's *Canon of Medicine*: 11th Century Rules for Assessing the Effects of Drugs.' *Journal of the Royal Society of Medicine* 102 (2): 78–80.
Pormann, Peter E. 2008. 'Medical Methodology and Hospital Practice: The Case of Tenth-century Baghdad.' In *In the Age of al-Farabi: Arabic Philosophy in the 4th/10th Century*, ed. Peter Adamson. Warburg Institute Colloquia, no. 12. London: Warburg Institute.
———., ed. 2011a. *Islamic Medical and Scientific Tradition*. Critical Concepts in Islamic Studies. 4 vols. Routledge: London.
———. 2011b. 'The Formation of the Arabic Pharmacology: Between Tradition and Innovation.' *Annals of Science* 68 (4): 493–515.
———. 2012. 'The Development of Translation Techniques from Greek into Syriac and Arabic: The Case of Galen's *On the Faculties and Powers of Simple Drugs, Book Six*.' In *Medieval Arabic Thought: Essays in Honour of Fritz Zimmermann*, eds. Rotraud Hansberger, Afifi al-Akiti, and Charles Burnett. Warburg Institute Studies and Texts, no. 4. London: Warburg Institute.
———. 2013. 'Qualifying and Quantifying Medical Uncertainty in 10th-century Baghdad: Abu Bakr al-Razi.' *Journal of the Royal Society of Medicine* 106 (9): 370–372.
———. 2017. 'Philosophical Topics in Medieval Arabic Medical Discourse: Problems and Prospects.' In *Philosophy and Medicine in the Formative Period of Islam*, eds. Peter Adamson and Peter E. Pormann. Warburg Institute Colloquia, no. 31. London: Warburg Institute.
———., ed. 2018a. *1001 Cures: Contributions in Medicine and Healthcare from Muslim Civilisation*. Manchester: Foundation for Science Technology and Civilisation.

———., ed. 2018b. *Cambridge Companion to Hippocrates*. Cambridge: Cambridge University Press.

Pormann, Peter E., and N. Peter Joosse. 2012. 'Commentaries on the Hippocratic *Aphorisms* in the Arabic Tradition: The Example of Melancholy.' In *Epidemics in Context: Greek Commentaries on Hippocrates in the Arabic Tradition*, ed. Peter E. Pormann. Scientia Graeco-Arabica, no. 8. Berlin: De Gruyter.

Pormann, Peter E., and Kamran I. Karimullah. 2017. 'The Arabic Commentaries on the Hippocratic Aphorisms: Introduction.' *Oriens* 45 (1–2): 1–52.

Pormann, Peter E., Samuel Barry, Nicola Carpentieri, Elaine van Dalen, Kamran I. Karimullah, Taro Mimura, and Hammood Obaid. 2017. 'The Enigma of Arabic and Hebrew Palladius.' *Intellectual History of the Islamicate World* 5 (3): 252–310.

al-Rāzī, Abū Bakr. 1955–75. *al-Kitāb al-Ḥāwī fī al-ṭibb*. Hyderabad: Maṭbaʿat Majlis Dāʾirat al-Maʿārif al-ʿUthmāniyya.

———. 1987. *al-Kitāb al-Manṣūrī fī l-ṭibb*, ed. Ḥāzim al-Ṣiddīqī al-Bakrī. Kuwait: Maʿhad al-Makhṭūṭāt al-ʿArabiyya.

Rosenthal, Franz. 1966. '"Life Is Short, the Art Is Long": Arabic Commentaries on the First Hippocratic Aphorism.' *Bulletin of the History of Medicine* 40 (3): 226–245.

Tibi, Selma. 2005. 'Al-Razi and Islamic Medicine in the 9th Century.' *James Lind Library Bulletin: Commentaries on the History of Treatment Evaluation*. Available at http://www.jameslindlibrary.org/articles/al-razi-and-islamic-medicine-in-the-9th-century/

Ullmann, Manfred. 2002. *Wörterbuch der griechisch-arabischen Übersetzungen des neunten Jahrhunderts*. Wiesbaden: Harrassowitz.

van der Eijk, Philip J. 1997. 'Galen's Use of the Concept of "Qualified Experience" in His Dietetic and Pharmacological Works.' In *Galen on Pharmacology: Philosophy, History and Medicine*, ed. Armelle Debru. Leiden: Brill.

———. 2005. *Medicine and Philosophy in Classical Antiquity: Doctors and Philosophers on Nature, Soul, Health and Disease*. Cambridge: Cambridge University Press.

———. 2016. 'On "Hippocratic" and "non-Hippocratic" Medical Writings.' In *Ancient Concepts of the Hippocratic*, eds. L. Dean-Jones and R. Rosen. Leiden: Brill.

Weisser, Ursula. 1997. 'Die Zitate aus Galens *de Methodo Medendi* im *Ḥāwī* des Rāzī.' In *The Ancient Tradition in Christian and Islamic Hellenism: Studies on the Transmission of Greek Philosophy and Sciences: Dedicated to H. J. Drossaart Lulofs on His Ninetieth Birthday*, eds. Remke Kruk and Gerhard Endress. CNWS, no. 50. Leiden: Research School CNWS.

**Professor Peter E. Pormann** teaches Classics and Graeco-Arabic Studies at the University of Manchester. His research investigates the transmission of Greek thought into the medieval and modern Arab world, with special focus on the history of medicine. He also works in the area of digital humanities, and collaborates with scientists, for instance in the area of palimpsest studies.

# Chapter 3
# The Piety of Health: The Making of Health in Islamic Religious Narratives

**Ahmed Ragab**

## 3.1 Introduction

What is health for pious Muslims? Scholarship on medicine and Islam and on Prophetic medicine has focused primarily on the spaces of concordance or disagreement between 'Islam,' often viewed from a purely legal perspective, and 'medicine,' almost always referring to learned Galenic medicine.[1] Absent from this picture is the myriad of ways that pious Muslims dealt and continue to deal with medicine and other healing arts beyond the dictates of the law. In this context, and outside the realm of legality, pious Muslims made choices and conceived of their lives in pietistic terms following at times the example of the Prophet, his Companions, and the Imams. While none of these acts was particularly or necessarily mandated, they represented behaviours that pious Muslims sought to emulate in order to achieve nearness to God. In this context, health acquires a different meaning, beyond what is legal or illegal, and conditions a series of behaviours, positions and predispositions.

In the beginning of a chapter dedicated to 'Asking God for Wellness (*al-ʿāfiya*),' the famous scholar and ascetic Hannād ibn al-Sarī (d. 243/858) cited the celebrated Follower[2] and *ḥadīth* reporter, Muṭarrif ibn ʿAbd Allāh ibn al-Shikhkhīr (d. 95/714)

[1] See, for instance, Rahman (1987); Dols (1988): 417–25; Pehro (1995); Stearns (2014): 49–80; Stearns (2011); Fancy (2013); Fancy (2009).

[2] A Follower (*tābiʿ*) is a designation of scholars and *ḥadīth* reporter who belonged to the first or second generations after that of the Prophet. This is in contradistinction to Companions (*ṣaḥābī*) which customarily referred to those who accompanied or knew the Prophet directly, or those who belonged in his generation. To be sure, the exact definition of Companions, and subsequently

A. Ragab (✉)
Johns Hopkins University, Baltimore, MD, USA
e-mail: ahmed_ragab@bbqplus.org


A. al-Akiti, A. I. Padela (eds.), *Islam and Biomedicine*, Philosophy and Medicine 137, https://doi.org/10.1007/978-3-030-53801-9_3

as saying: 'It is preferable to me to be healthy and grateful (to God), than to be sick and patient.'[3] Muṭarrif's remarks were not unique. In fact, he repeated a rather common Prophetic tradition (*ḥadīth*) that was attributed to the Prophet and to a number of Companions and Followers. Hannād's discussion of this *ḥadīth* was part of a longer conversation on health, which was often centred around this particular *ḥadīth*. For instance, the famous ascetic and *ḥadīth* reporter, Wakīʿ ibn al-Jarrāḥ (d. 197/813) reported two different versions of this *ḥadīth*, one of which was also attributed to Muṭarrif. Other scholars, such as Aḥmad ibn Ḥanbal (d. 241/855), also included a version of this *ḥadīth* in his book on asceticism (*Kitāb al-Zuhd*). Similarly, the prolific scholar Abū Nuʿaym al-Iṣfahānī (d. 430/1038) cited three different versions of this *ḥadīth* in his book *Ḥilyat al-awliyāʾ* (*The Adornment of the Saints*). While most of the *ḥadīth*'s versions circulating from the ninth century on were attributed to a number of Companions and Followers, another version directly attributed to the Prophet was also cited by *ḥadīth* compilers and scholars. In this version, such as the one reported by al-Ṭabarānī (d. 360/971) and others, a Companion mentioned his preference for health and gratitude to the Prophet. The Prophet commented in response, 'and so does the Prophet of God.'

This *ḥadīth* placed health in relation to three other categories, namely, gratitude, illness, and patience. In this formulation, health was conditionally accompanied by gratitude to God, who was perceived to be the ultimate giver of well-being. The couple of health and gratitude were understood in contradistinction to illness and the accompanying patience. While the contradiction between health and illness is rather obvious, and the resulting definition of health as the absence of illness is not particularly surprising, it is the relationship between gratitude and patience – and their relationship as a couplet with the couplet of health and disease – that remained key to the pietistic perception of health. In this view, illness was not simply an episode of pain and suffering but also a possibility for the production of new pietistic meanings through the diligent observance of patience and reliance on God. As I have shown elsewhere, illness, in this context, was understood in an ambivalent position. Pious Muslims were encouraged to seek cure but were also promised reward for their patience.[4] In the same context, health was construed in relation to a pietistic cosmology that rendered one's behaviours and perceptions of one's own body key to earning divine reward. In this view, the preference of health over illness was connected to the preference of one of two virtues that a pious Muslim needed to exercise: patience and gratitude. In the coming pages, this chapter investigates the meaning of health from a religious and pietistic perspective. It asks: How was health constructed within this pietistic cosmology? What narrative resources contributed to such construction? How did these pietistic discourses dictate (or attempt to dictate) pious Muslims' understanding of their healthy bodies?

---

Followers, changed over time and in relation to discussions of their intellectual and religious authority. See Khalek (2014): 272–294.

[3] Ibn al-Sarī (1985), 254–55.

[4] Ragab (2018), 2-5.

Scholarship on medicine and Islam, specifically on Prophetic medicine, has consistently focused on two areas of investigation. First, scholars have investigated the legal dimensions that conditioned and controlled medical practice, whether in the medieval, early modern, or in the contemporary periods. Here, scholars looked, for instance, at whether seeking cure was permissible, whether using prohibited materials, such as alcohol among others, was legally allowed, or whether non-Muslim physicians were afforded the same privileges and the same legal position as Muslim physicians.[5] In the same context, scholars investigated the legal regulations of medical practice and how Islamic law understood the responsibility of physicians. Second, scholars investigated the intersection of medical theory with Islamic doctrines and practices, looking for instance at potential contradictions and how religious scholars or Muslim physicians handled these different questions and contradictions.[6] Throughout, the main questions that have animated scholarship continue to be legally-focused.

Yet, and as I have argued elsewhere, another defining feature of the interactions between Muslim patients and physicians as well as between religious and medical knowledge and practice remains largely understudied: namely, the question of piety and pious practice.[7] Here, this investigation moves beyond the question of legality and permissibility to discussing how particular practices existed within a pious framework. I argue that, while the legality of specific acts was an important concern, pious commitment underwrote a larger variety of behaviours including seeking opinions on legality. In other words, it is this pietistic infrastructure that, in part, motivated Muslim patients and practitioners to seek legal opinions about their acts, to judge which opinions they can or should follow, and to ultimately decide whether or not to commit to these opinions. In this context, pious Muslim patients and medical practitioners are understood to act not only based on legal dictates but also in a manner that is partly motivated by commitment and piety as well as by their desire to lead a pious and proper life in the example of the Prophet, Imams, and their Companions.[8] The question of piety affords us a deeper understanding of the practice of pious Muslims as extending along a continuum rather than oscillating between two alternatives: legal and illegal; permissible and impermissible.

In this chapter, Muslim pieties are understood as partly relying on archives of *ḥadīths*, verses, and anecdotes, which provide the background for pietistic thought and practice. Scholars of *ḥadīth*, from the ninth century on, exhibited remarkable flexibility in relation to pietistic *ḥadīths* and narratives. While concerns about degrees of authenticity and reliability were often discussed in relation to *ḥadīths* with clear legal significance, scholars allowed for more flexible standards in relation to *ḥadīths* that engaged with pietistic questions, which were often termed *raqāʾiq* – a

---

[5] See, among many others, Rahman (1987) and Perho (1995).

[6] See, for example, Zinger (2016): 89–117; Lewicka (2014), 83–106.

[7] Ragab (2018), 2–5.

[8] In this vein, see Melchert (2011a): 345–359; Melchert (2011b): 283–300; Melchert (2002): 425–439; Yaldiz (2016); Salem (2016). For an overview of different works on piety, see Ragab (2018), 2–3.

term derived from this literature's goal of softening the heart (*tarqīq al-qulūb*).[9] Here, their main focus was on the socio-pietistic function that these *ḥadīths* played namely, providing for more religious commitment and inciting Muslims to inhabit a pietistic cosmology. The analysis of these *ḥadīths*, of how scholars selected and arranged them, and how some *ḥadīths* and anecdotes repeated over time, does not provide historical evidence as to the time of the Prophet or the early community – a claim that these scholars would not have made with any degree of certainty anyway. Instead, it provides us with a look at the discursive structure and key textual landmarks that defined how to live a pious life and that continued to be influential from the classical Islamic period into the present.

The chapter will investigate health at three different levels. First, I will look at health as a blessing, investigating how health was understood in relation to Divine intervention and care, and how pious Muslims related their healthy bodies to Divine will. Second, I will look at health as the absence of illness, further analysing how the category of health was perceived in relation to illness, as a calamity and as a conduit for forgiveness. Finally, health was also understood to be a process that required attention and care and relied on elaborate medical instructions for health preservation. Thus, in the chapter's final section, I look at health preservation from a pietistic perspective, exploring how religious and pietistic discourses contributed to the making of healthy bodies. The chapter seeks to uncover what health meant, what types of behaviours, habits and dispositions were constituted by this particular understanding of health at the intersection of medical and pietistic discourses.

As will become clear in the coming pages, this chapter deals primarily with a number of classical texts – that is texts produced in the early Islamic period by major authors who remain respected till today. These texts, despite addressing the concerns of their authors and their immediate audience, presented themselves, and were received as, distillations of eternal wisdom that is to be followed, emulated or, at least, contemplated by Muslims centuries beyond the time of their composition. The afterlife of these texts materialized in the Prophetic traditions and verses that they used and interpreted, and that continue to populate sermons and writings consumed by pious Muslims today. While contemporary pious Muslims certainly have different views and deal with new and different understandings of health and disease, the heritage produced and conveyed in these classical cornerstones of the tradition needs to be taken seriously, not as descriptions of the contemporary but as important influences on contemporary behaviour. In other words, this article offers an analysis of these classical writings as significant influences on healthcare seeking behaviour among Muslims till today.

---

[9] Brown (2011b): 1–52.

## 3.2 The Two Blessings: Health and Free Time

Wakīʿ ibn al-Jarrāḥ (d. 197/813) was a famous scholar and reporter of *ḥadīth*, who played a key role in the growing community of *ḥadīth* scholars in ninth-century Iraq. Himself a student of the venerated Sufyān ibn ʿUyayna (d. 198/814), Wakīʿ came to be known as one of the most knowledgeable and trustworthy scholars of his time. His associates included luminaries such as ʿAbd Allāh ibn al-Mubārak (d. 181/797), and his students included celebrated scholars such as Aḥmad ibn Ḥanbal, Hannād ibn al-Sarī, Ibn Abī Shayba (d. 235/849), and many others. Wakīʿ's book entitled *Kitāb al-Zuhd* (*The Book of Renunciation*) commences with two *ḥadīths* that define what *zuhd* or renunciation means as well as the importance of such virtue in a Muslim's life. In the first, the Prophet is reported to have said that no act or disposition in this world is better than renunciation. In the second, *zuhd* is defined as renouncing earthly goods and focusing on Divine favor.[10] Wakīʿ's book on *zuhd* was one of the earliest texts on the topic and had a profound influence on how contemporary and later scholars addressed the topic.[11] Owing in part to Wakīʿ's status and to the fact that his book was one of the earliest and most celebrated writings in the genre, the two framing Prophetic *ḥadīths* that opened the book were not only framing this text, but rather the entire genre.

Following these two Prophetic *ḥadīths*, and in the first chapter entitled 'the Prophet's exhortation on *zuhd*,' Wakīʿ listed a *ḥadīth* where the Prophet was reported as saying: 'There are two blessings of which most people are swindled: health and free time (*al-ṣiḥḥa wa-l-farāgh*).'[12] The *ḥadīth* referred to how people underestimated these two blessings and misused them because they were misguided, by their own hubris, as to their importance. Such neglect would ultimately lead these people to their demise. In his commentary on this *ḥadīth*, which also occurred in the *Ṣaḥīḥ* of al-Bukhārī (d. 256/870), Ibn Baṭṭāl (d. 449/1057) explained:

> Some scholars said that [the Prophet] wanted to alert his nation to the significance of these two blessings of health and self-sufficiency. That is because a person would not have free time, unless they are self-sufficient in terms of their livelihood. Thus, whoever God blesses with these two blessings should be careful not to waste them.[13]

In Ibn Baṭṭāl's view, health and free time were particularly significant because of how they provided the servant enjoying them with self-sufficiency and enabled them to perform more good acts that would bring them closer to God. As such, wasting such blessings and not realizing their importance was warned against by the Prophet.

[10] Ibn al-Jarrāḥ (1993), 43.

[11] Alongside Ibn al-Jarrāḥ's, the most celebrated books on *zuhd* were composed by his associates or students. These included Ibn al-Mubārak's book under the same title, which shared most of its traditions with Ibn al-Jarrāḥ's, as well as books by Wakīʿ and Ibn al-Mubārak's common students, such as Ibn Ḥanbal, Hannād ibn al-Sarī and Ibn Abī al-Dunyā (d. 281/894), and also books by later scholars who came from the same intellectual genealogy, such as Ibn Abī Ḥātim al-Rāzī (d. 327/938) and others.

[12] Ibn al-Jarrāḥ (1993), 44.

[13] Ibn Baṭṭāl (2003), 10:146.

Wakīʿ's text established a link between this particular *ḥadīth* and the question of *zuhd* or renunciation which other authors later followed. For instance, in al-Bukhārī's canonical collection, the *ḥadīth* was placed in the treatise on *riqāq* (often translated as exhortations).[14] Al-Bukhārī entitled the first chapter of this treatise 'No [Real] Life But the Life of the Hereafter.' He derived this phrase from the second *ḥadīth* listed in the same chapter, where the Prophet famously prayed for his Companions, 'O Lord! There is no [real] life but the life of the hereafter! (*lā ʿaysha illā ʿayshu l-ākhira*) O Lord! Mend [the affairs] of the Supporters and Emigres (*al-anṣār wa-l-muhājira*).' Al-Bukhārī chose to start his chapter with the 'two blessings' *ḥadīth*. Scholars have shown how al-Bukhārī, among other scholars of *ḥadīth*, deliberately arranged the *ḥadīths* in their books, and chose titles for their chapters in order to deliver specific messages to their readers.[15] Here, and as explained by Ibn Baṭṭāl, al-Bukhārī saw the 'two blessings' *ḥadīth* as connected to piety and renunciation creating, therefore, a link between enjoying these blessings and living a pious life.

Al-Tirmidhī (d. 279/892) similarly chose to start his discussion of *zuhd* with this *ḥadīth*, placing it as the first in his treatise on exhortations.[16] The last of the major Sunnī collections, which was composed by Ibn Mājah (d. 273/887), followed in the same *ḥadīth*.[17] He included the *ḥadīth* in his treatise of renunciation, but placed it in a chapter on 'wise sayings' in the middle of the treatise rather than in the beginning similar to other compilers.[18] In his treatise on preaching, where he included notes for preachers to use in their sermons, Ibn al-Jawzī (d. 597/1201) devoted a brief section to this *ḥadīth* explaining that the difference between the healthy and the sick is paramount, and that the *ḥadīth* invited people to reckon with the blessings of health and time and devote them to God in gratitude.[19]

In all these cases, and as the 'two blessings' *ḥadīth* continued to figure in writings on renunciation and other pietistic writing, 'health' acquired its defining character in the medieval Muslim pious cosmology. First, health was unambiguously defined as a blessing, which is given and endowed by God, rather than a natural state in which the human body simply existed. While health in the Galenic context, which dominated learned medical practice and was at the heart of these scholars' thinking about health and disease, was perceived as a balance between four humors, such balance was easily influenced by various environmental factors.[20] In this sense, health could not be simply assumed, but rather, it was an active state that required preservation and cultivation since the humoral balance was constantly under threat

[14] Al-Bukhārī (1981), 8:233 (*ḥadīth* no. 6412).

[15] Burge (2011).

[16] Al-Tirmidhī (1998). It is worth noting here that al-Tirmidhī chose to report the tradition in three different ways, the first of which was in a reporting by Ibn al-Mubārak, who included the tradition in his own book on *zuhd* as well.

[17] On Ibn Mājah's collection, see Brown (2011a): 169–181.

[18] Ibn Mājah (1998), 5:593 (*ḥadīth* no. 4170).

[19] Ibn al-Jawzī (1986b), 51–52.

[20] See, for instance, Bos (1994).

of change and disruption by wrong foods, drinks, habits, or by the environment.[21] Here, the link between health and free time is rather instructive. As seen before, free time, a seemingly negative state of being without distractions or occupations, was presented as a positive state of self-sufficiency – an active blessing that required gratitude and appreciation. Health, possibly a negative state of being without illness, was similarly presented as a positive state of maintaining the body's humoral balance and resisting the inevitable influences of the environment – an active blessing that also required gratitude and conditioned a particular pious disposition as will be seen below.

In the beginning of his book on medicine, *Luqaṭ al-manāfiʿ* (*The Gleanings of Benefits*), Ibn al-Jawzī explained the meaning of health and its importance:

> It is known that the body is composed of different humors, and built with opposing things. And that [the body's] proper condition is [achieved] by balancing its complexion. If the complexion is [balanced], health is achieved. And health is achieved by two means: giving the body what is good for it, and extracting harmful wastes from it. Know that health and wellness are the best blessings. As such, the wise (*al-ʿāqil*) need to be grateful for them and not to waste them.[22]

In Ibn al-Jawzī's view, health was a process that required keeping and protecting and could only be achieved by active intervention that protects the body and facilitates its normal action. Moreover, protecting health, and not wasting it, was seen as part of the gratitude and wisdom worthy of the pious believer.

In this context, al-Bukhārī's choice to follow the 'two blessings' *ḥadīth* with a *ḥadīth* that indicated that the only real life is in the hereafter and where the Prophet asked God to mend the affairs of his Companions affirmed the place of health within a pietistic cosmology and provided for a specific understanding of what Muslims needed to do in relation to their health. First, pious Muslims needed to accept a divine causality whereby health was endowed by God. Second, health, as a blessing similar to free time, was meant to provide an opportunity for pious Muslims to follow God's commandments in preparation for the afterlife. Health, in this context, is a means to a higher pietistic goal. As such, it becomes incumbent upon Muslims to protect their health and to perfect their bodies to use them for such important purpose. In the *Luqaṭ*, Ibn al-Jawzī followed his definition of health with the 'two blessings' *ḥadīth*. He then added another *ḥadīth*, where the Prophet was reported as saying:

> God [chooses] some servants, which he protects from being killed, from errors and from ills; he extends their lives in goodness, improves their earnings, keeps them alive in wellness, takes them to himself while they are well and on their beds, and gives them the standings of martyrs.[23]

---

[21] Pormann (2013); Graziani (1980). Galenic physicians also believed that some diseases can be contracted due to bad miasma, which further compounded the influence of environmental factors. See, for instance, Stearns (2011).

[22] Ibn al-Jawzī (2010), 62.

[23] Ibid., 62.

In this context, living a healthy life was a gift from God to a select few who were endowed with living a good life. At the end of his introduction, Ibn al-Jawzī added that the famous Follower Saʿīd ibn Jubayr (d. 95/714) explained that 'the bliss' in the verse, 'then you shall be questioned that day concerning true bliss,'[24] referred to health, further adding to the importance of exhibiting gratitude through proper behaviour and through the preservation of one's health.[25]

It is instructive to consider how this view of health, as a blessing, stands in an orthogonal relation to modern biomedical understandings of health. While health in modern biomedicine is seen primarily as a negative property – that is the absence of illness, it was seen in these text as a positive one – the presence of a specific blessing. The latter view renders the need to follow specific measures and to act in a particular way necessary to preserve and maintain health. Yet, the view from modern biomedicine also inherits the need to act in order to keep and maintain health, though for different reasons.

## 3.3 Health and Wealth

As explained before, the link between health and free time implied a connection between health and wealth, since free time was understood as referring to self-sufficiency. In his treatise on gratitude, *Risālat al-Shukr*, Ibn Abī al-Dunyā (d. 281/894) cited a saying by the well-respected Follower, Wahb ibn Munabbih (d. 114/732), who explained: 'The best blessings are three: the first is the blessing of Islam, without which no blessing is complete; the second is the blessing of wellness (*al-ʿāfiya*) without which there is no sweetness to life; and the third is freedom from want (*al-ghināʾ*) without which livelihood is not complete.'[26] Similarly, Ibn Abī al-Dunyā reported a prayer by the famous scholar al-Ḥasan al-Baṣrī (d. 110/728), where he commenced by thanking God for 'kin, wealth, and health.'[27] The same anecdote by Wahb was reported by several scholars and authors, as late as Ibn Qayyim al-Jawziyya (d. 751/1350), who cited the anecdote in his famous book *ʿUddat al-ṣābirīn* (*The Tools of the Grateful*). In all these cases, health was linked to wealth insofar that wealth was understood as freedom from want and not necessarily the accumulation of material goods.

This connection to wealth was particularly important as it allowed for explaining health in terms of the more-easily comprehensible wealth. For instance, Ibn Abī al-Dunyā, followed by Abū Nuʿaym al-Iṣfahānī, reported an anecdote about the famous mystic Yūnus ibn ʿUbayd (d. 139/756):

---

[24] Qur'an 102:8 (*al-Takāthur*).

[25] Ibn al-Jawzī (2010), 62.

[26] Ibn Abī al-Dunyā (1993), 67.

[27] Ibid., 13.

> A man came to Yūnus ibn ʿUbayd complaining of poverty. Yūnus asked him, 'would it satisfy you if you [trade] your eyesight for a hundred-thousand dirham? The man said 'No!' Yūnus: 'How about a hundred-thousand dirham for your hand?' The man said 'No!' Yūnus said, 'perhaps for your leg?' The man said 'No!' [...] Yūnus then said, 'Now, do you recognize God's blessings?' I see that you have hundreds of thousands of dirhams and you still complain of poverty.[28]

Here, the monetization of healthy body parts was not intended to place a particular value on these parts but rather to make the blessing of health more comprehensible by likening it to wealth. In the same vein, Ibn Abī al-Dunyā followed with a *ḥadīth* from the Companion Abū al-Dardāʾ (d. 32/652), who explained that 'health is the wealth of the body.'[29] Similarly, Ibn Abī al-Dunyā cited the Prophet-king David as saying, 'Health is the hidden kingdom.'[30] While health resided in the ambiguous sphere of positive and negative blessings, self-sufficiency and wealth were rather unambiguous as positive blessings that required particular modes of thanksgiving and of showing gratitude to God, which were explored and discussed briefly in these texts.

Ultimately, the proper pietistic response to all blessings was to express gratitude to God's blessings.[31] However, this gratitude was not simply a verbal act. It involved a number of actions and behaviours that were often specific to the particular blessing in question as will be seen below. For wealth, scholars explained that showing gratitude consisted of two main acts: exhibiting God's favour without boasting or pride, and spending this wealth in charity. For instance, Ibn Abī al-Dunyā cited the scholar al-Fuḍayl ibn ʿAyyād (d. 187/803) as saying, 'Part of gratitude is to mention the blessing.'[32] Similarly, al-Ḥasan al-Baṣrī was reported as instructing, 'Speak of [God's] blessings as speaking of them is [part of] thanking [God] for them.'[33] In another anecdote, the respected Companion ʿImrān ibn Ḥuṣayn (d. 52/672) was seen wearing a beautiful and expensive garment. When questioned about it, he explained, 'the Prophet said that, if God endows [a servant] with a blessing, He likes to see the effects of this blessing on his servant.'[34] In all of these cases, exhibiting wealth was conditioned by modesty and humility where the servant was not exhibiting God's blessings in order to boast but rather in recognition of his favour. As if to emphasize this particular restriction on pride and boastfulness, Ibn Abī al-Dunyā concluded his discussion of exhibiting wealth with a rather well-known *ḥadīth* where the Prophet was reported to have said, 'Eat, drink, and spend [in charity] without boastfulness or wastefulness. God likes to see the effect of His blessings on His servants.'[35]

---

[28] Ibid., 42.

[29] Ibid., 42.

[30] Ibid., 51.

[31] See Frenkel and Lev (2009).

[32] Ibn Abī al-Dunyā (1993), 29.

[33] Ibid., 21.

[34] Ibid., 27. This tradition was also reported by Ibn Ḥanbal and al-Tirmidhī.

[35] Ibid., 27–28.

At another level, expressing gratitude required the use of wealth for purposes sanctioned by God. In this context, and as shown before, creating a connection between health and wealth, or self-sufficiency, served two main purposes. The first was to further highlight the nature of health as a positive blessing that is endowed by God and not simply the absence of ills or diseases. The second is to link the practice of gratitude in relation to health to the more obvious and common practices of gratitude in relation to wealth. In this view, health was firmly situated within an ecology of blessings that conditioned modes of piety based primarily on gratitude.

## 3.4 Health and Forgiveness

In addition to wealth and self-sufficiency, health was also linked to forgiveness. In his famous book on renunciation, *Kitāb al-Zuhd*, Hannād ibn al-Sarī reported a *ḥadīth* where a man asked the Prophet about the best possible prayer. The Prophet replied, 'Ask God for [His] forgiveness, and for wellness in this life and the hereafter. If you are given these, you have won all.'[36] In this *ḥadīth*, which was also cited by al-Tirmidhī and Ibn Mājah, among others, the link between forgiveness (*ʿafw*) and wellness (*ʿāfiya*) was emphasized through the words' morphological proximity and their common root. Here, the coupling of the two served to emphasize the more general meaning of wellness as referring to both physical and spiritual wellness, which are manifest in God's forgiveness. At another level, unlike the connection between health and wealth, the connection between health and forgiveness was achieved not through similarity but rather through consistent pairing. In other words, health was not likened to forgiveness or equated to it in the way that it was likened and equated to wealth. Instead, it was a consistent coupling of health and forgiveness that solidified their connection. For instance, in Hannād's *Zuhd*, the relevant chapter where the previously mentioned *ḥadīth* cited was entitled 'A Chapter on Asking God for Wellness.' While all the *ḥadīths* reported in this chapter were related to physical health, they consistently connected health to asking for God's forgiveness. The first *ḥadīth* narrated a story of a man who prayed to God to punish him for his sins through illness and other calamities in this world. The man fell sick and was close to dying, when the Prophet explained to him, 'O man! You could not stand God's punishment! Instead say, "Our Lord, give us good in this world, and good in the world to come, and guard us against the chastisement of the fire",' citing a famous Qur'anic prayer.[37] The man kept repeating the verse and was healed.[38] In this *ḥadīth*, forgiveness was equated to health by recalling how illness was seen as a way to atone for sins and thus escape punishment in the hereafter. As I explained

[36] Ibn al-Sarī (1985), 256.

[37] Qur'an 2:201 (*al-Baqara*).

[38] Ibn al-Sarī (1985), 254. This tradition was reported in Ibn al-Jarrāḥ's and Ibn Ḥanbal's books on *zuhd*, among other similar writings.

elsewhere, illness was perceived to be a welcome sign of God's favour as one would withstand punishment in this world as a substitute for eternal punishment in the hereafter.[39] As such, asking for forgiveness became a conduit for health.

The other *ḥadīths* in Hannād's chapter linked forgiveness to health as two things that one needs to ask God for, similar to how the *ḥadīth* cited above indicated. Ibn Mājah, for instance, followed in the same vein by titling his chapter 'Asking God for Forgiveness and Wellness,' recalling the *ḥadīth* mentioned above.[40] This repeated linkage and the linguistic connection between the two words further solidified the central place of this *ḥadīth* within the repertoire of traditional and oft-repeated prayers that many authors and preachers continued to recite from the medieval period and well into the contemporary. Encouraging pious Muslims to ask for forgiveness as they ask for health also revealed a level of anxiety about the dangers of health. While different blessings, such as wealth, can be easily noticed and reckoned with allowing the pious Muslim to show gratitude, health was more ubiquitous in a manner that rendered the possibility of overlooking it or not performing the needed gratitude a more present possibility. This anxiety recalls the 'two blessings' *ḥadīth*, which also foregrounded the anxiety about not showing proper gratitude.

## 3.5 Health and Moderation

At another level, and as discussed before, the Galenic medical meaning of health, as an active state of balance that required care, attention, and preservation, engendered a layered perception of the society based on healthy habits. While health was possible and available for all, those who were learned and careful and who adhered to a life of moderation and balance were the ones who truly understood the meaning of health and were able to preserve it, from a medical perspective. This same discourse, which valued moderation and care, was also operative as a definition of piety, where the pious Muslim was one who adhered to a life of moderation and one of care and attention to one's behaviour.[41] In fact, both physicians and religious scholars deployed the term 'surveillance' (*murāqaba*) to refer to the proper attitude of healthy and pious people. Scholars recommended one to pay attention to one's body and soul, to question one's habits and practices, and to never do something simply out of convenience. In this sense, forgiveness was needed not only because one might underestimate the value of health and fail to show proper gratitude but also because such negligence, which was behind sins and errors, could lead to the deterioration of physical health. Forgiveness, for the spiritual sins against God, and the physical sins against one's own body and in turn also against God, was necessary to preserve health and also to account for it in this pietistic space.

[39] Ragab (2018), 90–105.

[40] Ibn Mājah (1998), 1265.

[41] Ragab (2018), 160–164.

Thinking about health as a positive blessing and not simply the absence of illness added significant texture to its meaning and to the perception of what healthy bodies meant. On one hand, health referred to the integrity of the body and the proper functioning of its different organs. As seen in the previously mentioned anecdote, where a scholar attempted to put prices on body parts, health was understood to refer to the absence of disability and the maintenance of physical integrity. Here, the functioning of the different senses, for example, was not understood as a default state from which disability deviated. Instead, it was seen as a blessing that is granted as a gift from absence.

For instance, in a famous prayer reported by Ibn Abī al-Dunyā and cited consistently afterwards, a Companion thanked God for 'clothing [us] after nakedness, guiding [us to Islam] after misguidedness, and granting us vision after blindness.'[42] Similar to how clothing was a gift as people are born naked, sight was seen as a gift as one was blind before birth, and because some animals were believed to be born blind. Moreover, the prayer connected *hudā* (Divine guidance to Islam) to vision, as the first indicated seeing right from wrong similar to how the latter meant the physical ability to see. Similarly, the lack of physical deformity was also a positive blessing that required consistent thanking and gratitude. Ibn Abī al-Dunyā reported that the Prophet prayed: 'Gratitude to God for forming my shape and fixing it, for honouring my face and beautifying it, and for making me a Muslim.'[43] Similar *ḥadīths* were reported by other Companions, where they thanked God for their appearance without deformity. This understanding of health as connected to the proper functioning of body parts allowed for detailed narratives about gratitude, which assigned specific pietistic acts to specific body parts. In an anecdote, which was reported by many authors in different versions, the Follower Abū Ḥāzim (d. 140/757) explained to a questioner the gratitude due for each body part. For hands, one should not steal or do harm; for ears, one should not repeat any malicious sayings that they hear; for the stomach, not to eat too much; for genitals, to practice chastity, etc.[44]

Apart from disability, health was understood to refer to the proper functioning of different organs. For instance, al-Bayhaqī (d. 458/1066) and Ibn Abī al-Dunyā, among others, reported that ʿAlī ibn Abī Ṭālib (d. 40/661), the Prophet's cousin and the first Shīʿī Imam, used to wipe on his belly after defecating and thank God before exclaiming, 'This [defecating] is such a blessing! If only God's servants knew to thank God for it!'[45] In an even more elaborate prayer connected to bodily functions, the Prophet was reported to have said: 'Whenever [the Prophet] Noah defecated, he would say, "Gratitude to God who blessed me by tasting [food], kept [the food's] benefits inside my body, and removed its harm from my body."'[46] In the same vein,

[42] Ibn Abī al-Dunyā (1993), 15.

[43] Ibid., 51.

[44] Ibid., 53. This was also reported by Abū Nuʿaym al-Iṣfahānī in his *Ḥilya*. The tradition was also reported by Ibn Qayyim in his *ʿUddat al-ṣābirīn,* in Ibn Qayyim al-Jawziyya (1989), 134.

[45] Ibn Abī al-Dunyā (1993), 14.

[46] Ibid., 52. This tradition was reported also by al-Kharāʾiṭī in his book on gratitude, among others as late as al-Suyūṭī (d. 991/1505) and beyond. In the same vein, Ibn Qayyim reported a tradition by

Ibn Abī al-Dunyā reported that the Prophet-king David asked God, '"what is your least blessings?" God replied, "O David! Breathe!" so he breathed. God said, "this is the least of my blessings on you."'[47]

As explained before, this concern about taking health for granted, and underestimating the most minor functions of the body, worked in tandem with the Galenic view of health as a state of balance, and with the consistent instructions given by physicians on how to keep one's health and well-being.[48] Keeping healthy required attention to bodily functions and to any minor changes or problems. Within the same ethos, giving God his due gratitude started with recognizing the different blessings manifested in bodily functions and then working to protect them and to use them for good. Together, medical and religious discourses served to generate habits of awareness of bodily functions which were necessary to protect the body from illness and to also render gratitude for the blessings of health.

In this context, it is important to underscore the expansive nature of gratitude as a pietistic practice. Gratitude, which was presented as a central quality of pious Muslims, included an elaborate set of acts that manifested across a pious Muslim's life. On the one hand, and as mentioned before, gratitude required showing God's blessing without boastfulness or waste. In relation to health, this included caring for one's appearance and outward health, and also protecting one's health as endangering oneself would be wasting God's blessing. On the other hand, gratitude for a particular blessing required using it to obey God's commandments. Similar to how wealthy Muslims were expected to spend money in charity, healthy pious Muslims were expected to utilize their organs and their health in doing good, as explained before.

At another level, proper gratitude was never possible. After all, scholars asserted that nothing a person could do would come close to repaying God or even properly thanking him. Many scholars reported that one of al-Ḥasan al-Baṣrī's acquaintances decided to be an ascetic (*tanassaka*), and in the process declared that he would not eat particular types of expensive food because, he explained, '[he] could not thank God enough for them.' Al-Ḥasan al-Baṣrī was rather indignant and responded, 'What a foolish man! And does he thank God enough for cool water?'[49]

Pious Muslims needed to reflect consistently on what was given to them in blessing. Such reflection, which was at the heart of gratitude, engendered specific mental habits of focus and self-awareness that came to be characteristic of learned culture in the medieval Islamic period. Here, however, this pietistic discourse aimed not only at learned elites but, intentionally, looked to extend the reach of this contemplative self-awareness to as many Muslims as possible. In this context, health,

---

'Ā'isha, the Prophet's wife, where she said, 'Any servant who drinks a sip of water that goes in the body with no harm, and comes out with no harm, is required to show gratitude,' Ibn Qayyim al-Jawziyya (1989), 144.

[47] Ibn Abī al-Dunyā (1993), 59–60.

[48] Al-Rāzī (1998).

[49] Ibn Abī al-Dunyā (1993), 33–34.

understood from the Galenic perspective, was a conduit for more piety because it provided opportunities for more reflection on divine blessings. At the same time, pietistic awareness and reflection were conduits for healthy behaviour in the Galenic sense as they conditioned a conscious awareness of one's body and one's behaviours.

Moreover, gratitude was also a blessing in itself. Scholars used the verse, 'If you are thankful, surely I will increase you, but if you are thankless, my chastisement is surely terrible,'[50] to explain that gratitude led to increase in different blessings. As such, the ability of a servant to persist in thanking God was a blessing because it yielded even more blessings. Ibn Abī al-Dunyā listed three consecutive *ḥadīths* that expressed how gratitude was a blessing. In the first, the Prophet explained, 'God never blesses a servant with gratitude and prevents him from increase because God said, "If you are thankful, surely I will increase you."'[51] Here, the *ḥadīth* used the term bless (*yarzuq*) to refer to gratitude as a conduit of more blessings. In the second *ḥadīth*, the Prophet was reported as directly praying for God to bless him with gratitude and proper worship. In all these cases, gratitude, with the attendant values of care for oneself and awareness of one's body, was a blessing that required prayer and gratitude in itself.

## 3.6 Health and Illness

Although health was consistently defined as a positive state and not simply the absence of illness, illness remained a key category in understanding health. As explained before, the preservation of health was a key role for physicians, who aimed to regulate what their patients ate and drank along with many other behaviours.[52] However, the physician's role in preserving health, though theoretically key, was rather rare in practice. Only physicians serving sovereigns or rich and elite clients, who were able to pay for physicians to monitor their health, were able to perform the tasks of health preservation with any regularity.[53] Another source of knowledge in relation to health preservation came from treatises composed by physicians and others which explained healthy habits and provided less wealthy readers with the resources to keep their bodies healthy.[54] However, even though these books were available to a wider audience, they remained confined to learned elites. On a more regular basis, the physician's and the patient's encounter with health and sickness happened at the moment of illness. Physicians encountered clients in the market and in hospitals when they had fallen sick and when their conditions have worsened and

[50] Qur'an 14:7 (*Ibrāhīm*).

[51] Ibn Abī al-Dunyā (1993), 11.

[52] See, for instance, Bos and Garofalo (2007): 43–95; Waines (1999): 228–240.

[53] See Brain (1977): 936–38; Nicolae (2012).

[54] Bos (1998): 365–375; Ragab (2015).

became significantly burdensome.[55] As such, pietistic literature engaged with health, both from the angle of preservation, and from that of illness and recovery.

As discussed elsewhere, pious Muslims were instructed to receive illness with patience and to view it as an opportunity, if not even a blessing from God, to repent for their sins avoiding punishment in the afterlife. The verse 'Whosoever does evil shall be recompensed for it'[56] seemed to have generated a series of discussions among Companions, Followers, and later scholars. Authors of *zuhd* texts explained that Companions, even as prominent as Abū Bakr (d. 13/634) – the Prophet's closest friend – were disconcerted by this verse as it meant to them that there was no chance of salvation in the afterlife. Since humans commit endless errors, punishment and eternal demise were assured. In these different accounts, the Prophet explained that such recompense included diseases and other calamities that befell the believers in this world rendering them safe from punishment in the afterlife. As such, illness was received with pietistic joy as a sign of God's forgiveness and was framed within narratives of patience and acceptance, which were necessary for God's reward to materialize.[57] This role of sickness in the pietistic cosmology posed important questions about the appropriateness of seeking cure and whether it was better for Muslims to wish for or withstand illness and not seek help in order to reap the benefits of patience.

Moreover, scholars also discussed the limits of medical intervention: if illness was predestined and ordained by God, what good could medicine do? And would seeking medicine become a way of shunning divine will and violating the principles of reliance on God (*tawakkul*)? As explained elsewhere, these questions were answered in two different ways. At the legal level, scholars affirmed the importance of seeking cure and how it was part of *tawakkul*. As such, there is little if any evidence of any legal opinion that prohibited or discouraged seeking cure.[58] At the pietistic level, which manifested in the genre of *raqāʾiq*, as explained before, pious Muslims were encouraged to hold both positions in pietistic tension that kept them constantly aware of their bodies and their attempt to get closer to God. In this context, health was understood as recovery from illness and was linked to questions of seeking cure and medical care.

## 3.7 Health and the 'Freedom' from Illness

Health was also the freedom (rather than recovery) from illness – a definition that manifested practically in discussions about the legality or the propriety of asking God for wellness and health with the attendant loss of the penance that illness

55 Millán (2004).

56 Qur'an 4:123 (*al-Nisāʾ*).

57 Ragab (2018), 100–102.

58 Ibid., 192–97.

provided. One *ḥadīth* stood as the anchor point in this debate. In this *ḥadīth*, the famous Follower and *ḥadīth* reporter Muṭarrif ibn ʿAbd Allāh was reported to have said, 'I prefer to be healthy and grateful, than to be sick and patient.'[59] Scholars reported a number of versions of this *ḥadīth*, in one of which a Companion (commonly referenced as Abū al-Dardāʾ) said the same to the Prophet and the Prophet responded, 'And the Prophet of God prefers health as well.' This *ḥadīth* was also part of a larger pietistic debate about which of the two virtues, patience and gratitude, occupied a higher position in the Muslim pietistic cosmology. In his book *ʿUddat al-ṣābirīn*, Ibn Qayyim al-Jawziyya dedicated two chapters to outlining the arguments for each side.[60] To be sure, Ibn Qayyim and those whom he reported from believed that both virtues were necessary for the spiritual well-being of pious Muslims. The argument, however, was a theoretical and literary one conditioned along the lines of the *faḍāʾil* (privileges) literature, where litterateurs discussed the privileges of certain people, places, or acts. Yet, when it came to health, the debate implied different sets of recommended acts: should one pray and wish for health, therefore preferring gratitude, or hope for illness and the attendant forgiveness, therefore opting for patience? Hannād ibn al-Sarī, among others, engaged with this question in his chapter on 'Asking God for Wellness,' where the Prophet was reported to advise against praying for illness to forgive sins, and instead encouraged asking for health and forgiveness.

At the conclusion of the second chapter, Ibn Qayyim followed previous scholars in attempting to reconcile the two virtues and explain that both gratitude and patience were indeed blessings that required gratitude, in themselves. That is to say that one's ability and commitment to showing gratitude and exercising patience was a divine gift of piety and sincerity that required further gratitude in themselves. Moreover, the blessings that required gratitude were in themselves a test that required patience and observance. Here, patience was not simply a mode of passive withstanding but rather an active act of accepting God's will and acting accordingly. Blessings, like health and wealth, were also trials that required withstanding because they came with the requirement of gratitude. Ibn Qayyim cited the famous Companion Ibn ʿAbbās (d. 68/687) as saying, 'hardship and well-being, health and sickness, wealth and poverty [...] are all trials [from God].'[61] In this context, health, understood as a trial in itself, was conceived as an equivalent of illness. Ibn Qayyim cited some 'good ancestors' as saying, 'Both believers and unbelievers can demonstrate patience in face of hardship. But only a true believer can be patient in face of health.'[62] Similarly, the Companion ʿAbd al-Raḥmān ibn ʿAwf (d. 32/652) lamented, 'We were tested with hardship and we were patient. We were then tested with good living and we were not [patient].'[63] Rendering health and other blessings as occasions for patience and observance served to reformulate living in wellness into a trial that

[59] Ibn Abī al-Dunyā (1993), 19.

[60] Ibn Qayyim al-Jawziyya (1989), 111–175.

[61] Ibid., 160.

[62] Ibid., 64.

[63] Ibid., 64.

required self-awareness and demanded pietistic observance. In this context, preferring illness to health or health to illness carried less significance. Patience and gratitude were to be held in pietistic tension as the pious Muslim continued to contemplate their behaviour in relation to their various conditions in life – not taking anything for granted but rather taking each occurrence as an occasion for observance.

Yet, health was also understood in a comparative perspective. Not all ills were alike and, therefore, a measure of health existed in some conditions that did not exist in others. I have discussed elsewhere how scholars explained that some diseases carried more weight than others and how certain afflictions guaranteed more reward because of the level of hardship.[64] Parallel to this discourse, scholars argued that pious Muslims needed to remember their well-being when encountering sick people. For instance, a scholar by the name of ʿAbd al-ʿAzīz ibn Abī Rawwād (d. 159/775)[65] reported that he met a friend of his who had a malignant ulcer in his hand. When his friend saw that Ibn Abī Rawwād was pained by its sight, he explained, 'Do you know the blessing that God bestowed on me by making this ulcer in my hand, when he could have made it in my pupil, or in my tongue or in my penis!'[66] In this account and similar other anecdotes, scholars engaged with the medical environment where perfect health was hardly possible, and where people became aware of their healthy bodies as they encountered or recovered from illness, or when they encountered other sick people. Here, the pietistic narrative allowed for redefining health on a continuum encouraging pious Muslims to be more reflective about their bodies in relation to others. Whether defined in active or passive terms, health conditioned a particular mode of observance, which was also a key component of both medical and pietistic discourses.

## 3.8 A Pious Healthy Body

As the report goes, Imam ʿAlī al-Riḍā (d. 203/818), the eighth Shīʿī Imam, was attending the court of the Abbasid caliph al-Maʾmūn (r. 198–218/813–833), when a discussion about medicine and preserving health took place. ʿAlī al-Riḍā, the then Shīʿī Imam for a faction of Imāmī shīʿites, had been named the heir to the Abbasid throne by al-Maʾmūn in a move that gave much hope to the Imam's supporters and led to divisions within the Abbasid household. He was summoned to al-Maʾmūn's court where he spent his remaining days before dying, as many believed al-Maʾmūn

[64] Ragab (2018), 105–107.

[65] There appeared to be a transcription error for the name of the scholar in the Damascus text: ʿAbd al-ʿAzīz ibn Abī *Dāwūd*. I am grateful to the editor, Afifi al-Akiti, who discovered this error and corrected it to Ibn Abī Rawwād – an early scholar and reporter of *ḥadīth* from Mecca. This is confirmed in another edition, namely the Meccan text [see Ibn Qayyim al-Jawziyya (2014), 268], as well as the equivalent narration found in Ibn Abī al-Dunyā (1993), 140, l. 5.

[66] Ibn Qayyim al-Jawziyya (1989), 139.

had poisoned him to escape the toxic political situation.[67] In this court meeting, ʿAlī al-Riḍā remained silent as the caliph debated with his physicians. When al-Maʾmūn asked him about his opinions, he explained that he had learned what was sufficient for him from the heritage of his ancestors – the Prophet and his family. Al-Maʾmūn asked ʿAlī al-Riḍā to write a treatise for him that addressed these questions. When completed, al-Maʾmūn admired the treatise so much that he had it written with gold water giving it the name *al-Risāla al-Dhahabiyya* (*The Golden Treatise*).[68]

While the treatise, attributed to Imam ʿAlī al-Riḍā, continues to survive and to inform important discussion about Islam and medicine in the Twelver context, its authorship is in doubt.[69] Regardless of its authorship, the treatise enjoyed the support of major figures in the Shīʿī community in Iraq during this period and represented rather unobjectionable issues that were accepted by the learned elite during this period.

As a treatise attributed to the Imam, it essentially functions as a single extended *ḥadīth* imbued with the Imam's authority. However, this long *ḥadīth* was deeply and unquestionably medical in nature. As explained before, the context described in the treatise was a medical setting with four of the most important physicians of the time in attendance. While Imam ʿAlī al-Riḍā claimed a different source of authority, namely that of the Prophet and his family, the content of the treatise relied heavily on Galenic medical knowledge. In fact, the proposition that medical knowledge derived from the Prophetic heritage was superior in authority while also similar in nature to medical knowledge derived from Galenic teachings was rather common in both Sunnī and Shīʿī works, such as those of Abū Nuʿaym al-Iṣfahānī, Ibn Qayyim al-Jawziyya, and physicians such as Ibn Ṭarkhān (d. 690/1291), and ʿAbd al-Laṭīf al-Baghdādī (d. 629/1231), among others.[70] For all of these authors, the source of Prophetic knowledge was divine and certain while that of Galenic physicians was built on human knowledge. While the two bodies of knowledge almost always seemed to agree, the difference in authority was unmistakable for pious and religious authors.[71]

Similar to *The Golden Treatise*, the famous Sunnī scholar and celebrated preacher Ibn al-Jawzī composed a medical text called *Luqaṭ al-manāfiʿ* (mentioned previously in Sect. 3.2).[72] He then wrote a summary of the *Luqat,* where he removed

---

[67] Yūsuf (1970). See Tor (2001): 103–128. See also, Crone and Hinds (2003), 94–98.

[68] Al-Riḍā (1982), 5–7.

[69] *The Golden Treatise* was not listed in any of the biographies of Imam ʿAlī al-Riḍā that were written close to the time of his death. Most notably, the treatise is absent from the *ʿUyūn akhbār al-Riḍā* by Ibn Bābawayh al-Qummī (1984), which is the most authoritative hagiography of the Imam owing to Ibn Bābawayh's important standing and his close association with the Imamate household. On Ibn Bābawayh (d. 381/991), see Ibn al-Nadīm (n.d.), 196. The treatise makes its first appearance in the biographical literature in Abū Jaʿfar al-Ṭūsī's (d. 460/1067) *Rijāl*, see al-Ṭūsī (1961). As such, the treatise appears to have become known and accepted as authentic between 990 and 1060.

[70] Ragab (2018), 187–191.

[71] Ibid., 46–87.

[72] Ibn al-Jawzī (2010).

much of the Prophetic materials that were included in the larger text making the summary's focus even more Galenic.[73] Both *The Golden Treatise* and the *Luqat* were deeply Galenic in their orientation – from their understanding of the body and its composition to their recommendations in terms of food, drink, and other healthy habits. Yet, neither of the two texts was a medical textbook, and their authors did not envision physicians or medical practitioners to be their main audience. Instead, they belonged to the self help or medical advice literature, where physicians and other learned authors provided advice on how one should take care of their bodies and preserve their health. The two texts were also invested in the religious authority of their authors, who added religious and pietistic undertones to their medical advice. These were not simply collections of medical recommendations similar to other recommendations offered by physicians. They were ones rooted in a pietistic narrative that advocated the importance of keeping one's body healthy as part of a religious comportment. The body portrayed in these texts, while almost wholly Galenic, was also a pious body – the responsibilities and the expectations related to behaviour were presented as those rooted in pietistic literature and invested in following the Prophet's and the Imam's example.

As such, it is unsurprising that both treatises spent time explaining the importance of health and its place in the pietistic cosmology. *The Golden Treatise* started with the famous *ḥadīth*: God has not created an illness without also creating a cure for it.[74] The *ḥadīth*, which commonly appeared in books of Prophetic medicine, served to provide a justification for the practice of medicine. Similarly, Ibn al-Jawzī started his treatise with the famous 'two blessings' *ḥadīth* mentioned earlier (Sect. 3.2). This was followed by a version of Muṭarrif's *ḥadīth* on preferring to be healthy and grateful. Ibn al-Jawzī chose to cite a version reported by Abū al-Dardā', who mentioned this preference to the Prophet who agreed: 'And the Prophet of God prefers health as well.'[75] With these *ḥadīths*, Ibn al-Jawzī recalled the previously discussed literature on health and its importance, and provided a justification for his book and for his inquiries on health and medicine.

However, as explained before, health was not a given that could be taken for granted. Instead, it required effort and cultivation. *The Golden Treatise* explained: 'The body is like a fertile, uncultivated land. If it is cared for with cultivation and irrigation, [...] its profit will increase and its produce will grow. If one ignores it, it will become corrupted and grass will claim it.'[76] Similarly, Ibn al-Jawzī explained that one had a religious obligation to care for one's own body so as to be fit for undertaking religious obligations: 'The protection of the inner [spiritual] core can only be achieved by caring for the apparent [physical] body. [This is why] the Prophet ordered his Companions to seek cure.'

[73] Ibn al-Jawzī (1986a).

[74] Al-Riḍā (1982), 10.

[75] Ibn al-Jawzī (2010), 61–62.

[76] Al-Riḍā (1982), 13–14.

Following Galenic thought, the body was deeply imbedded in, and connected to its environment. This was reflected in the recommendations related to different seasons. *The Golden Treatise* went into great detail outlining the best food and drink for each season and for each month of the year.[77] In all cases, moderation was the cardinal rule, helping to sustain the healthy body: 'especially when the body's [complexion] is moderate, then one should choose moderate diet and regiment for it.'[78] Both authors were clear on how moderation was connected to the Galenic understanding of the body's composition: 'Because God has built [human] bodies on four natures: blood, phlegm, yellow bile and black bile. Two are hot and two are cold. They were conversely matched so that they are hot and dry, hot and soft (*layyin*), cold and dry, and cold and soft.'[79]

Moderation required a keen sense of one's own body and an awareness of one's habits and behaviours. The pious learned reader needed not to blindly follow unhealthy habits but to continuously consider and reflect on their behaviours. In a rather stern tone, Imam ʿAlī al-Riḍā warned the caliph against settling into bad habits, and against trusting simple observation over intellectual reckoning:

> Never say: 'I have always done so and so and ate so and so and it never harmed me; or I have drunk so and so and it did not hurt me; or I have done so and so and I have not been ill. Those who say so, my lord, the Prince of the Believers, are like a beast that does not know what harms and what benefits it. [Consider that] if a thief is caught the first time he steals, was punished and never stole again, his punishment would be easier. However, [God] gives him time and power so he [steals] again, until he is caught with the biggest of thefts so he is mutilated, is severely humiliated; a result of his greed.[80]

The skepticism of personal and anecdotal experience is also a common Galenic theme, where Galenic physicians presented themselves as logical and rational practitioners compared to untrustworthy experimental practitioners, whose recommendations and prescriptions may work for some time but will then fail.[81] Similarly, pious Muslims were not supposed to simply trust in habits and common behaviours but to consult learned authorities and base their behaviours on their recommendations. In both cases, knowledge was key in providing and guiding one to the proper path.

Both authors, following in the footsteps of many others, painted a particular picture of the body which valued health and wellness, presenting these values as religiously motivated states of being. The attention to details concerning health preservation created a pietistic environment whereby caring for the body, preserving health, and treating diseases were part of a person's pietistic performance. This medico-pietistic performance was rooted in some of the same virtues that governed pietistic performances in other areas of a person's life and also intersected with the virtues that governed the life of the urban learned elites. In all of these cases, one

---

[77] Al-Riḍā (1982), 17–20.

[78] Ibn al-Jawzī (2010), 111.

[79] Al-Riḍā (1982), 48. Note the use of the word soft [*layyin*] as opposed to humid [*raṭīb*], which is more common in Galenic writings.

[80] Ibid, 66.

[81] Galen (1978).

needed to pay attention to their own bodies and their various activities. Similar to other forms of pietistic performances, this medical piety was based on self-reflection and constant observance and rooted in the practice of moderation and balance.

## 3.9 Conclusion

As shown in the previous pages, health was perceived to be primarily a divine gift and blessing that is endowed and accomplished in time and in contrast to a previous and a future potential state of lack of health. God was thanked for endowing one with eyesight after blindness, despite this blindness, in this case, being a largely intrauterine state. God was also thanked for keeping one healthy in anticipation of the inevitability of illness in human life. This view of health, as an active endowed state and not a passive default one, was perhaps inspired by, and in turn influenced, the Galenic view of health as a state of active balance that was constantly under threat. In both intertwined discourses, health was to be preserved and cultivated.

Such understanding led to two important dispositions: self-awareness and self-care. In both Galenic and pietistic contexts, pious Muslims were encouraged to pay attention to their bodies, the changes that happen to them, and the environment that surrounded them. They were also encouraged to exert intentional effort to protect their bodies and preserve their health as both a means to show gratitude, and in order to be able to do more good. As such, and as explained elsewhere, both medical and pietistic writings, not to mention philosophical and ethical writings as well, inscribed a particular mode of healthy and commendable behaviour – one that valued attention and awareness and emphasized one's control and responsibility for one's body. Far from asking whether maintaining health or seeking cure was legally acceptable or not, analysing pietistic writings show that Muslim pietistic writings conditioned particular modes of healthy behaviour, as understood within Galenic medical writings. These behaviours and dispositions constitute what can be described as a piety of health. In this context, health acquires a specific meaning within a pietistic cosmology, and piety is reframed and constructed along the lines of healthy and health seeking behaviour. Both health and piety become characters of upstanding individuals, who were the prototypical ideal figure in medieval Muslim society.

At the same time, this predisposition to healthy behaviour, or what I have termed a piety of health, interacted with complex views on illness and its own place within the pietistic cosmology. Illness was a conduit for forgiveness that was to be welcomed and accepted as a gift from God. The potential of forgiving sins as reward for patient endurance raised questions about whether Muslims should seek treatment or should simply opt for patience. As explained elsewhere, pietistic literature encouraged pious Muslims to maintain an ambivalent position, which acknowledged their weaknesses and need to seek cure, and, at the same time, wished for more ability to withstand and endure.[82] Health also figured within this pietistic geography. While

[82] Ragab (2018), 123–24.

health was indeed the opposite of illness, they were both divine gifts that could potentially turn into curses. Health that was not met with gratitude invited divine ire, and illness not followed by patience or accompanied by anger and contempt, negated reward and brought about God's wrath. In this pietistic context, illness and health functioned complementarily as ongoing states of potentiality that invited constant patience and gratitude, both of which emphasized the belief that God owned the body, endowed health and illness, and demanded one's gratitude and patience.

Looking at the pietistic literature is certainly not a substitute for a social history. There is no clear evidence that ordinary pious Muslims diligently followed the detailed dictates of pietistic writings or the requirements of the law. Moreover, it is difficult to see the influence of these texts beyond their own time, let alone into the contemporary. Finally, authors of pietistic writings spent most of their time, and most of the pages in their books, citing Prophetic *ḥadīths* rather than expressing their own views in their own words. While authors of pietistic writings indeed acted as compilers of Prophetic materials, their editorial voice, and the choices that they made, contributed to the construction of a pietistic archive – a series of well-known *ḥadīths* and anecdotes that became available to scholars and preachers and that conditioned how regular pious Muslims understood their religious obligations.[83] While these *ḥadīths* cannot inform us about the life and time of the Prophet, they provide us with a substrate for Muslim pietistic thought, which continues to be influential today. The texts discussed in this chapter continue to be printed, read, and regularly used by Muslim preachers and scholars today, informing how pious Muslims understand health and disease, the behaviours they take in relation to maintaining their health, and the concerns they have in this regard. Moreover, and at a constructive level, these texts provide the material for constructive Muslim ethic of health and for creating new understandings of health-seeking behaviour among contemporary pious Muslims.

## References

Abū Nuʿaym al-Iṣfahānī. 1997. *Ḥilyat al-awliyāʾ wa-ṭabaqāt al-aṣfiyāʾ*, ed. Muṣṭafá ʿAbd al-Qādir ʿAṭā. 12 vols. Beirut: Dār al-Kutub al-ʿIlmīyah.

Álvarez Millán, Cristina. 2004. 'Medical Anecdotes in Ibn Juljul's *Biographical Dictionary*.' *Suhayl: International Journal for the History of the Exact and Natural Sciences in Islamic Civilisation* 4: 141–158.

Bos, Gerrit. 1998. 'Ibn al-Jazzār on Medicine for the Poor and Destitute.' *Journal of the American Oriental Society* 118 (3): 365–375.

———. 1994. 'Maimonides on the Preservation of Health.' *Journal of the Royal Asiatic Society* 4 (2): 213–235.

Bos, Gerrit, and Ivan Garofalo. 2007. 'A Pseudo-Galenic Treatise on Regimen: The Hebrew and Latin Translations from Ḥunayn Ibn Isḥāq's Arabic Version.' *Aleph: Historical Studies in Science and Judaism* 7: 43–95.

[83] Burge (2011). See also, although in a different context, Hirschler (2006).

Brain, Peter. 1977. 'Galen on the Ideal of the Physician.' *South African Medical Journal* 52 (23): 936–938.

Brown, Jonathan A. C. 2011a. 'The Canonization of Ibn Mâjah: Authenticity vs. Utility in the Formation of the Sunni *Ḥadîth* Canon.' *Revue des mondes musulmans et de la Méditerranée* 129: 169–181.

———. 2011b. 'Even If It's Not True It's True: Using Unreliable Hadīths in Sunni Islam.' *Islamic Law and Society* 18 (1): 1–52.

al-Bukhārī. 1981. *Ṣaḥīḥ al-Bukhārī: The Translation of the Meanings of Ṣaḥīḥ al-Bukhārī, Arabic-English*, trans. Muhammad Muhsin Khan. 9 vols. Medina: Dar al-Fikr.

Burge, S. R. 2011. 'Reading Between the Lines: The Compilation of Ḥadīṯ and the Authorial Voice.' *Arabica* 58 (3): 186–188.

Crone, Patricia, and Martin Hinds. 2003. *God's Caliph: Religious Authority in the First Centuries of Islam*. Cambridge: Cambridge University Press.

Dols, Michael W. 1988. Review of *Islam and Medicine: Health and Medicine in the Islamic Tradition: Change and Identity*, by Fazlur Rahman. *History of Science* 26 (4): 417–425.

Fancy, Nahyan. 2009. 'The Virtuous Son of the Rational: A Traditionalist's Response to the *Falāsifa*.' In *Avicenna and His Legacy: A Golden Age of Science and Philosophy*, ed. Y. Tzvi Langermann. Cultural Encounters in Late Antiquity and the Middle Ages, no. 8. Turnhout: Brepols.

———. 2013. *Science and Religion in Mamluk Egypt: Ibn al-Nafīs, Pulmonary Transit and Bodily Resurrection*. Culture and Civilization in the Middle East. New York, NY: Routledge.

Frenkel, Miriam, and Yaacov Lev, eds. 2009. *Charity and Giving in Monotheistic Religions*. Studien Zur Geschichte und Kultur des Islamischen Orients, no. 22. Berlin: Walter de Gruyter.

Galen. 1978. *Kitāb Jālinūs fī firaq al-ṭibb lil-muta'ālimīn naql Abī Zayd Ḥunayn ibn Isḥāq al-'Ibādī*, ed. Muḥammad Salīm Sālim. Cairo: General Egyptian Book Organization.

Graziani, Joseph Salvatore. 1980. *Arabic Medicine in the Eleventh Century as Represented in the Works of Ibn Jazlah*. Karachi: Hamdard Academy.

Hirschler, Konrad. 2006. *Medieval Arabic Historiography: Authors as Actors*. London: Routledge.

Ibn Abī al-Dunyā. 1993. *al-Shukr li-Allāh*. Beirut: Mu'assasat al-Kutub al-Thaqafiyya.

Ibn Bābawayh al-Qummī, al-Shaykh al-Ṣadūq. 1984. *'Uyūn akhbār al-Riḍā*, ed. Ḥusayn al-A'lamī. 2 vols. Beirut: Mu'assasat al-A'lamī.

Ibn Baṭṭāl. 2003. *Sharḥ Ṣaḥīḥ al-Bukhārī*. Riyadh: Maktabat al-Rushd.

Ibn al-Jarrāḥ, Wakī'. 1993. *Ṣaḥīḥ Kitāb al-Zuhd*, ed. 'Abd al-Raḥman al-Faryawā'ī. Beirut: Mu'assasat al-Kutub al-Thaqafiyya.

Ibn al-Jawzī. 1986a. *al-Tadhkira fī l-wa'ẓ*. Beirut: Dār al-Ma'rifa.

———. 1986b. *al-Tibb al-Rūḥānī*. Cairo: Maktabat al-Thaqāfa al-Dīniyya.

———. 2010. *Luqaṭ al-manāfi' fī 'ilm al-ṭibb*, ed. Marzūq 'Alī Ibrāhīm. Cairo: Dār al-Kutub wa-l-Wathā'iq al-Qawmiyya.

Ibn Mājah. 1998. *Sunan Ibn Mājah*. 5 vols. Beirut: Dār al-Kutub al-'Ilmiyya.

Ibn al-Nadīm. n.d. *al-Fihrist*. Beirut: Dār al-Ma'rifa.

Ibn Qayyim al-Jawziyya. 1989. *Uddat al-ṣābirīn wa-dhakīrat al-shākirīn*, ed. Muḥyī al-Dīn Dīb Mittū. Damascus: Dār Ibn Kathīr.

———. 2014. *Uddat al-ṣābirīn wa-dhakīrat al-shākirīn*, ed. Ismā'īl ibn Ghāzī Marḥaba. Athār al-Imām Ibn Qayyim al-Jawziyya wa-mā laḥiqahā min a'māl, no. 15. Mecca: Dār 'Ālam al-Fawā'id.

Ibn al-Sarī, Hannād. 1985. *Kitāb al-Zuhd*, ed. 'Abd al-Raḥman al-Faryawā'ī. Kuwait: Dār al-Khulafā'.

Khalek, Nancy. 2014. 'Medieval Biographical Literature and the Companions of Muḥammad.' *Der Islam* 91 (2): 272–294.

Lewicka, Paulina. 2014. 'Medicine for Muslims? Islamic Theologians, Non-muslim Physicians and the Medical Culture of the Mamluk Near East.' In *History and Society During the Mamluk*

*Period (1250–1517)*, ed. Stephen Conermann. Studies of the Annemarrie Schimmel Research College, no. 1. Bonn: Bonn University Press.
Melchert, Christopher. 2011a. 'Aḥmad ibn Ḥanbal's *Book of Renunciation.*' *Der Islam* 85 (2): 345–359.
———. 2011b. 'Exaggerated Fear in the Early Islamic Renunciant Tradition.' *Journal of the Royal Asiatic Society* 21 (3): 283–300.
———. 2002. 'The Piety of the *Ḥadīth* Folk.' *International Journal of Middle East Studies* 34 (3): 425–439.
Nicolae, Daniel S. 2012. 'A Mediaeval Court Physician at Work: Ibn Jumayʿ's *Commentary on the Canon of Medicine.*' DPhil diss., University of Oxford.
Pehro, Irmeli. 1995. *The Prophet's Medicine: A Creation of the Muslim Traditionalist Scholars.* Studia Orientalia, no. 74. Helsinki: Finnish Oriental Society.
Pormann, Peter E. 2013. 'Qualifying and Quantifying Medical Uncertainty in 10th-century Baghdad: Abu Bakr al-Razi.' *Journal of the Royal Society of Medicine* 106 (9): 370–372.
Ragab, Ahmed. 2018. *Piety and Patienthood in Medieval Islam.* Routledge Studies in Religion. London: Routledge.
———. 2015. *The Medieval Islamic Hospital: Medicine, Religion and Charity.* Cambridge: Cambridge University Press.
Rahman, Fazlur. 1987. *Health and Medicine in the Islamic Tradition: Change and Identity.* New York, NY: Crossroad.
al-Rāzī, Abū Bakr. 1998. *Ṭabīb man lā ṭabīb la-hu, aw, Man lā yaḥduruhu al-ṭabīb*, ed. Muḥammad Rakābī al-Rashīdī. Silsilat Ṭibb al-Iʿshāb. Cairo: Dār Rakābī.
al-Riḍā, ʿAlī. 1982. *al-Risāla al-Dhahabiyya*, ed. Muḥammad Mahdī Najaf. Najaf: Maktabat al-Imām al-Ḥakīm.
Salem, Feryal. 2016. *The Emergence of Early Sufi Piety and Sunnī Scholasticism: ʿAbdallāh b. al-Mubārak and the Formation of Sunnī Identity in the Second Islamic Century.* Islamic History and Civilization, no. 125. Leiden: Brill.
Stearns, Justin K. 2014. 'All Beneficial Knowledge is Revealed.' *Islamic Law and Society* 21 (1–2): 49–80.
———. 2011. *Infectious Ideas: Contagion in Premodern Islamic and Christian Thought in the Western Mediterranean.* Baltimore, MD: John Hopkins University Press.
al-Tirmidhī. 1998. *al-Jāmiʿ al-kabīr.* 6 vols. Beirut: Dār al-Gharb al-Islāmī.
Tor, D. G. 2001. 'An Historiographical Re-Examination of the Appointment and Death of ʿAlī al-Riḍā.' *Der Islam* 78 (1): 103–128.
al-Ṭūsī, al-Shaykh al-Mufīd Abū Jaʿfar. 1961. *Rijāl al-Ṭūsī*, ed. Muḥammad Ṣādiq Āl Baḥr al-ʿUlūm. Najaf: al-Maktaba wa-al-Maṭbaʿa al-Ḥaydariyya.
Waines, David. 1999. 'Dietetics in Medieval Islamic Culture.' *Medical History* 43 (2): 228–240.
Yaldiz, Yunus. 2016. 'The Afterlife in Mind: Piety and Renunciatory Practice in the 2nd/8th- and Early 3rd/9th-century Books of Renunciation (*Kutub al-Zuhd*).' PhD diss., Utrecht University.
Yūsuf, ʿAbd al-Qādir Aḥmad. 1970. *al-Imām ʿAlī al-Riḍā Walī ʿAhd al-Maʾmūn.* Baghdad: Maṭbaʿat al-Maʿārif.
Zinger, Oded. 2016. 'Tradition and Medicine on the Wings of a Fly.' *Arabica* 63 (1–2): 89–117.

**Professor Ahmed Ragab** is a historian of science and medicine, and a trained physician. His research includes work on the history of medieval Islamic hospitals, and research on the epistemic authority of medieval Muslim women with a focus on women-reporters of prophetic traditions, and recent work on the history of temporality and disease.

# Chapter 4
# The Concept of a Human Microcosm: Exploring Possibilities for a Synthesis of Traditional and Modern Biomedicine

**Osman Bakar**

## 4.1 Introduction

The idea of 'human microcosm' as understood in traditional Islamic[1] civilization is important to its natural theology, but it is also known to have found scientific applications in many branches of knowledge, including medicine. In traditional Islamic thought, the concept of a human microcosm is denoted by the Arabic term *al-ʿālam al-ṣaghīr*, which literally means 'the small world.' It is rather noteworthy that this term itself is not found in the Qur'an, notwithstanding the centrality of the philosophical concept that it seeks to convey by virtue of its epistemic status as a core component in the web of ideas that define the Islamic *Weltanschauung* (worldview) in a complete and comprehensive manner. From the perspective of the Qur'an, apart from the concept of God or the Divine Reality and the concept of the universe or the cosmos, I would argue that there is no other concept that is as important and as far-reaching in its consequences and implications as the concept of the human microcosm.[2] The coinage of the term in question, *al-ʿālam al-ṣaghīr*, was apparently

[1] By 'traditional Islamic' is meant having the attribute of being in conformity with the Qur'an and Prophetic *ḥadīths* that found manifestations in Muslim life and thought since early Islamic history. The term refers to ideas and practices that are not time bound. It is thus different from the term 'classical Islamic' as used in this chapter, which refers to the Islamic epoch beginning from mid-eighth century till the end of the fifteenth century. The essence of Islamicity of ideas and practices is conformity either with the doctrine of Divine Unity (*al-tawḥīd*) or principles of the Sharīʿa, Islam's sacred law, or with both. For detailed discussions of this issue, particularly as applied to science, see Bakar (2008).

[2] Yet, despite its comprehensive and highly consequential epistemological role, this concept is almost forgotten, not only in the modern and postmodern West but also in the contemporary

O. Bakar (✉)
ISTAC-International Islamic University Malaysia, Kuala Lumpur, Malaysia
e-mail: osmanbakar@iium.edu.my


A. al-Akiti, A. I. Padela (eds.), *Islam and Biomedicine*, Philosophy and Medicine 137, https://doi.org/10.1007/978-3-030-53801-9_4

meant to convey a concept that would best capture the Qur'an's vision of the individual human reality viewed in all its dimensions. While this term is not found in the Qur'an, its full meaning is derived from this sacred book itself.[3] Interestingly, the term appears simple enough and yet it is deeply profound in its meaning.

The origin of the term is traditionally attributed to ʿAlī ibn Abī Ṭālib (d. 40/661), the cousin and son-in-law of the Prophet Muhammad, who was exceptionally noted for his penetrating insights on the inner mysteries of both (A) the macrocosm, that is, the outer universe or cosmos – external to human beings – and (B) the microcosm – the universe that resides within the human being. The term conveys the basic idea that the human constitution in its entirety essentially comprises elements from all of the *objective worlds* that form the macrocosmic universe. In short, a human being is a replica of the cosmos, which is complete in nature and form, but miniature in size. Thus, the often-heard expression, 'man is the universe in miniature.' By 'objective worlds' I mean: (1) the physical or corporeal/material world; (2) the psychic world; and (3) the spiritual or incorporeal/immaterial world that exists external to human beings but is perceptible to them through the use of the relevant cognitive faculties with which they have been naturally endowed.[4] These three worlds refer to the three fundamental states of objective existence that constitute the whole macrocosm.

In the cosmic domain, the psychic world may also be identified with what some classical Muslim experts, in both cosmology and psychology, referred to as the world of imagination or the imaginal world (*al-ʿālam al-khayālī*), which in ontological terms constitutes an intermediate reality between the spiritual and corporeal worlds.[5] In accordance with the microcosmic principle, the three worlds or realities

---

Muslim world. For this reason, I attempted to contribute in a humble way to the initiative taken thus far by only a few scholars to revive this traditional concept through my writings by raising the issue of its relevance to the advancement of knowledge in the contemporary world. My longest treatment of this concept may be found in Bakar (2016). In this chapter, however, I argue for the relevance of this concept to any serious attempt aimed at a knowledge-synthesis between traditional Islamic and modern biomedicine.

[3] I have provided detailed arguments and explanations to show that the idea of human microcosm in traditional Islamic thought has its basis in the Qur'an. See Bakar (2016), 105–193.

[4] The three worlds together – the physical, the psychic, and the spiritual – are qualitatively different from each other, yet ontologically related to form a unified system, and constitute the subject-matter of traditional cosmology and natural theology. The first two worlds are studied by both Islamic and modern Western cosmologists. Unlike Islamic cosmology, the latter do not consider the spiritual world as an integral part of the cosmos. In Islamic cosmology, the spiritual world is identified with the cosmic domain that is populated by the angels, which on the basis of the Qur'an and the Prophetic *ḥadīths* are characterized as creatures of light with divinely designated roles and functions in the natural and human worlds. In the scientific tradition of the *falsafa* and the *mashshāʾiyyūn* (Muslim Peripatetics), al-Fārābī (d. 339/950), for example, defines the angelic or purely spiritual world (*al-ʿālam al-malakī*) as the domain of separate intelligences (*ʿuqūl mufāriqa*). See Bakar (1998), 56, 98; and al-Fārābī (1985), 101–105.

[5] This intermediate domain or intermediary (*wāsiṭa*) is often referred to as *barzakh* (isthmus), which in its general sense is defined as anything that is situated between two other things. See Lane (1984), 1:187. Scientifically speaking, a *barzakh* between two adjacent substances becomes a

constituting the macrocosm or the objective universe also exist in the individual human being according to the same hierarchical order. As explained by Ibn al-ʿArabī (d. 638/1240),[6] perhaps the most creative and also the most prolific among Muslim cosmologists and psychologists to have ever lived, the imaginal world is situated between the purely spiritual and the physical worlds. He used the same terms, imagination (*khayāl*) and isthmus (*barzakh*) to refer to the domain that is intermediate between spirits and bodies within both the macrocosm and the microcosm.[7] By virtue of its intermediate character, the microcosmic imagination or equivalently termed the imaginal *barzakh* possesses a quality that combines the attributes of the spirit and of the body.[8] In postmodern science,[9] quantum physics seeks to better understand the reality of what is known in classical Islamic science as the macrocosmic imaginal *barzakh*, while neuroscience seeks to fathom into the reality of its microcosmic counterpart, including the mental states of existence. There is another dimension of the microcosmic *barzakh*, which is being investigated in modern and contemporary cell biology, particularly microbiology. More generally, it may be said that contemporary science is spending much of its resources to unravel the mysteries of two of the most important parts of the human microcosm, namely cerebral intelligence[10] and the molecular basis of life. Both parts are situated on the common borders of the imaginal and the physical worlds within the cosmos. In fact, both are of importance to contemporary medicine. The practical purpose of unravelling the mystery of cerebral intelligence is the pursuit of the creation of artificial intelligence (AI), while in the case of molecular basis of life, the pursuit of

---

necessity when no meeting between them is possible. The main property of a *barzakh* is that it combines the attributes of the two worlds or two substances between which it is situated. There can be many kinds of *barzakh* in the cosmos, and indeed in the whole of Reality.

[6] The most informative source on Ibn al-ʿArabī's life is perhaps his autobiographical work that is available in English translation. See Ibn al-ʿArabī (1988).

[7] For a good discussion of Ibn al-ʿArabī's treatment of the microcosmic and macrocosmic states of existence, especially the domain of imagination, see Chittick (1998), 331–339.

[8] It should be noted that this 'intermediate quality' that defines attributes of two different worlds is worth investigating, especially from the perspective of biomedicine.

[9] By postmodern science, I mean essentially the new physics founded in the 1920s embracing relativity, quantum mechanics, and particle physics and the new biology discovered at the turn of the present century comprising genomics, bioinformatics, and evolutionary genetics that both discarded the Newtonian paradigm. See Capra (1982). Some *scientists* have used the epithet 'postmodern' in reference to both the new physics and the new biology. See Carson (1995) and Theise (2006). For preliminary thoughts on possible syntheses between Islamic science, modern science, and postmodern science, see Bakar (2011, 2014, 2016, 2019).

[10] In Islamic science, the concept of cerebral intelligence in humans is to be understood as a contrast to cardiac intelligence that is associated with the cognitive function of the spiritual heart. Some authorities identify cardiac intelligence with the universal intellect (*al-ʿaql al-kullī*), the Latin *intellectus*, which is presented as 'the eye of the heart,' as distinct from reason (Latin: *ratio*) that cognizes objects indirectly such as through logical thinking. See al-Ghazālī (2007), 52–53; Schuon (2008), Chap. 1; and Bakar (1998), 194–195. The seat or locus of cerebral intelligence is the brain, whereas that of cardiac intelligence is the invisible heart. There are other species of intelligences, namely the angelic or incorporeal separate substances referred to earlier in note 4 above.

bioengineering enterprises. These pursuits, if not guided by ethics based on sound metaphysical principles, could have profound implications for the contemporary human condition.

The Qur'an provides precious data on the three qualitative worlds or states of cosmic existence just discussed. In the perspective of revealed epistemology as contained in the Qur'an, these data are said to be the most objective available to the human mind, since their source is believed to be supra-human or divine and thus to transcend the limitations of the empirical and rational data that are, by contrast, of human origin. One of the main features of human reason is its ability and capacity to derive new knowledge from both revealed and empirical data. The knowledge-synthesis of traditional Islamic and modern biomedicines that is proposed in this chapter is essentially a synthesis of revealed and scientific data pertaining to the human microcosm and its constituent parts, particularly the part that exists and functions as the isthmus between the physical body (*jism*) and the invisible soul (*nafs*).

## 4.2 The Human Microcosm as a Hierarchical and Integrated Living System

Islamic ontology and cosmology both depict the cosmos as a hierarchically ordered reality, but which they view from different perspectives and which they understand and interpret in quite different ways. *Ontology* has been defined as the study of being *qua* being.[11] In the light of its epistemological concern with the anatomy of being as implied by this definition, ontology may be said to be providing a qualitative differentiation of the world of objects through its fundamental classification of objects in the cosmos under three different qualities of being, namely the physical, the psychic, and the spiritual, as previously encountered. Beyond the cosmos, there is the Divine Reality, the absolute and infinite object or being that transcends all other objects and is absolutely spiritual in nature.[12] In the light of the nature of this absolutely spiritual being, the spiritual objects in the cosmos that are situated at the top of the ontological ladder are to be seen as relative in nature but as transcendent to the psychic and physical objects. And at another level, below the spiritual objects, are the psychic beings that are viewed as transcendent to the physical objects. The property of transcendence, which always involves a kind of 'creative jump,' is thus observable in several degrees in the relationship between the different states of being in the cosmos. This idea of 'relative transcendence' in its various degrees in the ontological relationship between two adjacent planes of cosmic objects that are

[11] In the history of Islamic thought, this particular branch of knowledge deals with *wujūd* ('being') and its hierarchical states.

[12] The spiritual objects in the cosmos, which traditionally are religiously referred to as angels and philosophically, by the *falsafa* and *mashshā'iyyūn* tradition, as separate substances or intellects, are relative realities when viewed in the light of the absolute and infinite Divine Reality.

qualitatively different from each other is posited in this philosophical-theological inquiry as having significant implications for the rational-empirical sciences, including the medical sciences. It is one of the objectives of this chapter to explore the idea of the psychic or imaginal domain that is transcendent to the physical reality and the meaning of this relative transcendence. The relation of relative transcendence in question is investigated within both the macrocosmic and microcosmic frameworks.

This ontological ladder may be viewed from the perspectives of both transcendence and immanence as these terms are theologically understood. In its transcendent mode, the ontological ladder links the various states of existence in an upward direction starting from the physical rung through the imaginal, right to the spiritual and beyond so as to constitute an ascending chain of being. In its immanent mode, the ontological ladder descends from the meta-cosmic or divine object through the various layers of beings right down to the lowest, which comprises the sensible objects, so as to constitute in turn a descending chain of being. A pertinent question to raise at this point is whether or not, when climbing the ontological ladder through its existential rungs, an observer of cosmic objects would see the same scenery and 'cosmic-scape' or have the same psychological experiences as when descending it. This is a complex question to answer. But perhaps it would be helpful to our search for answers if we were to formulate the problem in epistemological terms. In principle, an epistemological formulation of the problem is possible, since, as affirmed in classical philosophy, there is a relationship between the knower, who is the observer of the objects under study, and the object that is known. This relationship involves a progressive ascent of the knower's consciousness from the lower to the higher as symbolized by the ladder's consecutive rungs.

In epistemological, particularly methodological terms, there is a close analogy between the ascending and the descending ontological ladder bipolarity and the dualism that characterizes the Platonic descent of metaphysical 'Ideas' or Forms to the sensible objects and the Aristotelian ascent from the sensible to the metaphysical objects. The Platonic-Aristotelian epistemological bipolarity epitomizes two perennial approaches to the pursuit of knowledge discovery in the history of both Western and Islamic thought that are deemed opposite to each other in their points of departure and yet complementary to each other in their creative contributions to the advancement of the sciences. The two fundamental approaches in question are the metaphysical and the empirical. The Platonic metaphysical approach starts from the metaphysical 'ideas,' while the Aristotelian empirical approach starts from sense-knowledge (*maḥsūsāt*). As Seyyed Hossein Nasr has observed, the Platonic-Aristotelian epistemological tradition found an intellectual home in Islamic civilization, albeit in a philosophical setting that was in conformity with the synthetic spirit and character of this civilization. In his pioneering study on the cosmological schemes developed by the Ikhwān al-Ṣafā' (Brethren of Purity), who flourished in the tenth century,[13] and Ibn Sīnā (d. 428/1037), Nasr confirmed the highly visible

[13] On the identity of this philosophic-scientific fraternity and their encyclopaedic work, the *Rasā'il* (*The Epistles*), see Nasr (1978), 25–43.

presence of the Platonic-Aristotelian epistemological elements in their respective thought syntheses. The scientific dimension of each synthesis is waiting to be sorted out, and, if made available, could be of some significance to the scientific synthesis envisaged in this chapter.

An important dimension of the Islamic intellectual tradition, at least as it was during its most creative phase, and that includes the tenth and eleventh centuries, was its passion for knowledge-synthesis. Imbued with this spirit, Muslim inheritors of the Platonic, Neoplatonic and Aristotelian epistemological ideas succeeded in harmonizing and synthesizing them to produce several important schools of philosophy of science in Islamic civilization. Ibn Sīnā's Peripatetic (*al-mashshā'iy*) school and the Pythagorean-Hermetic school as represented by the Ikhwān al-Ṣafā' must be counted as among the most influential in eleventh-century Islam. Their intellectual legacies, especially their synthetic works, need to be revisited if we are contemplating the undertaking of a knowledge-synthesis enterprise in the context of the present state of human knowledge.[14]

As interpreted by al-Fārābī (d. 339/950) and like-minded Muslim philosophers, the Platonic Ideas became identified with the Qur'anic Divine Names and Qualities.[15] In later Islamic thought the harmony between the Platonic, Neoplatonic and Aristotelian methodological approaches to knowledge gained greater clarity and became further enhanced when Ibn al-ʿArabī introduced and articulated the principle of God's Self-Disclosure (*mutajalla*)[16] in his cosmology. This principle is understood as meaning that the cosmos and its contents are a wonderous and majestic display of the Divine Names and Qualities in their diverse modes of manifestation. In the light of the principle of *mutajalla*, one would be able to interpret the Platonic metaphysical approach to knowledge as the epistemological act of applying the ideas embodied in the Divine Names and Qualities to the natural and other cosmic phenomena. The cosmic qualities in general and the natural qualities in particular,

[14] Past Muslim philosophers offered a good insight into their attempts at a knowledge-synthesis in different branches of philosophy and science. For example, al-Fārābī formulated a theory of knowledge that harmonizes and synthesizes the epistemologies of Plato (d. *ca.* 347 BC) and Aristotle (d. 322 BC) within the *tawḥīdic* or monotheistic framework of Islam. See al-Fārābī (1907). Ibn Sīnā could explain many aspects of Aristotelian physics in the light of a metaphysics of love pervading the cosmos. See Ibn Sīnā (1945). Another philosopher, Quṭb al-Dīn al-Shīrāzī (d. 710/1311) found harmony between the metaphysics of light and optics. See Bakar (1998), 239–240. We could go on and on providing examples of knowledge-synthesis of varying degrees of complexity in various scientific disciplines in the history of Islamic civilization.

[15] For example, the Platonic idea of the Good would correspond to the Qur'anic *al-Raḥmān*, which is usually translated as 'the Most Gracious' but which essentially means the ultimate source of all that is good.

[16] In several of my writings I have referred to this important principle in its abbreviated form, namely the 'GSD Principle'. For example, Bakar, (2016), 19, 23 and 48, where the meaning and significance of the principle of *mutajalla* is emphasized, albeit in only a brief manner. I have long intended to explore the diverse applications of this principle to the study of the frontiers of knowledge in the sciences, particularly pertaining to the epistemological issues that I have raised in this chapter, but without really being able to embark on this enterprise. This current research provides a good opportunity to explore the scientific usefulness of this understudied metaphysical principle.

including the mathematical and the physical, that constitute the subject-matter of the cosmological and the natural sciences, may be viewed as the reflections of the corresponding Divine Qualities on the lower cosmic planes extending right down to the physical. Knowledge of the Divine Names and Qualities then becomes an important source of ideas for the scientific understanding of the physical and other cosmic qualities. In this way, empirical knowledge does not become detached from metaphysical knowledge.

Conversely, in the light of the same God's Self-Disclosure principle, one would be able to interpret the Aristotelian empirical approach to knowledge as the epistemological act of tracing physical qualities investigated in the empirical world to their metaphysical roots. This act involves the identification of Divine Qualities and Attributes and their associated Names that would best correspond to the physical qualities that are under study. The link between physics and metaphysics or between the scientific and the metaphysical is thus an integral component of Islamic epistemology, regardless of whether it is the Aristotelian or the Platonic epistemological approach that is being employed. Through the idea of cosmic phenomena as theophanies, namely as divine signs or manifestations in the visible external world as well as in the human souls,[17] the principle of God's Self-Disclosure thus ensures the preservation of the unity of science and religion. Neither religion nor science is sacrificed for the sake of the other. However, an outstanding issue to be addressed is: how best can the God's Self-Disclosure principle be utilized to realize a knowledge-synthesis such as the one we are now proposing in biomedicine?

As an academic discipline, *cosmology* is traditionally distinguished from ontology, although the philosophical link between the two is acknowledged. Cosmology has been defined as partly 'the scientific study of the form, content, organization, and evolution of the universe,' and partly 'the metaphysical study dealing with the origin and structure of the universe.'[18] It is quite clear from the given definition of cosmology that without the help of ontology as traditionally understood it would not be possible for us to have a whole picture of the structure of the universe. If the modern cosmos is found to lack a well-defined structure despite the great wealth of information about it that has been gathered by empirical cosmology, it is precisely because this cosmology has abandoned the idea of anatomy of beings as taught in traditional ontology. While ontology is basically concerned with the qualitative differentiation of the content of the cosmos, cosmology deals on the other hand with the cosmos' orderly system that necessitates the study of its form, content, organization, and history from its origin until the present. From the point of view of traditional cosmology, although the cosmos may be viewed as a total unitary system in the singular, it is known to comprise many subsystems, each with its own order, characteristics, and functions, which may be equated with what the Qur'an refers to

[17] This idea is emphasized in Qur'an 41:53 (*Fuṣṣilat*): 'We shall show them Our signs in the horizons (*al-āfāq*) and within their souls (*anfusihim*) until it becomes manifest to them that it is the truth.'

[18] Agnes and Guralnick (1999), 328.

as *al-ʿālamīn* ('the worlds'). This idea of hierarchical orderly subsystems in the macrocosm is important for our attempt to know its corresponding structure in the microcosm. It is within this microcosmic structure that fundamental issues pertaining to the current frontier knowledge in biomedicine are sought to be investigated.

The emergence of the human microcosm on the planet Earth occurs late in the history of the cosmos subsequent to the successive emergence of the mineral, plant and animal kingdoms. The idea of the human microcosm as a living system that is to contain and integrate all the cosmic elements, particularly of the mineral, plant, and animal kingdoms, dictates the historical appearance of the human species subsequent to all other species. In this respect, Islamic natural history concurs with the modern theory of biological evolution. However, the traditional idea of the human microcosm itself is in conflict with the conception of the human species as believed in modern evolutionary theory. Taking the symbolism of the human body as our guide, we may sympathetically go along with the Ikhwān al-Ṣafāʾ in advancing the idea that the cosmos is like the human body with a spirit or a soul.[19] The Ikhwān al-Ṣafāʾ and a number of other traditional Muslim epistemologists and spiritual authorities, including al-Ghazālī (d. 505/1111) and Ibn al-ʿArabī, maintained the idea of the cosmos as a living entity. This traditional idea of the cosmos as something that is alive is in stark opposition to the idea of a 'dead universe' that finds currency among many modern and contemporary scientists and thinkers.

According to the Ikhwān al-Ṣafāʾ, the universe or cosmos 'has one body in all its spheres, gradation of heavens, its generating elements and their productions,'[20] and it also has 'one soul whose powers run into all organs of its body, just like the man who has one soul which runs into all of his organs.'[21] It is the soul that animates the body, and this principle applies to both the macrocosm and the microcosm. Ibn al-ʿArabī strengthens the argument for a cosmos that is alive with his assertion that 'the Divine Spirit, which is the Breath of the All-Merciful (*nafas al-Raḥmān*), has been blown into everything in the cosmos' and the basic attribute of the spirit is life (*ḥayāt*).[22] The cosmological idea of the soul as the animating principle of the body or as the source of terrestrial life is closely related to the theological-metaphysical idea of the divine blowing of the Divine Spirit into the whole cosmos. In fact, the blowing of the Spirit into the whole cosmos is the root cause of the soul's animation of the body. Moreover, the cosmic effect of the divine act of blowing into the bodies something universal and undifferentiated that transcends particularization results in the differentiation and particularization of the souls. Thus, the divine blowing of the undifferentiated Spirit into the macrocosmic and microcosmic bodies explains why

[19] The Ikhwān al-Ṣafāʾ, an eleventh-century fraternity of scientist-philosophers, called the cosmos the great man (*al-insān al-kabīr*), since it has one body (*jism*) and one soul and mind (*nafs*). On this anthropological interpretation of the cosmos and the cosmological teachings of the Ikhwān al-Ṣafāʾ in general, see Nasr (1978), 44–104.

[20] Ibn al-ʿArabī is essentially saying the same thing when he says that 'the body of the cosmos comprises the bodies of its individual parts.' See Chittick (1998), 272.

[21] Nasr (1978), 67.

[22] Chittick (1998), 273.

there is multiplicity of souls and spirits, each being unique, which modern science finds mysterious and unexplainable. The same process of differentiation and particularization of the souls and spirits that is somehow influenced by the property of *preparedness*[23] to receive the undifferentiated Spirit attributable to the respective bodies further explains the hierarchical nature of the souls or life forms. The degree of preparedness varies from body to body. The traditional hierarchy of the mineral, plant, animal, and human souls is related to the process in question. In the case of human beings, each person is unique in the sense that his being is essentially determined by the unique way in which his differentiated soul enters into a relationship with his destined body. But as microcosmic beings, human persons bear within themselves a hierarchical and integrated structure of life forms.

## 4.3 The Traditional Perfect Man: The Meaning of the Human Prototype

According to a Prophetic *ḥadīth*, 'God created Adam in His Form (*ṣūra*).'[24] Islam thus shares with Judaism and Christianity the teaching that man is created in the image of God. When referring to God, what does the word 'Form' mean? According to the most authoritative traditional interpretations, the Divine Form refers to the Divine Qualities and Attributes that are absolute, infinite, eternal, and immutable. God created man as a theomorphic being. Man is endowed with qualities and attributes of such a nature that make him God-like. This is the meaning of his anthropological status as the image of God. We are therefore dealing here with what is perhaps the most important concept in spiritual anthropology. But being an image of the Divine Form, the resulting human form could only be relative in its nature. The relationship between the relative human form and the absolute Divine Form remains a mystery to the human mind, although quite miraculously the relative human intellect is somehow able to know the Absolute and the Infinite.

In principle, the divine image in man is total and integral, and not partial as characteristically found in the other creatures. Whether we are referring to the angels residing in the pure spiritual world or the animals in the physical world, the divine forms in these creatures are only partial. A total and integral image means that all divine qualities are present as reflections in human beings and thus in their relative forms. This divine image in its perfect human form, which may be described as the Primordial Reflection, is to serve as the original spiritual template or the prototype for the creation of the human species.[25] Religion teaches that this ideal human form

---

[23] Chittick adopts the term 'preparedness' to translate the Arabic term *istiʿdād* used by Ibn al-ʿArabī to describe the receptive property of each body in response to the divine blowing of the Spirit.

[24] See al-Bukhārī (1997), 8:1554 (*ḥadīth* no. 6227); and Muslim (2007), 7:237 (*ḥadīth* no. 7163). For interpretations of this *ḥadīth*, see Richter-Bernburg (2011) and Melchert (2011).

[25] The original spiritual template or the human prototype may be identified with the concept of *fiṭra* which both the Qur'an and a Prophetic *ḥadīth* identify as the original state of human nature. See,

is found in a particular category of people known as Prophets and saints, who have been described as individuals of extraordinary spiritual-intellectual genius. For ordinary people, the human form that defines their personhood varies from individual to individual to various degrees of perfection. Classical philosophy attributes this variation among human individuals to nature. This view is akin to Ibn al-ʿArabī's contention that the uniqueness of each human spirit or soul stems from the fact that it enters into a relationship with a unique body. The soul-body relationship in each human individual is unique. Ibn al-ʿArabī argues that it is bodies that divide the Universal Spirit into partial or particular (*juzʾī*) spirits.[26] The religious perspective on the meaning of the human person and the human condition that has just been outlined quite clearly calls for a comparative discussion of the subject with the contemporary scientific perspective. Tentatively speaking, I see the possibility of a promising synthesis of the religious and scientific perspectives on the subject of the human person.

As it exists in human individuals, the human form may be conceived and understood from several perspectives. From the psychological perspective that has to do with matters pertaining to the soul, the human form may be viewed in its various stages of growth and development. There is first of all the stage of the human form in potentiality, meaning that content-wise, the inborn qualities and traits in the human person, which are reflections of divine qualities and attributes, exist as human seeds that are awaiting development and growth for their actualization into real persons as conditioned by both internal and externals factors. A preliminary reflection seems to suggest that both natural and cultural factors are at play. The transformation of human seeds embedded in the *fiṭra* (primordial state) into real persons appears to be governed by a combination of biological (genetic) determinism and cultural and moral preferences. The interaction between the genetic makeup of the human form and spirituality appears to be particularly appealing to our mind. However, a detailed study of these possible factors and their dynamic interactions is obviously needed.

Then, there is the stage of the human form in actuality. This refers to the formative stage of the human person when he or she has come of age, which in Islam is traditionally identified with the age of puberty and simultaneously with the beginning of intellectual and moral discernment capacity in actuality. It is of much interest to many contemporary people that Islam defines the beginning of adulthood in rational and moral terms and their biological equivalents. The rational-moral terms refer to the capacity of the discerning reason (*ʿāqil bāligh*) to distinguish between right and wrong in the moral sense and thus to bear a legal responsibility. The biological terms in turn refer to the period of puberty in a person's life, which is a biological indicator of sexual maturity including the capacity for reproduction. It is quite clear that the Islamic and modern secular perspectives are at odds with each

for example, Qur'an 30:30 (*al-Rūm*): 'So set your face uprightly and steadily to the true religion. This is the natural disposition (*fiṭra*) God instilled in mankind.' The *ḥadīth*, 'Every child is born in a primordial state (*fiṭra*)', is found in al-Bukhārī (1997), 2:267 (*ḥadīth* no. 1385); and Muslim (2007), 7:32 (*ḥadīth* no. 6755). Abū Hurayra (d. 59/679), the sole narrator of this *ḥadīth*, linked it to the Qur'anic verse just quoted.

[26] Chittick (1998), 272.

other when it comes to the definition of legal majority and the choice of basis for its formulation. Generally, the Sharīʿa prefers a natural basis for the formulation of its legal-ethical rulings, meaning that its ethical-legal prescriptions are based on the 'nature of things.' On the other hand, the modern secular perspective prefers to employ social or cultural convention as the basis.

It is beyond the scope of concern of this chapter to go into a detailed discussion of the human form in potentiality and in its various stages of actuality. The above brief reference to this issue is meant to emphasize a number of salient points pertinent to the present study. First, to stress the unity of religion and science that is explicit in the interactions between the Sharīʿa and the natural order as illustrated, for example, in the definition of adulthood on the basis of biological considerations. Second, to highlight the need for a more critical interpretation of the significance of genetics for human behaviour. In the religious perspective, the genetic factor alone could not provide a sufficient basis for the understanding of human behaviour. Religion provides a broader view of the human person as made clear by its concept of the 'Perfect Man.'[27] It is in the light of this broader view that discussions should take place on the issue of the implications of advancements in genetics for the traditional understanding of the human person and human behaviour. And third, closely related to the second point, as part of an ongoing religion-science dialogue, to call on science to have a more sympathetic understanding of the non-scientific factors that influence and determine each individual's self-development, character traits and moral habits. Of particular relevance and importance is the traditional idea of the transformation of the 'divine seeds' implanted in human nature into their most developed forms, which philosophers and theologians called human virtues (*faḍāʾil*). In this light, human virtues, which constitute a special category of spiritual data in the complete profile of the human person, may be defined as perfect reflections of the divine qualities and attributes on the human plane.

## 4.4 Conclusion

In this discussion, traditional biomedicine refers primarily to what was cultivated and developed in Islamic civilization under the rubric of biological sciences and scientific medicine, especially as conceptualized and synthesized by Ibn Sīnā. In his treatise on the classification of the sciences, Quṭb al-Dīn al-Shīrāzī (d. 710/1311), a physician who was a follower of Ibn Sīnā's philosophy, treated medicine as a branch of applied biology in the same way agriculture was treated as one. Biology in turn

[27] As defined by Ibn al-ʿArabī, the term *al-insān al-kāmil*, literally 'the perfect man,' refers to someone who has reached the perfect stage of self-development to the point of possessing theomorphic human qualities that reflect the divine qualities in a total and integral manner and in perfect equilibrium. For detailed discussion of Ibn al-ʿArabī's conception of the Perfect Man, see Chittick (1989), 27–30.

was considered as a branch of the natural sciences.[28] In practice, however, medicine flourished as an independent science. With Ibn Sīnā, the relationship between biology and medicine, both conceptual and practical, was preserved. An interface between biology and medicine is visible in his synthesis, thereby allowing us to speak of a nascent biomedicine as a science in eleventh-century Islam. Medicine as theorized by him includes what is known in our time as biomedicine.[29]

This chapter proposes a new synthesis of traditional Islamic biomedicine and contemporary biomedicine. The nature of the synthesis task is epistemological. The challenge before the task is where and how to find an epistemological paradigm that would be viewed as broad enough to allow the two epistemologies to be integrated and be unified within itself. The main argument presented in this chapter is that the epistemology of Islamic biomedicine as theorized by Ibn Sīnā, if freshly interpreted, could be synthesized with contemporary biomedicine. In essential terms, the synthesis would involve the unification of the foundational elements of the 'soul biology' associated with the Avicennian biomedicine and those of the cell biology associated with contemporary biomedicine. Each biology has its own assumptions about the fundamental unit of life that need to be compared and contrasted. In furtherance of the envisaged synthesis, it would be necessary to undertake a comparative discussion of the two conceptions of biology.

'Avicennian biology,' largely of Aristotelian inspiration, is essentially what may be termed 'soul biology' inasmuch as it is centred on the idea of the soul (*nafs*) as the principle of life with its various powers or faculties (*quwwa*). In this particular biological perspective, every organism is considered as having a soul. Plants, animals, and humans all have souls but with different faculties. The more complex an organism is, the more faculties it would have. Ibn Sīnā's theory of plant, animal, and human souls illustrates a synthesis of ideas drawn from the metaphysics of life forms,[30] Neoplatonist conceptions of celestial souls and intellects,[31] Qur'anic cosmological ideas,[32] and traditional knowledge of biophysical properties of organisms accumulated and preserved in various civilizations. His own writings such as *The Metaphysics of the Healing* (*al-Shifāʾ: al-Ilāhiyyāt*),[33] itself a work of philosophical synthesis with scientific implications, provide clear evidence that it is the idea of the Divine Unity and its corollary, namely the idea of cosmic unity, that serve as the unifying theory for his knowledge-synthesis. In the light of this epistemological role attributed to the principle of Divine Unity, which is the core teaching of Islam, the new biology and medicine that resulted from the Avicennian synthesis may justifiably be characterized as Islamic.

---

[28] Bakar (1998), 254.

[29] Nasr (2003), 219–229 and Bakar (2008), 106–128.

[30] Nasr (1978), 252–253.

[31] Ibn Sīnā (2005), 326–338; Nasr (1978), 197–214.

[32] Bakar (2016).

[33] See Ibn Sīnā (2005); Nasr (2003), 184–229.

In previous sections in this chapter, the author has introduced a number of fundamental concepts that are considered as important for the purpose of securing a strong foundation for soul biology. These concepts are now recalled with the view of defining their respective epistemological functions as foundational elements of the soul biology. The first and most important of these concepts is the idea of the Universal Soul (*al-nafs al-kulliyya*), because of its proximity to the plant, animal and human souls that form the subject matter of this science. Next would be the idea of the human microcosm, since there is an analogy between the relation that exists between the Universal Soul and the Universe and the relation between the human soul and the human body. Detailed knowledge of the human microcosm in which are to be found several isthmuses (sing: *barzakh*) is assumed to be of importance to human biology itself. The other concepts are God's Self-Disclosure principle, human prototype and the ideal human or the Perfect Man, and the idea of relative transcendence, particularly as applied to the souls in terrestrial life. It is beyond the scope of this chapter to discuss in detail each of these fundamental concepts pertaining to the foundation of soul biology.

For the moment, suffice it to say that, based on the premise that some form of synthesis of traditional Islamic and contemporary biomedicines would be possible, the first major step towards its realization has been taken in this chapter in the form of identifying the key concepts that go into the foundation-making of soul biology. Further articulations of these ideas could come later on. The little remaining discussion in this conclusion is to point out the relevance of the Universal Soul to soul biology. The first foundational assumption of soul biology is that the Universal Soul is the cosmological source of the individual plant, animal, and human souls and it is what makes the Universe alive. In other words, the Universal Soul is the source or origin of terrestrial life forms, which are viewed as its activities. In this perspective of looking at the origin and meaning of life, the particular natures and characteristics of plants and animals are viewed as consequences of the special relationships into which plant and animal souls enter with their respective bodies. In each of these relationships it is the primacy of the soul over the body that is emphasized.

The incorporeality of the soul may not altogether present an insurmountable obstacle to the proposed synthesis as some would like to imagine. In traditional Islamic epistemology there is the long-established view that one can have knowledge of things in the invisible world by studying their properties and effects in the observable world. This doctrine is traceable to the Qur'an, which in many verses invite humans to reflect on God's observable signs in the natural world so that they may know His nature and reality, which is unobservable. Muslims apply this principle to various fields of study, including soul biology. Ibn al-ʿArabī was merely stating this commonly held view when he said that while the soul itself is invisible it does leave visible traces of its existence and activities in the body with which it is united.[34] The observable traces of the soul in question, of which there are plentiful, are open to empirical study. Historically, quite a wealth of scientific biological

[34] Chittick (1998), 280.

information was gathered over the centuries through studies pursued within the epistemological framework of soul biology. The achievements of soul biology were not only in the theoretical domain, but practical as well, notably in classical Muslim agriculture and medicine.

There is a good reason to believe that the epistemological gap between soul biology and the new century biology is narrowing. There is growing acceptance of the 'inductive' approach to knowledge of hidden causes through the empirical study of their effects such as found in contemporary studies on consciousness and intelligence. Such an approach is quite similar to the epistemological approach in soul biology. A broader acceptance in the contemporary scientific community of this epistemological approach would help generate greater sympathy for the perspectives of soul biology and thereby contribute to the realization of the particular knowledge-synthesis at hand. In the meantime, it may be a good idea to find answers to the question of when and why in scientific history soul biology was abandoned in favour of the Newtonian mechanistic worldview for biology. Real answers to this question could be helpful in resolving some of the issues that lie at the heart of the epistemological conflict between soul and modern biology.

## References


Agnes, Michael, and David B. Guralnick, eds. 1999. *Webster's New World College Dictionary*. 4th ed. New York, NY: Macmillan.

Bakar, Osman. 1998. *Classification of Knowledge in Islam: A Study in Islamic Philosophies of Science*. Cambridge: Islamic Texts Society.

———. 2008. *Tawhid and Science: Islamic Perspectives on Religion and Science*. Shah Alam: Arah Publications.

———. 1433/2011. 'Islamic Science, Modern Science, and Post-modernity: Towards a New Synthesis Through a *Tawhidic* Epistemology.' *Revelation and Science* 1 (3): 13–20.

———. 2014. 'From Secular Science to Sacred Science: The Need for a Transformation.' *Sacred Web: A Journal of Tradition and Modernity* 33: 25–49.

———. 2016. *Qur'anic Pictures of the Universe: The Scriptural Foundation of Islamic Cosmology*. Brunei: UBD Press.

———. 2019. 'Towards a Postmodern Synthesis of Islamic Science and Modern Science: The Epistemological Groundwork.' In *The Muslim 500: The World's 500 Most Influential Muslims, 2020*, ed. S. Abdallah Schleifer. Amman: The Royal Islamic Strategic Studies Centre: 197–201.

al-Bukhārī. 1997. *The Translation of the Meanings of Sahih Al-Bukhari*, trans. Muhammad Muhsin Khan. 9 vols. Riyadh: Darussalam.

Capra, Fritjof 1982. *The Turning Point: Science, Society, and the Rising Culture*. New York, NY: Bantam Books.

Carson, Cathryn. 1995. 'Who Wants a Postmodern Physics?' *Science in Context* 8 (4): 635–655.

Chittick, William C. 1989. *The Sufi Path of Knowledge: Ibn al-'Arabi's Metaphysics of Imagination*. Albany, NY: SUNY Press.

———. 1998. *The Self-Disclosure of God: Principles of Ibn al-ʿArabī's Cosmology*. Albany, NY: SUNY Press.

al-Fārābī. 1325/1907. *Kitāb al-Jamʿ bayn raʾyay al-ḥakīmayn Aflāṭūn al-ilāhī wa-Arisṭūṭālīs* [The Book of Synthesis of the Views of the Two Sages: the divine Plato and Aristotle]. Cairo: Maṭbaʿat al-Saʿāda.

———. 1985. *Al-Farabi on the Perfect State: Mabādi' ārā' ahl al-madīna al-faḍila*, ed. and trans. Richard Walzer Oxford: Clarendon Press.
al-Ghazālī. 2007. *The Wonders of the Heart*, trans. Walter James Skellie. Kuala Lumpur: Islamic Book Trust.
Ibn al-ʿArabī. 1988. *Sufis of Andalusia: The Rūḥ al-Quds and al-Durrat al-Fākhirah*, trans. R. W. J. Austin. London: Routledge.
Ibn Sīnā. 1945. A Treatise on Love by Ibn Sina [*Risāla fī al-ʿishq*], trans. Emil L. Fackenheim. *Mediaeval Studies* 7: 208–228.
———. 2005. *The Metaphysics of the Healing* [*al-Shifāʾ: al-Ilāhiyyāt*], trans. Michael E. Marmura. Provo, UT: Brigham Young University Press.
Lane, E. W. 1984. *An Arabic-English Lexicon*, rev. ed. 2 vols. Cambridge: Islamic Texts Society.
Melchert, Christopher. 2011. 'God Created Adam in His Image.' *Journal of Qur'anic Studies* 13 (1): 113–124.
Muslim ibn al-Ḥajjāj. 2007. *English Translation of Sahih Muslim*, trans. Nasiruddin al-Khattab. 7 vols. Riyadh: Darussalam.
Nasr, Seyyed Hossein. 1978. *An Introduction to Islamic Cosmological Doctrines: Conceptions of Nature and Method Used for Its Study by the Ikhwān al-Ṣafāʾ, al-Bīrūnī and Ibn Sīnā*, rev. ed. Boulder, NY: Shambhala.
———. 2003. *Science and Civilization in Islam*. Cambridge: Islamic Texts Society.
Richter-Bernburg, Lutz. 2011. 'God Created Adam in His Likeness' in the Muslim Tradition.' In *The Quest for a Common Humanity: Human Dignity and Otherness in the Religious Traditions of the Mediterranean*, eds. Katell Berthelot and Matthias Morgenstern. Leiden: Brill.
Schuon, Frithjof. 2008. *The Eye of the Heart: Metaphysics, Cosmology, Spiritual Life*. Bloomington, IN: World Wisdom Book.
Theise, Neil D. 2006. 'Implications of Postmodern Biology for Pathology: The Cell Doctrine.' *Laboratory Investigation* 86 (4): 335–344.

**Dato' Dr Osman Bakar** is Emeritus Professor of Philosophy of Science at University of Malaya and Al-Ghazali Chair of Islamic Thought at ISTAC-International Islamic University Malaysia. He was formerly Distinguished Professor at Sultan Omar Ali Saifuddien Centre for Islamic Studies, Universiti Brunei Darussalam and Malaysia Chair of Southeast Asian Islam at the Prince Talal al-Waleed Centre for Muslim-Christian Understanding, Georgetown University. Dato' Dr Bakar is author and editor of 38 books and numerous articles on various aspects of Islamic thought and civilization, particularly Islamic science and philosophy. He is listed in *The Muslim 500: The World's 500 Most Influential Muslims* since 2009. His best-selling book is *Classification of Knowledge in Islam*, first published in 1992 and which has been translated into several languages. His latest book is *Islam and Confucianism: A Civilizational Dialogue* (co-editor, 2019, new edition).

# Chapter 5
# Islamic Ethics in Engagement with Life, Health, and Medicine

**Adi Setia**

## 5.1 Introduction

To frame the discourse, we may note that salient aspects of modern medicine pose serious intellectual and ethical challenges to the Islamic value system and its definition of 'medicine' (*ṭibb*)[1] itself, and, consequently, its conception of life, health, disease and general well-being. These challenges, which are largely generated by the current hegemony of the biomedical paradigm in modern western medicine,[2] need to be systemically engaged with first and foremost at the conceptual and

[1] In the Islamic medical tradition, *ṭibb* (medicine) has generally been defined as a vocation (*kasb*) that integrates art (*ṣināʿal-ʿamal*) and science (*ʿilm*) in the service of preserving and restoring bodily health (*ṣiḥḥa*); e.g., as can be gleaned from Ibn Hindū (2011), 3–6; see also, Hussain (2015), xv-xvii, for a good elegant elucidation as to why medicine, properly conceived, is at once, art, science and vocation.

[2] For a discussion of the nature of this hegemony, see Weber (2016): 1–2; for a case study of the impact of this hegemony, see Mohyuddin et al. (2004): 59–67.

A. Setia (✉)
Worldview of Islam Research Academy, Kuala Lumpur, Malaysia
e-mail: adisetiawangsa@gmail.com



A. al-Akiti, A. I. Padela (eds.), *Islam and Biomedicine*, Philosophy and Medicine 137, https://doi.org/10.1007/978-3-030-53801-9_5

scientific level of first principles (*uṣūl*),[3] theories and methodologies,[4] and then, at the pragmatic level of ethico-moral conduct[5] and legal praxis.[6]

Such a constructive engagement can and should be carried out by (1) drawing pertinent insights from the rich history of the theologico-scientific[7] engagement of the *ḥukamā'*[8] and *mutakallimūn*[9] (including the *fuqahā'*)[10] with the received Greek medico-philosophical tradition;[11] (2) a thorough critical familiarity with the current profound and wide-ranging critique and rethinking of the premises, methods, practices, and even social and institutional culture of modern, western medicine;[12] and (3) cross-cultural and comparative religious perspectives on healing and medical ethics.[13] Aspects of how this systemic engagement is to be undertaken are outlined here by, *inter alia*, looking critically (albeit briefly) into current debates over medical education, iatrogenesis, medical monopoly, medicalization of health, animal testing (or vivisection), biotechnology and genetic engineering.

It concludes with a proposal for an Islamic Medical Research Programme (IMRP)[14] that is informed and guided by critical, constructive engagement with both traditional Islamic and modern medicine. Hence, instead of a largely *ad hoc*,

---

[3] The question of 'first principles' here refers to the axiomatic bases (tacit or explicit) of any systematic intellectual inquiry into the sciences, including those pertaining to religious, ethical and moral issues. It bears relation also to the traditional ten foundational principles or aspects (*al-mabādi' al-ʿashara*) of any discipline that are to be considered upon embarking on it so as to acquire a clear idea of its scope and nature; see Haleem (1991): 5–41.

[4] I have in mind here the Lakatosian concept of 'methodology of scientific research programmes,' which I find to be most in congruence with the nature of scientific research in Islamic intellectual history, see Setia (2017a), 23–52; and Lakatos (1978).

[5] On the relation between religion and ethics in Islam, see al-Attas (1976); and al-Attas (1995), 41–90.

[6] Specifically, the axio-teleology of ethico-legal praxis, see al-Būṭī (1966), cited and discussed in Setia (2016), 127–157. The term 'axio-teleology' refers to the ultimate moral direction and purpose of ethics, law, science and medicine.

[7] The conjuctive term 'theologico-scientific' here refers to the critical integration of Hellenistic philosophy and science into the framework of Islamic natural theology; see Setia (2005).

[8] Adamson and Pormann (2017).

[9] For example, see Mohaghegh (1988): 207–212; Mohaghegh (1993); and Schwarb (2017), 104–169; cf. Setia (2005), 127–151.

[10] As reflected in say, al-Suyūṭī in his *Ṭibb al-nabawī* and Ibn Nafīs in his *Sharḥ Tashrīḥ al-Qanūn*, but see specifically Shihadeh (2013), 135–174.

[11] And also to a significant extent, Indian, Persian, indigenous Arabian healing tradition, and even Chinese; see Oliver Kahl (2007), 2–3; Heydari et al. (2015): 363; Maidin (2018), 8–9. The qualifying term 'medico-philosophical' refers to the fact that traditionally medicine has always been treated as part of natural philosophy and its application to healing.

[12] Marcum (2008); cf. Illich (1976); Robin (1984); Le Fanu (2011).

[13] Veatch (2000); cf. Tarakeshwar, Stanton, and Pargament (2003): 377–394.

[14] This is conceived as part of an overarching Islamic Science Research Program (ISRP), see Setia (2017a), 93–101. The concept of 'research programme' here largely follows Imre Lakatos' notion of 'methodology of scientific research programmes' (MSRP); for MSRP as applied to medical research, see Cabaret and Denegri (2008): 501–505.

intellectually impoverished 'fire engine' legalistic and *fatwā*-issuing culture that simply reacts hastily to whatever challenges posed by some new-fangled biomedical developments (such as gene therapy[15]), the *generative*[16] IMRP integrates into its *hardcore* axio-teleological first principles as informed by the worldview of Islam,[17] such that it leads to systematic, *prospective* research into treatment and healing modalities that are *intrinsically* sound ethically, epistemically and medically.[18]

## 5.2 The Question of First Principles

The position that this chapter takes is that medicine is concerned with the truth insofar as it pertains to the application of useful knowledge to attain beneficial results relevant to the preservation of health or its restoration after illness, and the prevention of disease. Its *telos* is, as Dr Edmund Pellegrino puts it, the caring of the physician for the patient's healing.[19]

This definition of medicine which focuses on the physician's care for the patient as *individual person*, based as it were on the rational or philosophical aspects of Hippocratic-Aristotelian-Galenic virtue-based medical ethics, dovetails very well with that of the Islamic medical tradition, in which *ṭibb* (medicine) has generally been defined as a vocation (*kasb*) that integrates art (*ṣināʿal-ʿamal*) and science (*ʿilm*) in the service of preserving and restoring the bodily health (*ṣiḥḥa*) of the patient,[20] where health here is understood as referring to a state of equilibrium, moderation and balance in bodily functions and movements.[21] For Ibn Hindū (d. 423/1032), 'Health is the condition of the body when all its functions follow a normal course … Disease is an abnormal condition of the human body, which causes

[15] A good critical survey of the medical and ethical debate over gene therapy is Kelly (2007).

[16] Following Lakatos, the qualifier 'generative' or 'progressive' as opposed to 'degenerative' or 'regressive' refers to the nature of a scientific research programme that is, *inter alia*, making progress in developing new theories and hypotheses that can predict and account for facts not accountable in competing research programmes, thus *productive* of new cognitive and empirical content that further enriches and fleshes out the programme rather than merely increase the stock of linguistic interpretations or reinterpretations.

[17] See al-Attas (1995), 1–40.

[18] Further elaboration on the IMRP will have to be the subject of a separate paper.

[19] Pellegrino (1998): 315–336, cited in Marcum (2008), 6–7. A similar focus on caring for the patient is articulated in Williams (2005), 6.

[20] Ibn Hindū (2011), 15–16; cf. al-Rānirī (2018), 97.

[21] Ibn Hindū (2011), 8–9 and 21–22.

harm to the body's functions.'[22] Ibn Sīnā (d. 428/1037) in his *Canon of Medicine* (*al-Qānūn fī al-ṭibb*) gives a similar definition.[23]

This is obviously in broad accord with the much more ambitious definition given by the World Health Organization (WHO): 'Health is a state of complete physical, mental and social well-being and not merely the absence of disease or infirmity.'[24] Guaranteeing 'complete' social well-being as implied by the WHO definition can very well run the risk of compelling medicine to become sociology and much else besides (such as conflating health with medicalization or even 'disease mongering').[25] Without going into too much pedantic comparative analysis of the merits and demerits of the Islamic and WHO definitions, for our purpose here we may opt to focus on health as constituted by the *functional integrity* of the body as the minimalist definitional common ground that gives a more realistic and pragmatic rather than an utopian understanding of what medicine can or cannot do as a distinct field of human endeavour.[26]

Being critically particular about definitions (and thereby *conceptualizations*) may seem trivial to many in the current hegemony of the biomedical (or biomechanical) model of medicine,[27] but if doctors and medical researchers fail to be critically conscious and articulate about their definitional and conceptual commitments[28] in relation to the various scientific and operational aspects of healthcare, they risk reducing the rich, social ecological meaning of medicine as the science, art and vocation of healing the patient to the mechanical techniques of applied biology.[29] With a view towards reducing this risk and recovering the original multi-layered meaning of medicine by encouraging a healthy dialectical engagement with that multi-layeredness, what follows are some preliminary, somewhat rambling thoughts on first principles as they relate to medicine and healthcare.

---

[22] Ibid., 69.

[23] Ibn Sīnā (2013), 34–35.

[24] World Health Organization (2006).

[25] An interesting critique of the WHO definition is Huber et al. (2011): 1–3. See also, Moynihan, Heath, and Henry (2002): 886–891; and Casell (2004).

[26] The basic idea here is that once the patient as person is restored to optimal functioning then he or she can be more ready to tackle the ills of society or improve their own fortunes in society.

[27] A wide-ranging critique of the biomechanical model is Kriel (2000); see also, Wade and Halligan (2004): 1398–1401.

[28] Ibn Hindū (2011) devotes the last and longest chapter of his *Miftāḥ* to the definitions of medical terms, 43–99. For a modern discussion, see Caplan, McCartney, and Sisti (2004).

[29] See Grzywacz and Fuqua (2000): 101–115.

## 5.3 Axiological Commitments

We may begin by briefly making a distinction between epistemic (or cognitive and methodological) and ethical values even while recognizing and acknowledging the manner in which the one may presuppose, entail or overlap with the other, as has been elaborated at some length by al-Ghazālī (d. 505/1111). To paraphrase Honerkamp, al-Ghazālī juxtaposes epistemological principles within a semantic field governed by ethical concepts thereby rendering the pursuit of knowledge as an inherently critical and ethical undertaking.[30] Here, it will suffice us to observe in passing that the intellectual integrity of a science is but a function of the ethical propriety of the scientist as knowing subject and moral agent, who must not only observe accurately but also report and act honestly. In the case of physicians and medical researchers, this means in practice cultivating *personal* vocational commitment[31] to the care of patients, and avoiding conflict of interest.[32]

If this principle of intellecto-ethical integrity is compromised (say, by the practice of medical ghost writing)[33] then much of the scientific and medical journal industry that underpins, say, the so-called evidence-based medicine (EBM)[34] approach of the Cochrane Collaboration will be in vain.[35] Therefore, scientific knowledge is very much as personal and subjective as it is impersonal and objective.[36] In relation to medicine (*ṭibb*) in the Islamic tradition, these questions of medical axiology[37] have been elaborated at some length by, among others, al-Rūḥawī (*ca.* 9th cent.) in his well-known treatise on the *Ethics of the Physician* (*Ādāb al-ṭabīb*).[38]

Epistemic or intellectual value pertains to knowing what is true or is actually the case. This knowledge is ascertained through the various methods of discovery and justification normally accepted and applied in scientific research, i.e., research pertaining to any systematic field of study in either the natural or social sciences.[39] In the case of the knowledge of medicine, this is ascertained according to the *ḥukamāʾ* and *aṭibbāʾ* (philosophers and physicians) of yore by means of observation,

---

[30] Al-Ghazālī (2015).

[31] Personal vocational commitment arises from finding both personal meaning and social relevance in one's occupation; see Schumacher (1979); and Lahham (2013).

[32] On this danger, see Rodwin (2011); see also, Lo and Field (2009).

[33] Gøtzsche et al. (2009): 122–125.

[34] A critical appraisal of EBM is Howick (2011).

[35] For the website: www.cochrane.org. A recent board crisis has raised questions about Cochrane's integrity and freedom from conflict of interest, especially in its funding sources; see Gøtzsche (2019).

[36] See Polanyi (2015); cf. Jenkins (1981). An application of Polanyi's notion of 'personal knowledge' to medical practice is McHugh and Walker (2015): 577–585; cf. Henry (2010): 292–297; and Jha (1998): 547–568.

[37] For a discussion, see Marcum (2008), 189–205.

[38] See al-Rūḥāwī (1991); see also, Levey (1967).

[39] For an overview of the methodologies of research in the Islamic tradition, see al-Nashshār (1983).

experience, experimentation, intuition,[40] examination and reliance on expert and trustworthy authority.[41] All these are well in accord with the basic parameters of Islamic epistemology[42] and have their analogues in modern scientific epistemology and methodology,[43] which are beyond the remit of this chapter to elaborate in any detail.

Ethical value pertains to the imperative of good and right conduct in appropriate response to true knowledge; hence, the principle of *iqtiḍā' al-'ilm al-'amal* (knowledge mandates action).[44] Knowing what a thing is or consists of in reality is prior to or a prerequisite for deciding on the appropriate course of action in respect thereof, hence the dictum that a statement (*kalām*) or judgement (*ḥukm*) about something is a function of the understanding or conceptualization (*taṣawwur*) of its essence or real nature (*māhiyya*).[45]

How one ought to act or conduct oneself towards something is dependent on what one reliably knows about it and about how it relates to other things in a given context. The human mind organizes out of relevant facts and information knowledge it recognizes to be valid and true and then *acknowledges* that truth by actualizing it in attitude and conduct. Hence, knowledge in the mind is actualized as *adab* (virtuous comportment) in the manner one relates in conduct to oneself, other people, the general environment and to God.[46] In this respect, Islamic medical ethics is a creative integration of formal legal rulings (*fiqh*) into the virtue ethical conceptual and practical framework of *adab*, in which knowledge serves a clear moral purpose (*maqṣid*).[47] As al-Attas puts it succinctly, '*Adab* is right action that springs from self-discipline founded upon knowledge whose source is wisdom.'[48] The Islamic value system as a whole seamlessly integrates cognitive values into ethical values, and hence knowledge, insofar as it is true,[49] must necessarily include moral purpose

---

[40] A modern medical analogue is P. B. Medawar (2009); cf. Braude (2012); Quirk (2006).

[41] A discussion of medical epistemology is in Ibn Hindū (2011), 23–30; see also, 'Abd Allāh (2017), 2–3; Setia (2003), 165–214. Cf. Montgomery (2006).

[42] An exposition is Ismail (2002).

[43] I have in mind, especially, Lakatos (1978).

[44] This is actually the title of a book by al-Khaṭīb al-Baghdādī (d. 463/1071).

[45] Al-Ghazālī (2015), 23.

[46] Al-Attas (1995), 16–20.

[47] For an elaboration, see Sartell and Padela (2015): 756–761. A comprehensive philosophical exposition of *adab* virtue ethics is al-Attas (1980), which is largely inspired by the *Iḥyā'* and other works of al-Ghazālī.

[48] Al-Attas (1995), 16.

[49] We shall not here digress into discussing the various theories of truth (and related theories of meaning and reality), but it suffices here to say that in general the Islamic viewpoint on the matter is that the pragmatic and correspondence theories of truth are to be integrated into an over-arching, *transcendent* coherence theory of truth (understood as the Islamic vision of truth and reality) grounded in Revelation. For an involved discussion of truth, facts, meaning and reality within the conceptual framework of the worldview of Islam, see al-Attas (1995), 123–135.

activating right action as *adab*.[50] Inasmuch as true knowledge demands as its right or due (*ḥaqq*) right action (*ʿamal ṣāliḥ*), then, *to know is to be what you know*.[51]

This principle of *adab* is important because questions of ethics (including questions of formal legal rulings that may proceed therefrom) that arise in response to a particular situation must already assume that its cognitive value or content has been determined in order for those questions to be resolved satisfactorily. If that assumption is unexamined or mistaken, then that response would be in vain, misplaced or faux, i.e., responding to a pseudo or misconceived problem. Hence, if the epistemic status or cognitive content of a medical issue is yet to be established, then ethico-legal (*fiqh*) questions regarding it do not arise, and even if they should arise, their resolutions are to be put in abeyance (*tawaqquf*) until such time as when a proper, thorough disinterested scrutiny (*tabayyun*)[52] of that issue is completed and concluded. This issue of the intimate link between the cognitive and the ethical is of paramount importance for evidence-based medicine, given recent disclosure that 'most published research findings are false':

> There is increasing concern that most current published research findings are false. The probability that a research claim is true may depend on study power and bias, the number of other studies on the same question, and, importantly, the ratio of true to no relationships among the relationships probed in each scientific field. In this framework, a research finding is less likely to be true when the studies conducted in a field are smaller; when effect sizes are smaller; when there is a greater number and lesser preselection of tested relationships; where there is greater flexibility in designs, definitions, outcomes, and analytical modes; when there is greater financial and other interest and prejudice; and when more teams are involved in a scientific field in chase of statistical significance. Simulations show that for most study designs and settings, it is more likely for a research claim to be false than true. Moreover, for many current scientific fields, claimed research findings may often be simply accurate measures of the prevailing bias.[53]

Generally, physicians have both a cognitive and moral obligation to apply well-honed critical thinking skills in their clinical practice,[54] and to identify and weed out as far as possible the 'fifty cognitive and affective biases in medicine.'

Another consideration to bear in mind in this regard is that of the relation between ethics and techniques. Given that *the end does not justify the means*,[55] it follows that the techniques or methods designed and applied to the solution of a well-defined

---

[50] Ibid., 16.

[51] Or: *al-ḥaqqu min ḥaqqihi an yataḥaqqaqa taḥaqquqan* (the truth as its due is to be actualized).

[52] That is, one that is not motivated by extra-medical or extra-scientific considerations such as commercial or political interests, but is focused on tackling cognitive problematics intrinsic to the issue at hand.

[53] Ioannidis (2014): 1–6. A book length treatment for tackling bias in biomedical research is Rothstein, Sutton, and Borenstein (2005).

[54] Groopman and Hartzband (2011); and Montgomery (2006).

[55] That is, if the ends are moral, then the means must also be moral, a key first principle of virtue ethics. This is in contrast to the tendency in bioethics, constrained as it were to serve open-ended biomedical progress, in which the utilitarian-consequentialist ethos predominates leading to the justification of even clearly immoral means (such as vivisection or animal testing) in terms of some self-proclaimed individual or societal good.

problem must embody and realize in themselves ethical values. Since all techniques are conceptualized and invented by technologists, and all technologists are individual human beings having moral agency and hence *personal* ethical commitments, it stands to reason that these commitments are expressed tacitly or explicitly in the very conceptualization and development of new technologies. Technologists as moral agents deploy their personal ethical commitments in the very act of making decisions as to why and which particular techniques or applications should be invented and how these are to be formulated, developed and actually deployed. To the extent that they are conscious decision makers and to that extent they exercise foresight into the consequences, intended or unintended, good or bad, of the techniques and methods they have brought into existence, they are responsible and accountable for those consequences. As Mario Bunge points out,

> …the technologist must be held not only technically but also morally responsible for whatever he designs or executes: not only should his artefacts be optimally efficient but, far from being harmful, they should be beneficial, and not only in the short run but also in the long term.[56]

As for the Islamic point of view on this question (as articulated by, among others, al-Ghazālī), praiseworthy technologies (*ṣināʿāt maḥmūda*) are those that serve to realize the duty of sufficing the public good (*farḍ al-kifāya*) through the cultivation of the wholesome vocations (*makāsib ṭayyiba*) by which the affairs of the world are put in good order (*mā yatarattabuʿalayhi maṣāliḥ al-dunyā*). It goes without saying then that those technologies, techniques and methods that bring about disruption or even destruction (*fasād*, *mafāsid*) to the good ordering of people's lives are blameworthy (*madhmūma*) and censured in the Revealed Law (*al-Sharīʿa*).[57] This means that ethical considerations come into play not only at the downstream level of application in the actual therapeutical deployment of biomedical techniques or results of clinical trials, but also at the midstream and upstream levels of their design, fabrication and deployment in research, including the whole process of decision-making these involve.

This issue of the increasing divergence between medical ethics and the techniques of biomedical technology and genetic engineering (with its problematic underlying commitment to genetic reductionism)[58] is such that the latter now largely defines the parameters of the problematic context within which the former is to exercise its evaluative prerogative, while the very possibility of these techniques and parameters being themselves subject to moral analysis (due to biosafety[59] and

[56] Bunge (1975): 69–79.

[57] Al-Ghazālī (2015), 38–39 and 78–86. Here, I translate *sharīʿa* as Revealed Law (i.e., revealed in the Qur'an and Sunna) to contrast it with *fiqh*, which refers to the particular rulings derived therefrom through a process of legal reasoning guided by *uṣūl al-fiqh* (principles of jurisprudence).

[58] See Carrier and Finzer (2006); and van Regenmortel (2004a, b).

[59] Burrows (2001b).

similar concerns about potential hazards)[60] is overlooked, ignored or even dismissed outright in public discourse as 'irrational.'[61] This problem of divergence between technics and ethics has also become acute, for instance, in the current era of big data research in the sciences, including medicine, with its tendency to overlook or downplay the reality that ethics concern human rather than machine agency and accountability.[62] The biomechanical model of medicine tends to marry biological to technological determinism, and it is both unintellectual and unethical to allow this double-determinism to subvert the traditional Islamic understanding of human nature, namely that man is a free moral agent capable of choice (*ikhtiyār* = to choose for the better) and hence of responsibility and accountability for the consequences of his actions.[63]

Hence, if ethics is to be taken seriously then it has to be taken *structurally* as a proactive point of departure and applied consistently throughout the 'value chain' of any medical procedures and techniques, from upstream to midstream to downstream, otherwise ethics runs the risk of becoming a mere afterthought, an *ad hoc*, overly reactive though necessary appendage to an essentially amoral structure in which the technical systemically overrides the ethical by *subsuming* it, as in the manner the biomedical now subsumes the bioethical. So, we either insist on, and submit to the principle that the ethical leads the technical, or we surrender to the crass consequentialist utilitarianism of the hegemony of the technical over the ethical, in which the role of ethics is reduced to the sorry task of mopping up as best as it can the ever mounting moral debris spawned by the run-away tyranny of technique. Hence, it is important to make ethical awareness and commitment integral to the initial development of bio-techniques in order to 'recognize and anticipate potential risks and unintended consequences.'[64]

To sum up, the basic axio-epistemic framework[65] guiding this enquiry into Islamic ethical engagement with modern medicine is that the technical is to be in accord with the ethical so as to embody and realize it, and that moral conduct is to be in appropriate response to the ascertained, multidimensional reality of a given medical situation. The call here is for the creative integration of virtue ethics with critical realism[66] in order to realize afresh a systematic medical ethics that truly

[60] Regal (1998). In general, since the 1970s, the rest of the world, especially Europe and Japan, has followed the lead of the United States in policy-framing relating to biotechnology due to its geopolitical and economic hegemony.

[61] Burrows (2001a), 244. A fuller treatment is Rose and Rose (2014).

[62] A general, introductory discussion of the problem is Markham, Tiidenberg, and Herman (2018): 1–9.

[63] Al-Attas (1995), 143–176.

[64] Vayena et al. (2015): 1; cf. Norman, Aikins, and Binka (2011): 115–124.

[65] I.e., cognitive (or epistemic) and ethical value system.

[66] Bhaskar (2008).

informs and guides the field of medicine as science and art,[67] as well as *vocation*.[68] This means that we need to *subsume bioethics into medical ethics*.

## 5.4 Teleological Commitments

The ethical considerations outlined above are of pertinence to what is called virtue ethics, namely the understanding that, through the conscious inculcation of virtuous character traits (*makārim al-akhlāq*), a good person will be a good doctor who will practice good medicine and develop a good relationship with his or her patient. Instead of regarding any particular action (and by extension, technique) to be ethical or otherwise in reference to some imperative, principle or consequence external to the content of character of the moral agent, virtue ethics focuses systemically on the personal integrity of the physician or medical researcher inasmuch as he or she possesses the faculty for choice and foresight (*ikhtiyār*), namely, the capacity to tell right from wrong and choose and act accordingly by exercising their moral agency in a given healthcare context. The idea here is that prudent decisions, right actions and thereby appropriate techniques embodying the virtues will naturally or normally arise from persons who comport themselves virtuously, thereby leading to the production and deployment of virtuous sciences, virtuous technologies and virtuous vocations.[69]

A corollary of this is that good people will see it to be their personal responsibility to take due care in the maintenance of their good health as a virtue in itself, and if nevertheless they should fall sick, they will make it a point to be good patients careful to follow the instructions of good doctors in the framework of a virtuous doctor-patient relationship. In short, for medicine to serve its purpose, both doctors and patients as moral agents exercising moral agency need to observe medical ethical decorum, or to be more specific, the personal and interpersonal ethics pertinent to the maintenance or recovery of health and the pre-emption of disease.[70] What guides that relationship is the end or purpose of medicine – the healing bond. Hence, we can agree with Dr Pellegrino that, 'Medicine in its function as medicine resides in the making of a prudent healing decision for a specific person.'[71]

Needless to say, it is also the personal responsibility of people *before* they fall ill to cultivate the prudential foresight necessary for acquiring an adequate degree of cognitive discernment to tell true physicians from charlatans, and this in turn requires of them the acquisition of the virtue of knowledge as it pertains to the

[67] Panda (2006): 127–138.

[68] Laurel (2018), 126–131. For the notion of virtuous vocational individuals constituting the vocational society, see Lahham (2013).

[69] A good short overview is in Walker (2010), 1–2.

[70] Sobree (2018), 23–34.

[71] Cited in Marcum (2008), 307.

nature of the medical vocation sufficient enough for them to tell the difference between doctors practicing vocational integrity and those concerned with narrow commercial returns in their clinical practice or afflicted otherwise with conflict of interest. Abū Bakr Rābiʿ al-Akhwinī al-Bukhārī (d. 371/983), student of the famed Abū Bakr al-Rāzī (d. *ca.* 313/925), is of the view that just as people are expected to know the basics of Revealed Law so as to safeguard their spiritual health, so too they are expected to know the basics of medicine to safeguard their bodily health from destruction at the hands of quack doctors.[72] As Dr Eugene D. Robin has so forthrightly put it,

> As a patient you influence your doctor by your attitude, by your expectations, and by the degree to which you take responsibility for your own treatment. The greater the interest on the part of patients, the more aware the medical system will become of the need to correct its flaws.[73]

This sentiment of taking a certain degree of personal responsibility for one's health is quite in accord with that expressed in the traditional *ṭibb nabawī* (Prophetic medicine) texts.[74]

Virtue ethics in Islam overlaps with what has been called divine-command (or religious deontological) ethics, since the Qur'an and Sunna command believers to cultivate both personal and social virtues (*faḍāʾil, makārim al-akhlāq*) by patterning themselves on the ethico-moral comportment of the Prophet, peace and blessings of Allāh be on him.[75] Both concern too teleological ethics,[76] namely, the cultivation of the good life leading to enduring happiness (*saʿāda*),[77] and the attainment of divine pleasure (*marḍātillāh*); and in the case of medicine as such, the maintenance and attainment of health and well-being as part and parcel of realizing that good life.[78] This fits very well into the notion of *ḥifẓ al-nafs*, the preservation of life, one of the five *maqāṣid*, or overriding objectives of the Revealed Law.[79]

In general, it can be said that in Islam, virtue ethics translates into *adab* (virtuous comportment), divine-command (as religious deontological) ethics into *fiqh* (ethico-legal rules of conduct), and teleological ethics into *maqāṣid* and *maṣāliḥ* (objectives and benefits) discourses. In this integrative, transcendental ethical vision rooted in and derived from the primordial Covenant (*al-mīthāq*) between God and man, the notion of utility (*manfaʿa, maṣlaḥa*) and thereby self-interest (*maṣlaḥa nafsiyya*) is at once de-secularized and re-sacralized through its systematic reconceptualization

---

[72] In al-Akhwinī al-Bukhārī's *Hidāyat al-mutaʿallimīn*, as cited in Rahman (1989), 39 and 136 n. 28.

[73] Robin (1984), 177.

[74] For example, Ibn Qayyim al-Jawziyya (2003), 121 and 124–130 (on the imperative of seeking and identifying good doctors); cf. Fries and Vickery (2017).

[75] See al-Ghazālī (2019).

[76] For a study, see Shihadeh (2006).

[77] Al-Attas (1995), 91–110.

[78] Ibn Hindū (2011), 17.

[79] Padela (2018), 121–132.

within the framework of an expanded,[80] spiritual psychology of the self and a vision of the soul's transcendent identity and destiny.[81]

It is in the light of these axio-teleological commitments that the *ḥukamā'* and *aṭibbā'* of yore are in accord on the definition of medicine in terms of its *telos* or goal (*maqṣid* or *ghāya*), namely, medicine as the science of the preservation of health, the prevention of disease and the restoration of health should it be lost.[82] And if this should beg the question of what is the goal of health, they further say that it is so that one cultivates soundness of both body and mind in order to render worship (*'ibāda*) to Allāh in the most optimal manner. Hence, the *telos* of medicine is health (*ṣiḥḥa*), and the *telos* of health in turn is the good life (*ḥayāt ṭayyiba*) lived in private and in public in perpetual mindfulness (*taqwā*) and remembrance (*dhikr*) of the Creator.[83] This religiously rooted teleologico-virtue ethics underpinning Islamic medicine critically subsumes within its framework the core ethical substance of the Hippocratic-Aristotelian-Galenic medico-virtue ethical system that it finds accord with,[84] and thereby it is not at all unexpected that one finds much concord between it and the Christian scholastic virtue ethics underpinning Edmund Pellegrino's philosophy of medicine.[85]

The Islamic ethico-scientific engagement with modern bioethics and medical ethics in general will have to argue for and insist on the revival and re-articulation of this historical cross-cultural, virtue ethical common ground[86] of departure if any meaningful progress is to be made in the *systemic* resolution of any medico-ethical and healthcare issues in a manner that is faithful to the worldview of Islam.[87] Minus this shared, objective medico-ethical conceptual point of departure for dialogue, the alternative will be surrendering to an ever shifting moral relativism and arbitrary subjective consequentialist utilitarianism, which is, in fact, not really an alternative for conscientious Muslims who care for their belief and value system and the manner it should impact on their understanding of their transcendent identity and destiny as individuals and as communities, inasmuch as this understanding pertains to the domain of healthcare.

---

[80] That is, expanded beyond the ego.

[81] Al-Attas (1995), 143–176.

[82] Ibn Sīnā (2013), 35–36.

[83] Ibn Hindū (2011), 15–16; al-Suyūṭī (2015), 6–7; Ibn Qayyim al-Jawziyya (2003), 11–16; and Ibn Jumayy (1983), 8–9.

[84] For example, Abū al-'Alā ibn Jābir al-Baṣrī, *al-Bayān fī tashrīḥ al-abdān*, cited in Jamal (2018), 74. For the Arabo-Islamic reception to the Hippocratic *Aphorisms*, see Pormann (2017): 412–415 and see also, Chap. 2, 'Medical Epistemology in Arabic Discourse: From Greek Sources to the Arabic Commentary Tradition,' by Pormann in this book; for a good modern discussion on the Hippocratic *Oath*, see Jotterand (2005): 107–128; and also Miles (2004).

[85] See Pellegrino and Thomasma (1993).

[86] Baltussen (2015), 47–66.

[87] An introductory outline of this worldview is in al-Attas (1995), 1–39.

## 5.5 Cosmological Commitments

The human being as microcosm reflects the macrocosm, which is the universe, and both points to the reality of their Creator.[88] The cosmos or universe is seen as *niʿam āfāqiyya* or the divine blessings manifest externally in the cosmic horizons, while the *niʿam anfusiyya* are the divine blessings manifest internally in the constitution of man himself. The whole universe is thus understood as having been created to facilitate (*taskhīr*) the blossoming of human life on earth that they may show gratitude to their Creator.[89]

In Islamic cosmology, nature is then ultimately only a symbolic form manifesting divine creativity at the level of phenomenal sensible reality. Instead of an unconscious 'event —> event' causality giving rise to emergent meaning and order, there is rather at every instant a self-expressing intelligent 'agent —> event' causality, such that events as are but intertwining networks of causes and effects brought about in relatively stable conjunction by a transcendent knowing and willing agent.

Consequently, things in the world are not independent, self-subsisting, self-organizing essences having persistence in absolute time and space, but rather they perish upon coming into existence and are continually being recreated by the Creator, hence the absence of a necessary connection between cause and effect in the processes of nature. Everything, from the tiniest particular part to the greatest universal whole, is *both* proximately and ultimately caused by Allāh alone, continuously and at every instant. The implication of such a cosmology is that ontologically causes and effects are created and correlated within an order or integral system in which the causes are but concomitant conditions for the effects. This order or integral system is perceived through scientific observation and inquiry as natural patterns and regularities, as so-called 'laws of nature,' which in reality are but expressions of God's 'manner of creation' or His 'custom' (*sunnat Allāh*). God creates both causes and effects and connects them together within a dynamic unified network of events, processes and relations.

Scientists, including physicians and medical researchers, perceive, describe and account for aspects of this total integral system in terms of a certain lineal spatio-temporal order of priority and posteriority governing natural entities and processes, some of which they posit as antecedent 'causes' for others, the consequent 'effects,' whereas in reality all causal efficacy lies with God alone. Causes and their perceived effects are, in the final analysis, only more or less stable intertwining networks of probabilistic conjunctions, associations and correlations.[90] For all practical purposes, this cosmological vision poses no problem for applying broad principles of

[88] See Chap. 4, 'The Concept of a Human Microcosm: Exploring Possibilities for a Synthesis of Traditional and Modern Biomedicine,' by Osman Bakar in this book.

[89] Setia (2004).

[90] Setia (2003): 179–187.

methodological naturalism[91] in medical research and healthcare as the *methodological common ground* of both Islamic and modern, western medicine, thus allowing for their mutual engagement. This is because Islamic teachings do accord due consideration to the observed regularities in the phenomena of nature as a guide to decision and action in the pragmatic dimensions of life, including healthcare.

The conclusion from this cosmological vision is that natural laws and regularities – including those that obtain in medical phenomena – are not inherent, necessary properties of natural phenomena, but are properties designed for and imposed on the natural world (*taskhīr*)[92] by a Unique, Transcendent Intelligent Being of Knowledge, Will and Power – properties which are somehow perceived and correlated by the human mind in terms of causes and their effects through its committed involvement in the systemic study of nature. Hence, though Islamic teachings (as expressed in the *ṭibb nabawī* texts) do encourage believers to seek medical treatment and pursue healthcare, ultimately Muslims believe in the transcendental truth of the Qur'anic verse, 'When I fall sick, He heals me.'[93]

## 5.6 Ontological Commitments

The term ontological here refers to what is understood to be extra-mentally and existentially real or existing (*ḥaqīqī, wujūdī*) about the nature of man (*ṭabīʿat/ḥaqīqat al-insān*), and by extension, the nature of his health and sickness. Although medicine as such is concerned with bodily health and wellness, it has also to take into consideration that the patient *qua* human being is at once biological, psychological, and social, as well as spiritual, intellectual, emotional and religious (i.e., personally committed to a set of values rooted in belief in a Transcendent Reality). This holistic consideration has been referred to in current parlance as the biopsychosocial perspective[94] that the patient is much more than their biophysical disease or biomedical symptoms. In other words, the patient as well as the state of his health or illness are not reducible to, and hence *transcend*, the biomechanical aspects of the functional integrity of his body.[95]

---

91 Methodological naturalism as a research strategy *per se* is the practical commitment in scientific and medical research to opt for explanations in terms of some regularities or patterns in nature or culture, regardless of one's philosophical or theological commitment; see the critical discussion in Okello (2015).

92 On *taskhīr*, or the divine subjection of nature for the benefit of man, see Setia (2004): 7–32.

93 Qur'an 26:80 (*al-Shuʿarāʾ*).

94 Engel (1977): 129–136; see also, Frankel, Quill, and McDaniel (2003); and White (2005). For good examples of Muslim doctors' engagement with the biopsychosocial model, see Chap. 7, 'Where the Two Oceans Meet: The Theology of Islam and the Philosophy of Psychiatric Medicine in Exploring the Human Self,' by Asim Yusuf and Afifi al-Akiti; and Chap. 8, 'Muslim Values and End-of-Life Healthcare Decision-making: Values, Norms and Ontologies in Conflict?' by Mehrunisha Suleman; both in this book.

95 Cf. Chishti (1985), 11–38; Ahn et al. (2006); Knox (2010).

The very notion of the ethical, as outlined above, already assumes that man, as moral being and thus moral agent, is possessed of a cognitive mind (*ʿaql*), understood as a spiritual (i.e., non-material) substance inhering in the heart (*qalb*), which is the spiritual organ of cognition by which the rational soul (*al-nafs al-nāṭiqa*) recognizes and distinguishes truth from falsehood. Here, the real existence of the soul or mind is affirmed as an autonomous substantive entity distinct from the physical brain and body, and not a mere epiphenomena or emergent property of the latter; on the contrary, *the mind controls the brain*. Therefore, ethics as it pertains to personal conduct and evaluation of right and wrong is grounded in a psychology of the nature and scope of the intellect by means of which man apprehends his relation to himself, to fellow human beings, to God and to the world.[96]

In practical healthcare terms, this would mean that medicine is less concerned about treating or managing the disease or pathological condition than caring for and healing the patient *qua* physical body yet spiritual being; and that the patient's subjective experience of his illness is just as significant as the doctor's objective diagnosis of it, such that the former goes into informing the latter. Hence, the wisdom necessary for efficacious application of medical knowledge is obtained from years of caring for patients as persons with *real* non-physical feelings, beliefs and aspirations, and not simply as just so many diseased somatic parts impacted by this or that pathogens that are in turn further reduced to their biomolecular and biochemical states, processes and structures. This also entails that physicians cannot allow themselves to be reduced to mere bio-technicians whose access to their understanding of what ails their patients are largely impersonally mediated by biomedical tests, instruments and machines.[97]

The growing realization over the past two decades or so that medical reality or the reality of the factors leading to health or illness is much too multi-layered and systemically complex to be exhausted by the currently dominant biomechanical model of healthcare has led to the rise, articulation and institutionalization of alternative healthcare paradigms and frameworks which are nonetheless just as evidence-based[98] and clinically successful or even more so than the currently dominant biomedical model. This *critical realism*[99] as applied to medical practice and research can only serve to help conscientious physicians, specialists and medical researchers to be further committed to realizing the moral imperative of maximizing care and

[96] See al-Attas (1993). For a wide-ranging discussion of the relationship between self, mind and the brain largely compatible with traditional Islamic faculty psychology, see Popper and Eccles (1985); Beauregard and O'Leary (2007). See also, Chap. 7, 'Where the Two Oceans Meet,' by Asim Yusuf and Afifi al-Akiti in this book.

[97] A relevant discussion is Montgomery (2006); and Groopman (2007).

[98] See, for instance, the journal *Evidence-Based Complementary and Alternative Medicine*: https://www.hindawi.com/journals/ecam/

[99] Critical realism is an approach in philosophy of science that shows that reality or what exists cannot be reduced or restricted to, or exhausted by whatever we can know about it through our methods, models and theories; for what is real and existing is always much more than what we can ever know about it.

minimizing harm by acquiring the cognitive capacity to choose the best or most optimal amongst competing healthcare paradigms, like those that come under the rubric of what is called complementary and alternative medicine (CAM).[100]

To conclude, it is always important for doctors and medical researchers to be sufficiently trained to give due, critical realist consideration to the ontological status of the concepts, terms and processes invoked in the course of describing or explaining the state of health or sickness of the patient.[101]

## 5.7 Bioethics Versus Medical Ethics

Medical ethics can be understood as that branch of ethics that is concerned with ethico-moral issues that arise in the course of clinical practice and research, and, as such, it has a rich and long intellectual and civilizational history.[102] In contrast, bioethics – or more accurately, *the ethics of the biomechanical model of medicine* – is a new, largely post-WWII discourse that is primarily motivated by and concerned with the moral, legal and political implications of the rapid developments in biomedical and biotechnological sciences (such as genetics) over the past few decades and their possible or actual applications to medical research and clinical practice. Due to the current dominance of the biomedical paradigm in healthcare protocols, there is a growing tendency for bioethics to dominate and even supplant medical ethics. Bioethics is a very broad subject that is concerned with the moral issues raised by developments in the biological sciences more generally.[103] However, insofar as these developments impact for good or bad on medical practice and research, bioethics has to be seen as subsumable under the overarching conceptual framework of medical (or *healthcare*) ethics.

Now, given all the above considerations in respect of first principles, there is much that can be criticized about the current reduction of medical ethics to bioethics and then to ultra-utilitarian, consequentialist *principlism*.[104] It is further deplorable to observe the largely unthinking and hence *tacit* reception of this reductionism by many writers, Muslims and non-Muslims, as well evidenced by their largely uncritical appending of the qualifier 'Islamic' to the term 'bioethics,'[105] hence unwittingly legitimizing it as congenial to the worldview of Islam. Even cursory research into

---

[100] Tataryn (2004).

[101] A good, wide ranging discussion is Caplan, McCartney, and Sisti (2004).

[102] Baltussen (2015), 47–66.

[103] Williams (2005), 9–10.

[104] A critique of principlism is Traphagan (2013).

[105] For instance, Mohammed Ali Al-Bar and Hassan Chamsi-Pasha, *Contemporary Bioethics: Islamic Perspective* (2015). The title of the book itself is telling in the manner bioethics is taken for granted as largely unproblematic at core, while the role of Islamic ethics and law is basically to comment on it and maybe mollify some of its more unpalatable aspects; it never really asks the important question of why bioethics was generated in the first place, by whom and for what ultimate purpose. This core uncritical attitude is also discernible in Abdulaziz Sachedina, *Islamic Biomedical Ethics: Principles and Applications* (2009) and others, amongst the numerous papers

the background of the rise of bioethics and the current marginalization, even eclipse, of medical ethics will show that the former is largely a narrow politically and then commercially driven consequentialist utilitarian ethics formulated in haste to respond to the rapid rise of the biomedical and biotechnological (including genetic engineering) paradigm in medical research and its commercial promise for the private corporatization of healthcare.

Although at its inception the term 'bioethics' connotes the imperative of the ethico-moral attitude towards *all* life forms and their ecosystems (hence in effect synonymous with *ecological ethics*),[106] its discursive scope was later reduced to purely the consideration of the ethical implications and impact of the rise of the biomedical paradigm in medical research and clinical practice. Hence, although the original term was retained, it has since been largely taken to specifically refer to biomedical ethics. In short, bioethics is official shorthand for *biomedical* ethics to concord with the molecular biological and biochemical turn in medical research and practice.

The dominance of biomedicine and the concomitant utilitarian bioethical discourse that it generated has largely displaced the notion of traditional virtue-based medical ethics with its more holistic concern with the proper personal relationship between physician and patient as it pertains to palliative care and the healing process. Now however, the focus is on treating the disease and its symptoms by utilizing various biomedical technologies developed from the technical disciplines of microbiology, genetics, biotechnology and biochemistry. This conceptual shift in focus from patients as persons to diseases as microbiological phenomena resulted also in the axiological shift from medical ethics to biomedical ethics and thence to bioethics.[107]

These developments which occurred over several decades post WWII (especially from the 1970s onwards) have caused many philosophers of medicine as well as practicing doctors to express concern that this techno-scientific turn in modern medicine has diverged so far from the *art and vocation* of medicine that the physician risks being reduced from wise doctor to bio-technician or even drug dispenser. This development has been detrimental to the cultivation of the capacity for and practice of clinical judgement among physicians, nurses and medical professionals in general.[108] For the medical vocation to recover its original ethico-cognitive physician-patient relationship as a key element in palliative care and the healing process, there is an urgent need to revive the concept of 'medical ethics' as the overarching axiological discursive framework subsuming within its fold *as sub-ethical categories* such specialized ethics as biomedical ethics, nursing ethics, medical professional ethics and medical research ethics.

---

and monographs on the subject of Islamic bioethics I have had the opportunity to peruse in the course of researching the issue for this chapter.

[106] Goldim (2009): 377–80.

[107] See the important overview of the history and nature of bioethics in Irving (2002), 1–84.

[108] Relevant discussions in Kienle and Kiene (2011); Groopman (2007); and Montgomery (2006).

*Fuqahā'* and *muftīs* sitting on the various global, regional and local *fiqh* and *fatwā* councils simply cannot go on conducting themselves, wittingly or unwittingly, as procedural bureaucrats, largely signing forms and papers in moving the whole bioethical and hence biomedical process along, all the while assuming that whoever has *originally* set the agenda has done it rightly with the purest of intentions for the progress of objective medical science and the best of aspirations for the well-being of humanity. Sadly to say, recent well-documented exposé of the political economic underbelly of the modern medical industrial complex provides compelling reasons to question such innocent, misplaced assumptions.[109]

## 5.8 Case Examples

What follows are outlines of some selected case examples serving to illustrate briefly the manner in which the conceptual matter of first principles explored above is to be translated into an integrative ethical engagement with the whole structure of biomedicine that underpins the bioethical discourse, instead of the currently reactive and intellectually shallow *fiqho-legalistic* approach that takes for granted as largely unproblematic current norms in biomedical research and clinical practice.

***Animal Testing*** The prominent Italian doctor, professor and medical researcher from Milan, Pietro Croce[110] (as well as many others)[111] has tackled the problem of live animal experimentation (or vivisection) from the scientific, methodological and medical rather than from the ethico-moral point of view. He highlights the increasing dangers to human health resulting from the animal experimenter's unexamined and unproven assumption that the biological systems of the various test animal species and human beings are sufficiently similar for valid biomedical translation from the former to the latter. He provides for the medical researcher an introduction to the range of alternative scientific methods, including epidemiological research, computer simulation and *in vitro* techniques.

In this regard it should be noted too that in the Islamic tradition of pharmacology (*'ilm al-ṣaydala* or *al-adwiya*), prospective medicinal drugs are to be tested on

[109] Brown (1979); Fisher (2011); Doyal and Pennell (1991).

[110] Croce (1999). He sets out with detailed argumentation and documentation the pseudo-scientific nature of animal experimentation in general, by drawing detailed attention to several cases in point such as the pseudo-scientific nature of most cancer research, birth defects due to thalidomide and the vivisective approach to surgical training, and then proceeds to explain many proven and promising methodological alternatives to vivisection.

[111] Such as in Greek and Greek (2000).

human subjects, for animal testing would produce unreliable results.[112] 'Unreliable results' is in fact quite an understatement here, for patients and research volunteers are easily exposed to serious harms and even death resulting from the *systemic* biases, flaws and failures *inherent* in preclinical animal research. These include:

(1) Bias and poor practice in research methodology and data analysis
(2) Lack of transparency in scientific assessment and regulation of the research
(3) Long-term denial of weaknesses in cross-species translation
(4) Profit-driven motives overriding patient interests
(5) Lack of accountability of expenditure on animal research
(6) Reductionist-materialism in science which tends to dictate scientific inquiry and control the direction of funding in biomedical research.[113]

Many have argued that an ethical attitude towards animal welfare would *a priori* preclude them from being subjects of life experimentations that distress, harm, maim or kill them. This ethical preclusion is reinforced by the fact that *medically and scientifically* animal trials have no relevance for human healthcare. Hence, animal experiments in biomedical research are *both* unscientific as well as unethical. In fact, the immoral and unethical nature of animal experimentation is amplified by its pseudo-scientific nature, since it would be unethical to waste precious research resources into pursuing a methodology that has so clearly proven to be both mistaken and unproductive, *even if* no suffering and death was inflicted on the test animals.

From the above scientific and ethical considerations, it should be quite obvious that the *fiqh* argument regarding the lesser of two harms, namely, that since human subjects would be harmed in experiments, wouldn't animal models be better since one must reject harm, would not be applicable at all, since there is no scientific basis for the animal models anyway. Hence, invoking the fact that animal trials come before human trials in contemporary medicine precisely for this reason of the lesser harm is misplaced since the reasoning itself is scientifically baseless.[114]

Apart from the well-known concern for animal welfare in the Islamic ethical and cultural tradition, the rights of kept animals are also formally well protected in Islamic jurisprudence (*fiqh*).[115] Given both the immoral and pseudo-scientific nature

[112] See Shaffri (2018), 108, specifically citing MS no. 19 (IAMM 2016.11.11) from the Islamic Arts Museum Malaysia entitled *Ṭibb al-adwiya* ascribed by a certain Khuzr ibn Mubārak al-Mutaṭabbib. Editor's note: see Ibn Sīnā's arguments against animal testing in Chap. 2, 'Medical Epistemology in Arabic Discourse: From Greek Sources to the Arabic Commentary Tradition,' by Peter E. Pormann in this book.

[113] Green (2015): 1–14; see also, Ioannidis (2012): 1–4; and Akhtar (2015): 407–419.

[114] Arguments, such as from gene knockout models to simulate human physiology, or from genetic and other sciences showing similarities in drug effect, are invalid here because they already assume the prior validity of results from animal trials, which is precisely the assumption contested here. Given the foundational epistemic and ethical objections to animal trials, such arguments need to be re-examined. Critical discussions in this regard include von Scheidt et al. (2017); Eisener-Dorman, Lawrence, and Bolivar (2009); see also, the 'Knockout Mice Fact Sheet' issued by the National Human Genome Research Institute (USA) (2015): https://www.genome.gov/about-genomics/fact-sheets/Knockout-Mice-Fact-Sheet.

[115] Furber (2015); see also, Foltz (2006); Masri (2007).

of animal experimentation and animal testing, it would be intellectually, morally and legally imperative to pursue viable alternatives and/or to create them. All ethically humane and truly scientific methods of biomedical research to replace the intolerable cruelty and wastefulness of pseudo-scientific vivisection are certainly well in accord with the philosophy of medicine in Islam.[116]

***Biotechnology and Genetic Engineering*** The past three decades or so have also witnessed rising wide-ranging criticism over the hyperbolic, pseudo-scientific claims and promises of biotechnology and genetic engineering to promote healthcare and food security.[117] Many studies have documented the global negative impact of the present-day overly-commercialized model of biotechnology/genetic engineering (BT/GE) research on medicine, agriculture and rural agrarian economies. They call into question the scientific integrity of the overly optimistic claims of BT/GE to enhance food production and overcome diseases, including treating genetic disorders.[118] While these critiques fall short of advocating a wholesale abandonment of the BT/GE programme, they do emphasize that it is high time for scientists and medical researchers in the public interest to apply the precautionary principle of biosafety first in order to do a systemic, disinterested review of BT/GE, including a thorough scrutiny (*tabayyun*) of all its theoretical assumptions, research methods, objectives and overall agenda.

Unfortunately, current *fiqh* debates and rulings on biomedical interventions resulting from BT/GE are overly caught up in dealing in a haphazardly *ad hoc* manner with the endless ethico-legal enigmas generated by these biotechnological and genetic engineering interventions in clinical practice. Consequently, there is little or no intellectually detached and systemic investigation into the provenance and nature of the underlying technology itself,[119] in terms of its very scientific integrity or lack thereof or even in terms of its actual medical or palliative efficacy.[120] If BT/GE 'is, like any technology, a social creation that reflects the interests and perceptions of its creators' and funders,[121] the medical and healthcare community would be duty-bound to find out and know if these interests and perceptions are benign or otherwise, science-driven or finance-driven, especially in the light of what we now do

[116] Bakar (1999), 103–130; and see also his chapter on 'Islam and Bioethics,' in Bakar (1999), 173–200.

[117] See, for instance Brian Tokar (2001), 1–16. On the largely speculative and pseudo-scientific nature of current research in medical genetics, see Ioannidis et al. (2001): 306–309; Ioannidis (2007): 203–13; Ioannidis (2013): 1–2; Roberts et al. (2012); and Kaplan (2013).

[118] Robinson, Antoniou, and Fagan (2015)

[119] Such as gene therapy and its tacit assumption of genetic reductionism; a critique is Strohman (2003): 169–191.

[120] A particular case in point is the scientific and ethical issues pertaining to genetic medical treatment for mitochondrial diseases as lucidly discussed in Zoloth (9 February 2015).

[121] Brian Tokar (2001), 67–68.

know about the techno-scientific and socio-historical development, and the political economy, of BT/GE.[122]

In many respects BT/GE encapsulates the intellectual conceit and big business tyranny of a run-away technology that has gone way off-track in its unthinking eagerness to reduce all life to a set of objects and codes to be taken apart and reconfigured just so that it can be patented (a.k.a., commercially monopolized), repackaged and sold in the name of scientific and medical advancement for some pre-conceived greater good of society. It is a technology that has to be done simply because it can be done and society will, whether it likes it or not, simply have to adjust or even transform altogether its age-old values and traditions to the coercive absoluteness of the ever-shifting consequentialist-utilitarian ethos of mainstream bioethics. The more we look into it, the more we are brought to the conclusion that bioethics was invented to make the world safe for biotechnology and the genetic manipulation of life forms for private profit.[123]

***Other Ethico-Legal Concerns*** Here I would like to outline briefly the ethico-legal dimensions of current debates over issues pertaining to medical education and research, iatrogenesis, patents and biomedical monopoly, and the medicalization of health.

(1) Medical education, research and funding: In general, mainstream medical schools do not train their students in nutrition and dietary therapy,[124] which are foundational to preventive healthcare,[125] and there is relatively little funding for research in these areas, especially under the current hegemony of high-tech interventive biomedicine and biotechnology. This deplorable medical educational framework results in a systemic, *de facto*, and, arguably, unprincipled and unethical preference for expensive high-tech biomedical interventive over *non-invasive* preventive therapy, and in the diversion of precious resources from research into low-tech primary healthcare.[126] They also do not educate medical students in philosophy and history of medicine, not even history of Islamic medicine in the case of Muslim universities. Such an education in what is called the *medical humanities*[127] would have inculcated a healthy dose of critical attitude towards the promises and limits, and the benefits and risks of modern

---

[122] Drucker (2015), 9–60. Although the focus of the book is on the genetic engineering of food, the underlying systemic problems also apply to medical genetics, especially given the intimate relation between good nutrition and good health, as shown in Chap. 3 of Drucker's book, 'Disappearing a Disaster: How the Facts About a Deadly Epidemic Caused by a Genetically Engineered Food Have Been Consistently Clouded,' 61–86.

[123] A discussion is Coletta (2000).

[124] Mogre et al. (2018): 2–11.

[125] Pellegrino (1974), 19–38.

[126] Kriel (2000), 34–35.

[127] Bleakley (2015); Cole, Carlin, and Carson (2014); Epstein (2017).

western medicine, as well as an intellectual exposure to and familiarity with well-proven alternative healthcare modalities.[128]

(2) Iatrogenesis: The term refers to diseases or adverse effects caused to patients due to the individual random mistakes or carelessness of their doctors (or their nurses); or due to 'systematic errors incorporated into medical practice,' in which case Dr Robin calls it iatroepidemics.[129] Many studies have shown that mishaps even deaths due to iatrogenesis have occurred all too frequently in hospitals.[130] Without going into detail into the various clinical practice contexts in which iatrogenesis (such as adverse effects of prescription drugs) occurs, suffice to say that it is only ethical for the healthcare system to openly recognize and acknowledge the high incidence of iatrogenesis and take concrete steps to minimize if not eliminate them altogether.[131]

(3) Patents and biomedical monopoly (*iḥtikār*) by private, pharmaceutical corporations: The basic premise of intellectual property rights and the granting of patents as protection and execution of those rights is that for medical science to progress in overcoming ever more new diseases, it is imperative for biomedical researchers and corporations to have exclusive ownership of their biomedical discoveries and their potentially profitable commercialization in order to recover their financial investment in them. But this premise has lately come under intense, detailed scrutiny.[132]

Specifically in this context, the main problem is that this commercial framework as applied to healthcare has led in fact to a global monopolistic commodification of health to maximize corporate profits from out of people's concern for their well-being and their fear of illness and disease. In many cases, even biomedical discoveries in research carried out at publicly funded universities and government medical research institutes have been allowed to be privatized for the sake of the corporate bottom-line. The monopolistic nature of patent laws and licensing rights have been shown to lead (i) to exorbitant prices for much needed drugs, (ii) actual stifling of further useful research into realizing the full medical potential of the patented discovery, (iii) global phenomena of biopiracy euphemized as bioprospecting, and (iv) overall socio-economic inequality in people's access to affordable and reliable healthcare services. It is clearly immoral to have a legal and regulatory regime in place that encourages or even protects monopolistic commercial practices that result in high prices for basic goods and services that are needed by people on a daily basis, like food, and, in this case, access to affordable healthcare for society as a whole.[133]

---

[128] Such as those comprehensively surveyed in some detail in Diamond (2001).

[129] Robin (1984), 65–86.

[130] Milligan (1998): 46–67.

[131] For a detailed multi-layered investigation, see Sharpe and Faden (1998); Gussak et al. (2017).

[132] Kinsella (2015); Boldrin and Levine (2008).

[133] A critical overview of the issue is Gold et al. (2009): 1–5; see also, Johnston (2008), 93–96.

(4) Medicalization of health: The state of being in overall good health and well-being should be the normal state of affairs amongst individuals and communities in any society, and illness should thus only be a medical situation requiring in-patient hospitalization in relatively rare cases. Hence, the first line of defence against disease and loss of health lies in taking personal responsibility for one's dietary habits and lifestyle.[134] This will result in fewer or even no visits to doctors, medical clinics or hospitals and thereby less exposure to iatrogenesis resulting from invasive tests and treatments, many of which are completely unnecessary. However, the currently overly commercialized biomedical paradigm of healthcare tends to medicalize completely healthy people, through unnecessary tests, screenings and check-ups, leading to 'disease mongering,'[135] and thus '*making patients out of normal human beings*.'[136] If health is an individual virtue as well as a public good, then health is or should be the normal state of affairs, but if health is medicalized and thus commodified through the corporatization of biomedicine then illness and disease will be the new norm.[137]

## 5.9 Conclusion

If the ethical enigmas brought into stark relief from these robust debates on the scientific and ethical aspects of biomedicine are rooted in the very institutional structures and/or research programmes underpinning it, then the current reactive *fatwā*-issuing activities of *fiqh* councils in the course of resolving these enigmas will only serve to encourage the generation of more of the same. Such a situation will in effect reinforce the validity and legitimacy of those institutional structures and research programmes, thereby rendering what is de facto *de jure* through unthinking, mechanical *fatwā*-issuing. That is the inevitable pitfall of narrow, formal *fiqho*-legalism when it is harried by the rush of biotechno-innovations into shallow formal casuistic evaluations and justifications without prior proper conceptualization and identification of medical problems and their contexts, despite the legal maxim that the legal evaluation of a problem is but a function of its cognitive conceptualization. Hence, *epistemic-cognitive mis-conceptualization leads to ethico-legal mis-evaluation.*

In the deluge of ever novel biotechnological interventions in institutionalized healthcare generating ever more moral problems impacting on Muslims that demand

[134] In the Islamic medical tradition good eating from good cooking contributed to good health; see Nasrallah (2018), 144–149; cf. Ibn Qayyim al-Jawziyya (2003), 22–24 and 29–30. In general, a balanced nutritious diet is considered the first line of defence against illness and disease thereby pre-empting medicalization as far as possible.

[135] Moynihan, Heath, and Henry (2002); Wolinsky (2005); Payer (1992); and Moynihan and Cassels (2008).

[136] Robin (1984), 119–148.

[137] A recent overview is Clark (2014): 1–6.

urgent *fatwās* (formal juristic rulings) for their resolutions, current *fiqh* of medicine and its practitioners, the *fuqahā'*, as well as Muslim 'bioethicists,' will need to stand back and decide if their job is to be mere reactive ethico-legal apologists, even enablers and justifiers of the results of biomedical science, or to say, 'Enough is enough,' and set about to embark on creative work in articulating a proactive *deep-fiqh* of medicine, one that is systematic and rigorous enough to generate a *long term medical research programme* that consciously takes the Islamic axio-telelogical value system as its core point of departure.

A proactive deep-*fiqh* of medicine will entail the conceptualization of an Islamic Medical Research Programme (IMRP)[138] along Lakatosian lines that is informed and guided by critical, constructive engagement with both tradition and modernity, taking as its cue the engagement that is reflected in, say, the *ṭibb nabawī* texts,[139] and in the grand critical synthesis of the Avicennan *Canon of Medicine*, including the post-Ghazālian responses to that *Canon* on the part of the *mutakallimūn*.[140] Instead of a largely *ad hoc* 'fire engine' ethics that simply reacts hastily to whatever challenges posed by some new-fangled biomedical developments in modern western medicine, such a *generative* research programme will lead to a revived autonomous Islamic Medicine capable of generating effective treatment and healing modalities that are *intrinsically* sound ethically and epistemically, and thereby free Muslims from the unceasing onslaught of medico-moral dilemmas imposed on them by a run-away biotechnologization of medicine and healthcare.[141]

## References

Abdel Haleem, M. A. S. 1991. 'Early Islamic Theological and Juristic Terminology: *Kitāb al-Ḥudūd fi'l-Uṣūl* by Ibn Fūrak.' *Bulletin of the School of Oriental and African Studies* 54 (1): 5–41.

'Abd Allāh, Ḥakīm. 2017. *Khazīnat al-Insān: Perbendaharaan Manusia* [Treasury of Humankind], eds. Sarah Syazwani Shaifuddin and Naseer Sobree. Kitab Perubatan Melayu [Series on Malay Medicine]. Kuala Lumpur: Akademi Jawi Malaysia.

Adamson, Peter, and Peter E. Pormann, eds. 2017. *Philosophy and Medicine in the Formative Period of Islam*. Warburg Institute Colloquia, no. 31. London: Warburg Institute.

Ahn, Andrew C., Muneesh Tewari, Chi-Sang Poon, and Russell S. Phillips. 2006. 'The Limits of Reductionism in Medicine: Could Systems Biology Offer an Alternative?' *PLoS Medicine* 3 (7): e209.

Akhtar, Aysha. 2015. 'The Flaws and Human Harms of Animal Experimentation.' *Cambridge Quarterly of Healthcare Ethics* 24 (4): 407–419.

---

[138] See n. 14 above.

[139] I have in mind in particular al-Suyūṭī's *Ṭibb al-Nabī* (*Prophetic Medicine*). A brief overview of the *ṭibb nabawī* tradition is in Barakat (2018), 56–57.

[140] See Setia (2012), 25–73. This call for contemporary Muslim theologians to engage in 'new dialectics' and/or '*Kalām* of the Age' is precisely that which Afifi al-Akiti invites us to heed in his important article, see al-Akiti (2010), 119–134.

[141] Details of this research programme will understandably be the subject of a separate paper.

al-Akiti, Afifi. 2010. 'The Negotiation of Modernity Through Tradition in Contemporary Muslim Intellectual Discourse: The Neo-Ghazālian, Attasian Perspective.' In *Knowledge, Language, Thought and the Civilization of Islam: Essays in Honor of Syed Muhammad Naquib al-Attas*, eds. Wan Mohd Nor Wan Daud and Muhammad Zaini Uthman. Kuala Lumpur: UTM Press.
al-Attas, Syed Naquib. 1976. *Islām: The Concept of Religion and the Foundation of Ethics and Morality*. Kuala Lumpur: ABIM.
———. 1980. *The Concept of Education in Islām*. Kuala Lumpur: ABIM.
———. 1993. *The Nature of Man and the Psychology of the Human Soul*. Kuala Lumpur: ABIM.
———. 1995. *Prolegomena to the Metaphysics of Islām: An Exposition of the Fundamental Elements of the Worldview of Islām*. Kuala Lumpur: ISTAC.
Bakar, Osman. 1999. *The History and Philosophy of Islamic Science*. Cambridge: Islamic Texts Society.
Baltussen, Han. 2015. '"Hippocratic" Oaths: A Cross-Cultural Exploration of Medical Ethics in the Ancient World.' In *The Frontiers of Ancient Science: Papers in Honor of Heinrich von Staden*, eds. B. Holmes and K. D. Fischer. Berlin: De Gruyter.
al-Bar, Mohammed Ali, and Hassan Chamsi-Pasha. 2015. *Contemporary Bioethics: Islamic Perspective*. New York, NY: Springer.
Barakat, Heba Nayel. 2018. 'Prophetic Medicine: *al-Tibb al-Nabawi*.' In *Al-Tibb: Healing Traditions in Islamic Medical Manuscripts*, eds. Lucien de Guise and Siti Marina Mohd. Maidin. Kuala Lumpur: Islamic Arts Museum Malaysia.
Beauregard, Mario, and Denyse O'Leary. 2007. *The Spiritual Brain: A Neuroscientist's Case for the Existence of the Soul*. New York, NY: HarperOne.
Bhaskar, Roy. 2008. *A Realist Theory of Science*. London: Routledge.
Bleakley, Alan. 2015. *Medical Humanities and Medical Education: How the Medical Humanities Can Shape Better Doctors*. London: Routledge.
Boldrin, Michele, and David K. Levine. 2008. *Against Intellectual Monopoly*. Cambridge: Cambridge University Press.
Braude, Hillel D. 2012. *Intuition in Medicine: A Philosophical Defense of Clinical Reasoning*. Chicago, IL: University of Chicago Press.
Brown, E. Richard. 1979. *Rockefeller Medicine Men: Medicine and Capitalism in America*. Berkeley, CA: University of California Press.
Bunge, Mario. 1975. 'Towards a Technoethics.' *Philosophic Exchange* 6 (1): 69–79.
Burrows, Beth. 2001a. 'Patents, Ethics and Spin.' In *Redesigning Life?: The Worldwide Challenge to Genetic Engineering*, ed. Brian Tokar. London: Zed Books.
———. 2001b. 'Safety First.' In *Redesigning Life?: The Worldwide Challenge to Genetic Engineering*, ed. Brian Tokar. London: Zed Books.
al-Būṭī, Saʿīd Ramaḍān. 1966. *Ḍawābiṭ al-maṣlaḥa fī al-sharīʿa al-Islāmiyya*. Damascus: al-Maktabat al-Umawiyya.
Cabaret, J., and G. Denegri. 2008. 'The Scientific Research Programmes of Lakatos and Applications in Parasitology.' *Parasite* 15 (3): 501–505.
Caplan, Arthur L., James J. McCartney, and Dominic A. Sisti, eds. 2004. *Health, Disease and Illness*. Washington, DC: Georgetown University Press.
Carrier, Martin, and Patrick Finzer. 2006. 'Explanatory Loops and the Limits of Genetic Reductionism.' *International Studies in the Philosophy of Science* 20 (3): 267–283.
Casell, Eric J. 2004. *The Nature of Suffering and the Goals of Medicine*. 2nd ed. New York, NY: Oxford University Press.
Chishti, Hakim Moinuddin. 1985. *The Book of Sufi Healing*. New York, NY: Inner Traditions.
Clark, Jocalyn. 2014. 'Medicalization of Global Health 1: Has the Global Health Agenda Become Too Medicalized?' *Global Health Action* 7 (1): 1–6.
Cole, Thomas R., Nathan S. Carlin, and Ronald A. Carson. 2014. *Medical Humanities: An Introduction*. Cambridge: Cambridge University Press.
Coletta, Raymond. 2000. 'Biotechnology and the Creation of Ethics.' *McGeorge Law Review* 32 (1): 89–110.

Croce, Pietro. 1999. *Vivisection or Science?: An Investigation into Testing Drugs and Safeguarding Health*. London: Zed Books.
Diamond, W. John. 2001. *The Clinical Practice of Complementary, Alternative, and Western Medicine*. New York, NY: CRC Press.
Doyal, Lesley, and Imogen Pennell. 1991. *The Political Economy of Health*. London: Pluto Press.
Drucker, Steven M. 2015. *Altered Genes, Twisted Truth: How the Venture to Genetically Engineer Our Food Has Subverted Science, Corrupted Government, and Systematically Deceived the Public*. Salt Lake City, UT: Clear River Press.
Eisener-Dorman, Amy F., David A Lawrence, and Valerie J Bolivar. 2009. 'Cautionary Insights on Knockout Mouse Studies.' *Brain, Behavior, and Immunity* 23 (3): 318–324.
Engel, George L. 1977. 'The Need for a New Medical Model: A Challenge for Biomedicine.' *Science* 196 (4286): 129–136.
Epstein, Ronald. 2017. *Attending: Medicine, Mindfulness and Humanity*. New York, NY: Scribner.
*Evidence-Based Complementary and Alternative Medicine*. Available at https://www.hindawi.com/journals/ecam/
Fisher, Jill A. 2011. *Medical Research for Hire: The Political Economy of Pharmaceutical Clinical Trials*. New Brunswick, NJ: Rutgers University Press.
Foltz, Richard C. 2006. *Animals in Islamic Tradition and Muslim Cultures*. Oxford: Oneworld.
Frankel, Richard M., Timothy E. Quill, and Susan H, McDaniel, eds. 2003. *The Biopsychosocial Approach: Past, Present, Future*. New York, NY: University of Rochester Press.
Fries, James F., and Donald M. Vickery. 2017. *Take Care of Yourself: The Complete Illustrated Guide to Self-Care*. 10th ed. Boston, MA: Da Capo Press.
Furber, Musa. 2015. *Rights and Duties Pertaining to Kept Animals: A Case Study in Islamic Law and Ethics*. Abu Dhabi: Tabah Foundation.
al-Ghazālī. 2015. *The Book of Knowledge* [Book 1 of the *Iḥyāʾ ʿulūm al-dīn*], trans. Kenneth Honerkamp. Louisville, KY: Fons Vitae.
———. 2019. *The Ethics of Prophethood and the Courtesies of Living* [Book 20 of the *Iḥyāʾ ʿulūm al-dīn*], trans. Adi Setia. Louisville, KY: Fons Vitae.
Gold, E. Richard, Warren Kaplan, James Orbinski, Sarah Harland-Logan, and Sevil N-Marandi. 2009. 'Are Patents Impeding Medical Care and Innovation?' *PLoS Medicine* 7 (1): 1–5.
Goldim, José Roberto. 2009. 'Revisiting the Beginning of Bioethics: The Contributions of Fritz Jahr (1927).' *Perspectives in Biology and Medicine* 52 (3): 377–380.
Gøtzsche, Peter C. 2019. *Death of a Whistleblower and Cochrane's Moral Collapse*. Copenhagen: People's Press.
Gøtzsche, Peter C., Jerome P Kassirer, Karen L. Woolley, Elizabeth Wager, Adam Jacobs, Art Gertel, and Cindy Hamilton. 2009. 'What Should Be Done to Tackle Ghostwriting in the Medical Literature?' *PLoS Medicine* 6 (2): 122–125.
Greek, C. Ray, and Jean Swingle Greek. 2000. *Sacred Cows and Golden Geese: The Human Costs of Experiments on Animals*. New York, NY: Continuum.
Green, Susan Bridgwood. 2015. 'Can Animal Data Translate to Innovations Necessary for a New Era of Patient-Centred and Individualised Healthcare?: Bias in Preclinical Animal Research.' *BMJ Medical Ethics* 16 (53): 1–14.
Groopman, Jerome. 2007. *How Doctors Think*. Boston, MA: Houghton Mifflin.
Groopman, Jerome, and Pamela Hartzband. 2011. *Your Medical Choices: How to Decide What Is Right for You*. Melbourne: Scribe Publications.
Grzywacz, Joseph G., and Juliana Fuqua. 2000. 'The Social Ecology of Health: Leverage Points and Linkages.' *Behavioral Medicine* 26 (3): 101–115.
Gussak, Ihor, John B. Kostis, Giovanni Campanile, and Ibrahim Akin, eds. 2017. *Iatrogenicity: Causes and Consequences of Iatrogenesis in Cardiovascular Medicine*. New Brunswick, NJ: Rutgers University Press.
Henry, Stephen G. 2010. 'Polanyi's Tacit Knowing and the Relevance of Epistemology to Clinical Medicine.' *Journal of Evaluation in Clinical Practice* 16 (2): 292–297.

Heydari, Mojtaba, Mohammad Hashem Hashempur, Mohammad Hosein Ayati, Detlev Quintern, Majid Nimrouzi, and Seyed Hamdollah Mosavat. 2015. 'The Use of Chinese Herbal Drugs in Islamic Medicine.' *Journal of Integrative Medicine* 13 (6): 363–367.

Howick, Jeremy. 2011. *The Philosophy of Evidence-based Medicine*. Oxford: Wiley.

Huber, Machteld, J. André Knottnerus, Lawrence Green, Henriëtte van der Horst, Alejandro R. Jadad, Daan Kromhout, Brian Leonard, Kate Lorig, Maria Isabel Loureiro, Jos W. M. van der Meer, Paul Schnabel, Richard Smith, Chris van Weel, and Henk Smid. 2011. 'How Should We Define Health?' *British Medical Journal* 343 (7817): 1–3.

Hussain, Abdul Ghani. 2015. *MSS 2999 Kitab Tib: A Modern Medical Insight into and Interpretation of a Malay Medical Manuscript*. Kuala Lumpur: Forest Research Institute Malaysia.

Ibn Hindū. 2011. *The Key to Medicine and a Guide for Students* [*Miftāḥ al-ṭibb wa-minhāj al-ṭullāb*], trans. Aida Tibi and Emilie Savage-Smith. Reading: Garnet.

Ibn Jumayy. 1983. *Treatise to Ṣalāḥ al-Dīn on the Revival of the Art of Medicine* [*al-Maqālat al-Ṣalāḥiyyah fī iḥyā' al-ṣināʿat al-ṣiḥḥiyya*], ed. and tr., Hartmut Fähndrich. Abhandlungen für die Kunde des Morgenlandes, no. 46.3. Wiesbaden: Steiner.

Ibn Qayyim al-Jawziyya. 2003. *Healing with the Medicine of the Prophet*, trans. Jalal Abu al-Rub. Riyadh: Darussalam Publications.

Ibn Sīnā. 2013. *Avicenna's Medicine: A New Translation of the 11th-Century Canon with Practical Applications for Integrative Health Care*, trans. Mones Abu-Asab, Hakima Amri, and Marc S. Micozzi. Rochester, VT: Healing Arts Press.

Illich, Ivan. 1976. *Medical Nemesis: The Expropriation of Health*. New York, NY: Pantheon Books.

Ioannidis, John P. A. 2005. 'Why Most Published Research Findings Are False.' *PLoS Medicine* 2 (8): 696–701.

———. 2007. 'Non-replication and Inconsistency in the Genome-Wide Association Setting.' *Human Heredity* 64 (4): 203–213.

———. 2012. 'Extrapolating from Animals to Humans.' *Science Translational Medicine* 4 (151): 1–4.

———. 2013. 'This I Believe in Genetics: Discovery Can Be a Nuisance, Replication Is Science, Implementation Matters.' *Frontiers in Genetics* 4 (33): 1–2.

———. 2014. 'How to Make More Published Research True.' *PLoS Medicine* 11 (10): 1–6.

Ioannidis, John P. A., Evangelia E. Ntzani, Thomas A. Trikalinos, and Despina G. Contopoulos-Ioannidis. 2001. 'Replication Validity of Genetic Association Studies.' *Nature Genetics* 29 (3): 306–309.

Irving, Diane N. 2002. 'What Is Bioethics?' In *Life and Learning X: Proceedings of the Tenth University Faculty for Life Conference*, ed. Joseph W. Koterski. Washington, DC: University Faculty for Life.

Ismail, Mohd Zaidi. 2002. *The Sources of Knowledge in al-Ghazali's Thought: A Psychological Framework of Epistemology*. Kuala Lumpur: ISTAC.

Jamal, Farida. 2018. 'Anatomy and Physiology in Medieval Islam.' In *Al-Tibb: Healing Traditions in Islamic Medical Manuscripts*, eds. Lucien de Guise and Siti Marina Mohd. Maidin. Kuala Lumpur: Islamic Arts Museum Malaysia.

Jenkins, David O. 1981. '*The Ethical Dimension of Personal Knowledge*.' PhD diss., Loyola University.

Jha, S. R. 1998. 'The Tacit-Explicit Connection: Polanyian Integrative Philosophy and a Neo-Polanyian Medical Epistemology.' *Theoretical Medicine and Bioethics* 19 (6): 547–568.

Johnston, Josephine. 2008. 'Intellectual Property and Biomedicine.' In *From Birth to Death and Bench to Clinic: The Hastings Center Bioethics Briefing Book for Journalists, Policymakers, and Campaigns*, ed. Mary Crowley. Garrison, NY: The Hastings Center.

Jotterand, Fabrice. 2005. 'The Hippocratic Oath and Contemporary Medicine: Dialectic Between Past Ideals and Present Reality?' *Journal of Medicine and Philosophy* 30 (1): 107–128.

Kahl, Oliver. 2007. *The Dispensatory of Ibn al-Tilmīdh: Arabic Text, English Translation, Study and Glossaries*. Leiden: Brill.

Kaplan, Jonathan Michael. 2013. *The Limits and Lies of Human Genetic Research: Dangers for Social Policy*. London: Routledge.
Kelly, Evelyn B. 2007. *Gene Therapy*. Westport, CT: Greenwood Press.
Kienle, Gunver S., and Helmut Kiene. 2011. 'Clinical Judgement and the Medical Profession.' *Journal of Evaluation in Clinical Practice* 17 (4): 621–627.
Kinsella, N. Stephan. 2015. *Against Intellectual Property*. Auburn, AL: Ludwig von Mises Institute.
Knox, Sarah S. 2010. *Science, God and the Nature of Reality: Bias in Biomedical Research*. Boca Raton, FL: Brown Walker Press.
Kriel, Jacques. 2000. *Matter, Mind and Medicine: Transforming the Clinical Method*. Amsterdam: Rodopi.
Lahham, Karim. 2013. *The Vocational Society*. Abu Dhabi: Tabah Foundation.
Lakatos, Imre. 1978. *The Methodology of Scientific Research Programmes*. Cambridge: Cambridge University Press.
Laurel, Jane Dominic. 2018. 'Medicine As Sacred Vocation.' *Baylor University Medical Center Proceedings* 31 (1): 126–131.
Le Fanu, James. 2011. *The Rise and Fall of Modern Medicine*. Rev. ed. London: Hachette.
Levey, Martin. 1967. 'Medical Ethics of Medieval Islam with Special Reference to al-Ruhāwī's *Practical Ethics of the Physician*.' *Transactions of the American Philosophical Society* 57 (3): 1–100.
Lo, Bernard, and Marilyn J. Field, eds. 2009. *Conflict of Interest in Medical Research, Education, and Practice*. Washington, DC: National Academies Press.
Maidin, Siti Marina Mohd. 2018. 'The Spread of Medical Knowledge in the Islamic World.' In *Al-Tibb: Healing Traditions in Islamic Medical Manuscripts*, eds. Lucien de Guise and Siti Marina Mohd. Maidin. Kuala Lumpur: Islamic Arts Museum Malaysia.
Marcum, James A. 2008. *Introductory Philosophy of Medicine: Humanizing Modern Medicine*. Berlin: Springer.
Markham, Annette N., Katrin Tiidenberg, and Andrew Herman. 2018. 'Ethics as Methods: Doing Ethics in the Era of Big Data Research: Introduction.' *Social Media + Society* 5 (3): 1–9.
Masri, Basheer Ahmad. 2007. *Animal Welfare in Islam*. Markfield: Islamic Foundation.
McHugh, Hugh Marshall, and Simon Thomas Walker. 2015. 'Personal Knowledge in Medicine and the Epistemic Shortcomings of Scientism.' *Journal of Bioethical Inquiry* 12 (4): 577–585.
Medawar, P. B. 2009. *Induction and Intuition in Scientific Thought*. London: Routledge.
Miles, Steven H. 2004. *The Hippocratic Oath and the Ethics of Medicine*. Oxford: Oxford University Press.
Milligan, Frank. 1998. 'The Iatrogenic Epidemic.' *Nursing Standard* 13 (2): 46–47.
Mogre, Victor, Fred C. J. Stevens, Paul A. Aryee, Anthony Amalba, and Albert J. J. A. Scherpbier. 2018. 'Why Nutrition Education is Inadequate in the Medical Curriculum: A Qualitative Study of Students' Perspectives on Barriers and Strategies.' *BMC Medical Education* 18 (26): 1–11.
Mohaghegh, M. 1988. 'The *Kitāb al-Shukūk ʿala Jālinus* of Muhammad ibn Zachariya al-Razi.' *Medical Journal of the Islamic Republic of Iran (MJIRI)* 2 (3): 207–211.
———. ed. 1993. *Kitāb al-Shukūkʿalā Jālīnūs lil-Ṭabīb al-Faylasuf Muḥammad ibn Zakariyā al-Rāzī*. Kuala Lumpur: ISTAC.
Mohyuddin, Anwaar, Mamonah Ambreen, Juhi Naveed, and Danish Ahmad. 2004. 'World System Analysis of Biomedical Hegemony.' *Advances in Anthropology* 4 (2): 59–67.
Montgomery, Kathryn. 2006. *How Doctors Think: Clinical Judgement and the Practice of Medicine*. Oxford: Oxford University Press.
Moynihan, Roy, and Alan Cassels. 2008. *Selling Sickness: How the World's Biggest Pharmaceutical Companies are Turning Us All Into Patients*. New York, NY: Greystone Books.
Moynihan, Roy, Iona Heath, and David Henry. 2002. 'Selling Sickness: The Pharmaceutical Industry and Disease Mongering.' *British Medical Journal* 324 (7342): 886–891.
al-Nashshār, Alī Sāmī. 1983. *Manāhij al-baḥth ʿinda mufakkirī al-Islām wa-naqd al-muslimīn lil-manṭiq al-arisṭuṭālīsī*. 4th ed. Cairo: Beirut: Dār al-Nahdat al-ʿArabiyya.

Nasrallah, Nwal. 2018. 'Eating and Good Health in Medieval Islam.' In *Al-Tibb: Healing Traditions in Islamic Medical Manuscripts*, eds. Lucien de Guise and Siti Marina Mohd. Maidin. Kuala Lumpur: Islamic Arts Museum Malaysia.

National Human Genome Research Institute. 2015. 'Knock Out Mice Fact Sheet.' Available at https://www.genome.gov/about-genomics/fact-sheets/Knockout-Mice-Fact-Sheet.

Norman, Ishmael, Moses Aikins, and Fred Binka. 2011. 'Ethics and Electronic Health Information Technology: Challenges for Evidence-Based Medicine and the Physician-Patient Relationship.' *Ghana Medical Journal* 45 (3): 115–124.

Okello, Joseph B. Onyango. 2015. *History and Critique of Methodological Naturalism*. Eugene, OR: Wipf and Stock.

Padela, Aasim I. 2018. 'Social Responsibility and the Moral Obligation toward Providing Healthcare: An Islamic Ethico-Legal Analysis.' In *Religious Perspectives on Social Responsibility in Health: Toward a Dialogical Approach*, eds. Joseph Tham, Chris Durante, and Alberto García Gómez. New York, NY: Springer.

Panda, S. C. 2006. 'Medicine: Science or Art?' *Mens Sana Monographs* 4 (1): 127–138.

Payer, Lynn. 1992. *Disease Mongers: How Doctors, Drug Companies and Insurers Are Making You Feel Sick*. New York, NY: Wiley.

Pellegrino, Edmund D. 1974. 'Preventive Healthcare and the Allied Health Professions.' In *Review of Allied Health Education: 1*, ed. Joseph Hamburg. Lexington, KY: University Press of Kentucky.

———. 1998. 'What the Philosophy of Medicine Is.' *Theoretical Medicine and Bioethics* 19 (4): 315–336.

Pellegrino, Edmund D., and David C. Thomasma. 1993. *The Virtues in Medical Practice*. Oxford: Oxford University Press.

Polanyi, Michael. 2015. *Personal Knowledge: Towards a Post-critical Philosophy*. Enlarged ed. Chicago, IL: University of Chicago Press.

Popper, Karl R., and John C. Eccles. 1985. *The Self and Its Brain*. Berlin: Springer.

Pormann, Peter E. 2017. 'The Hippocratic Aphorisms in the Arabic Medical Tradition.' *Aspetar: Sports Medicine Journal* 6: 412–415.

Quirk, Mark. 2006. *Intuition and Metacognition in Medical Education*. New York, NY: Springer.

Rahman, Fazlur. 1989. *Health and Medicine in the Islamic Tradition: Change and Identity*. New York, NY: Crossroad.

al-Rānirī, Nūr al-Dīn. 2018. *Bustān al-Ṣalāṭīn,* trans. Naseer Sobree. Penang: Baytul Hikma.

Regal, Philip J. 1998. *A Brief History of Biotechnology Debates and Policies in the United States*. Edmonds, WA: Edmonds Institute.

Roberts, Nicholas J., Joshua T. Vogelstein, Giovanni Parmigiani, Kenneth W. Kinzler, Bert Vogelstein, and Victor E. Velculescu. 2012. 'The Predictive Capacity of Personal Genome Sequencing.' *Science Translational Medicine* 4 (133): 133ra58.

Robin, Eugene D. 1984. *Matters of Life and Death: Risks vs. Benefits of Medical Care*. Stanford, CA: Stanford Alumni Association.

Robinson, Claire, Michael Antoniou, and John Fagan. 2015. *GMO Myths and Truths*. London: Earth Open Source.

Rodwin, Marc A. 2011. *Conflicts of Interest and the Future of Medicine: The United States, France and Japan*. Oxford: Oxford University Press.

Rose, Hilary, and Steven Rose. 2014. *Genes, Cells and Brains: The Promethean Promises of the New Biology*. London: Verso.

Rothstein, Hannah R., Alexander J. Sutton, and Michael Borenstein, eds. 2005. *Publication Bias in Meta-Analysis: Prevention, Assessment and Adjustments*. Chichester: Wiley.

al-Rūḥāwī, Isḥāq ibn ʿAlī. 1991. *Ādāb al-ṭabīb*, eds. Kamāl al-Sāmarrāʾī and Dāwūd Salmān ʿAlī. Baghdad: Dār al-Shuʾūn al-Thaqāfiyya.

Sachedina, Abdulaziz. 2009. *Islamic Biomedical Ethics: Principles and Applications*. Oxford: Oxford University Press.

Sartell, Elizabeth, and Aasim I. Padela. 2015. '*Adab* and Its Significance for an Islamic Medical Ethics.' *Journal of Medical Ethics* 41 (9): 756–761.

Schumacher, E. F. 1979. *Good Work*. New York, NY: Harper and Row.

Schwarb, Gregor. 2018. 'Early *Kalām* and the Medical Tradition.' In *Philosophy and Medicine in the Formative Period of Islam*, eds. Peter Adamson and Peter E. Pormann. Warburg Institute Colloquia, no. 31. London: Warburg Institute.

Setia, Adi. 2003. 'Al-Attas's Philosophy of Science: An Extended Outline.' *Islam and Science* 1 (2): 165–214.

———. 2004. '*Taskhīr*, Fine-tuning, Intelligent Design and the Scientific Appreciation of Nature.' *Islam and Science* 2 (1): 7–32.

———. 2005. 'The Theologico-Scientific Research Program of the Mutakallimūn: Intellectual Historical Context and Contemporary Concerns with Special Reference to Fakhr al-Dīn al-Rāzī.' *Islam and Science* 3 (2): 127–151.

———. 2012. '*Kalām Jadīd*, Islamization, and the Worldview of Islam: Applying the Neo-Ghazālian, Attasian Vision.' *Islam and Science* 10 (1): 25–73.

———. 2016. 'Freeing *Maqāṣid* and *Maṣlaḥah* from Surreptitious Utilitarianism.' *Islamic Sciences* 14 (2): 127–157.

———. 2017a 'Islamic Science as a Scientific Research Program.' In *Studies in the Islam and Science Nexus*. Vol. 1 of *Islam and Science: Historical and Contemporary Perspective*, ed. Muzaffar Iqbal. 4 vols. London: Routledge.

———. 2017b 'Three Meanings of Islamic Science: Towards Operationalizing Islamization of Science.' In *Studies in the Islam and Science Nexus*. Vol. 1 of *Islam and Science: Historical and Contemporary Perspectives*, ed. Muzaffar Iqbal. 4 vols. London: Routledge.

Shaffri, Mohd Affendi Mohd. 2018. 'Pharmacy and Its Offshoots.' In *Al-Tibb: Healing Traditions in Islamic Medical Manuscripts*, eds. Lucien de Guise and Siti Marina Mohd. Maidin. Kuala Lumpur: Islamic Arts Museum Malaysia.

Sharpe, Virginia A., and Alan I. Faden. 1998. *Medical Harm: Historical, Conceptual and Ethical Dimensions of Iatrogenic Illness*. Cambridge: Cambridge University Press.

Shihadeh, Ayman. 2006. *The Teleological Ethics of Fakhr al-Dīn al-Rāzī*. Leiden: Brill.

———. 2013. 'A Post-Ghazālian Critic of Avicenna: Ibn Ghaylān al-Balkhī on the *Materia Medica* of the *Canon of Medicine*.' *Journal of Islamic Studies* 24 (2): 135–174.

Sobree, Naseer. 2018. *Risalah Ilmu Perubatan: Sebuah Integrasi Antara Perubatan Greek-Arab dan Perubatan Moden* [An Epistle on the Science of Medicine: Integration of Arabo-Greek and Modern Medicine]. Penang: Darul Hikma.

Strohman, Richard C. 2003. 'Genetic Determinism as a Failing Paradigm in Biology and Medicine: Implications for Health and Wellness.' *Journal of Social Work Education* 39 (2): 169–191.

al-Suyūṭī, Jalāl al-Dīn. 2015. *Medicine of the Prophet,* trans. Cyril Elgood, ed. Ahmad Thomson. London: Ta Ha.

Tarakeshwar, Nalini, Jeffrey Stanton, and Kenneth I. Pargament. 2003. 'Religion: An Overlooked Dimension in Cross-Cultural Psychology.' *Journal of Cross-Cultural Psychology* 34 (4): 377–394.

Tataryn, Douglas J. 2004. 'Paradigms of Health and Disease: A Framework for Classifying and Understanding Complementary and Alternative Medicine.' *Journal of Alternative and Comparative Medicine* 8 (6): 877–892.

Tokar, Brian, ed. 2001. *Redesigning Life?: The Worldwide Challenge to Genetic Engineering*. London: Zed Books.

Traphagan, John W. 2013. *Rethinking Autonomy: A Critique of Principlism in Biomedical Ethics*. Albany, NY: SUNY Press.

van Regenmortel, Marc H. V. 2004a. 'Reductionism and Complexity in Molecular Biology.' *EMBO Reports* 5 (11): 1016–1020.

———. 2004b. 'Biological Complexicity Emerges from the Ashes of Genetic Reductionism, Reductionism and Complexity in Molecular Biology.' *Journal of Molecular Recognition* 17 (3): 145–148.

Vayena, Effy, Marcel Salathé, Lawrence C. Madoff, and John S. Brownstein. 2015. 'Ethical Challenges of Big Data in Public Health.' *PLoS Computational Biology* 11 (2): 1–7.

Veatch, Robert M. 2000. *Cross-Cultural Perspectives in Medical Ethics*. 2nd ed. London: Jones and Barlett.

von Scheidt, Moritz, Yuqi Zhao, Zeyneb Kurt, Calvin Pan, Lingyao Zeng, Xia Yang, Heribert Schunkert, and Aldons J. Lusis. 2017. 'Applications and Limitations of Mouse Models.' *Cell Metabolism* 25 (2): 248–261.

Wade, Derick T., and Peter W. Halligan. 2004. 'Do Biomedical Models of Illness Make for Good Healthcare Systems?' *British Medical Journal* 329: 1398–1401.

Walker, Rebecca L. 2010. 'Virtue Ethics and Medicine.' *Lahey Clinic Journal of Medical Ethics* 17 (3): 1–2.

Weber, Daniel. 2016. 'Medical Hegemony.' *International Journal of Complementary and Alternative Medicine* 3 (2): 1–2.

White, Peter, ed. 2005. *Biopsychosocial Medicine: An Integrated Approach to Understanding Illness*. Oxford: Oxford University Press.

Williams, John R. 2005. *Medical Ethics Manual*. Ferney-Voltaire: World Medical Association.

Wolinsky, Howard. 2005. 'Disease Mongering and Drug Marketing.' *EMBO Reports* 6 (7): 612–614.

World Health Organization (WHO). 2006. *Constitution of the World Health Organization: Basic Documents*. 46th ed. Geneva. World Health Organization.

Zoloth, Laurie. 9 February 2015. 'Reaching the Limits of Genetic Medicine: British MPs Have Voted to Allow Three-parent Babies To Be Created.' *Cosmos*. Available at https://cosmosmagazine.com/society/reaching-limits-genetic-medicine.

**Dr Adi Setia** was an Associate Professor of Islamic Economics at the Center for Advanced Studies in Islam, Science and Civilization (CASIS), University of Technology, Malaysia. Prior to this role, he was an Associate Professor of History and Philosophy of Science at the Faculty of Science and later at the Faculty of General Studies at the International Islamic University Malaysia (IIUM).

# Part II
# The Meaning of Life and Death

# Chapter 6
# When Does a Human Foetus Become Human?

**Hamza Yusuf**

*Do not sever the bonds of the womb.* [Qur'an 4:1 (*al-Nisā'*)]

*Do not kill your children from fear of poverty.* [Qur'an 17:31 (*al-Isrā'*)]

*On the Day when the one buried alive will be asked for what sin was she killed.* [Qur'an 81:8–9 (*al-Fajr*)]

*Marry and be fruitful, for I will be proud of the multitudes of my community of believers on the Day of Judgment.* [Prophet Muhammad]

*To die by other hands more merciless than mine.*
*No; I who gave them life will give them death.*
*Oh, now no cowardice, no thought how young they are,*
*How dear they are, how when they first were born;*
*Not that; I will forget they are my sons.*
*One moment, one short moment—then forever sorrow.* [Euripides' *Medea*]

## 6.1 Introduction

In English, the term we define ourselves with, *human being*, emphasizes 'being' over doing. It is not our actions that mark us as humans but our mere being. When, then, do we come to be? When does that being we identify as human first become human? The answer is consequential for many reasons, not the least of which is that our nation's foundational document states that all human beings are 'endowed by their Creator with certain unalienable rights' that include the rights of 'life, liberty, and the pursuit of happiness.' The question of when human life begins stubbornly

This chapter is a revision of an article that first appeared in the journal *Renovatio*. See Yusuf (2018).

H. Yusuf (✉)
Zaytuna College, Berkely, CA, USA
e-mail: hyusuf@zaytuna.edu



A. al-Akiti, A. I. Padela (eds.), *Islam and Biomedicine*, Philosophy and Medicine 137, https://doi.org/10.1007/978-3-030-53801-9_6

remains a central point of contention in the debate, now raging for half a century, regarding the ethics of abortion. The Supreme Court made its decision, but for many, it is far from a settled matter.

Beyond our borders, meanwhile, induced abortion rates are increasing in developing nations, despite declining slightly in developed nations; an estimated one-quarter of all pregnancies worldwide end in abortion.[1] The debate over abortion still rages across parts of Europe and remains contentious in North Africa, the Middle East, Asia, as well as Central and South America. While the Catholic Church continues to prioritize abortion as an egregious social ill, for many, abortion has become an acceptable option for dealing with unwanted pregnancies. Increasingly, some Muslims are adding their voices to the conversation – some even supporting legalization in areas where abortion remains illegal.

Given this global trend, it becomes all the more urgent to re-examine the normative view of infanticide and abortion in the Islamic legal tradition, which relies on the Qur'an, Prophetic tradition, and scholastic authority for its proofs.

Abortion derives from the Latin word *aboriri*,[2] meaning 'to perish, disappear, miscarry.'[3] The verb to abort is both intransitive (meaning to 'miscarry' or 'suffer an abortion') and transitive ('to effect the abortion of a foetus').[4] In standard English, we also use the word to connote the failure of something, as 'an aborted mission' – something that ends fruitlessly. As a noun, abortion means 'the expulsion of a foetus (naturally or esp. by medical induction) from the womb before it is able to survive independently, esp. in the first 28 weeks of a human pregnancy.'[5]

Historically, civilizations and religious traditions often grouped abortion with infanticide – defined as 'the killing of an infant soon after birth' by the *Oxford Modern English Dictionary*. Indeed, even some modern philosophers link abortion and infanticide by arguing for what they euphemistically term 'after-birth abortions.'[6] Reviewing the sordid history of infanticide since the Axial Age[7] and how the different faith traditions inspired a change in attitudes about both practices helps set the stage for understanding the Islamic ethical vision toward abortion, which depends ultimately, as we'll see, on the central question of when human life begins. The

[1] Guttmacher Institute (2020): www.guttmacher.org/fact-sheet/induced-abortion-worldwide

[2] Herbermann et al. (1907), 1:46.

[3] Barnhart et al. (1988), 4. According to Chambers, the word came into use in 1580. The first use of 'abortionist,' one who performs an abortion, was in 1872.

[4] Thompson (1996), 3.

[5] Ibid., 508.

[6] Two philosophers, Alberto Giubilini and Francesca Minerva, argued in the *Journal of Medical Ethics* that 'when circumstances occur "after birth" such that they would have justified abortion, what we call 'after-birth abortion' (killing a new-born) should be permissible.' See Giubilini and Minerva (2013): 261–263. Also, see Saletan 2012).

[7] The Axial Age is a term first used by the German philosopher, Karl Jaspers (d. 1969), characterizing the period from the eighth to the third century BCE. Jaspers argued that 'the spiritual foundations of humanity were laid simultaneously and independently in China, India, Persia, Judea, and Greece. These are the foundations upon which humanity still subsists today.' See Jaspers (2003), 98.

Mālikī legal school – or the Way of Medina,[8] as it was known – offers modern Muslims a definitive response rooted in the soundest Islamic methodology to a seemingly intractable problem vexing our world today.

## 6.2 Infanticide and Abortion in Pre-modern Civilizations

Arguably, the justifications proffered for infanticide approximate those proposed for abortions, although significant differences remain. A striking aspect of both infanticide and abortion, however, is their apparent historical universality. Historian Anne-Marie Kilday[9] quotes Michelle Oberman, author of *When Mothers Kill*: 'Infanticide was common among early people, particularly insofar as it enabled them to control population growth and to minimize the strain placed on society by sickly newborns.'[10] Kilday continues:

> In the main, therefore, there have been two contexts for child murder throughout history: first, the killing of what were considered to be 'defective' offspring, and, second, the killing of 'normal' but unwanted children. The exposure and/or infanticide of sickly or disabled infants was an accepted feature of ancient Greco-Roman cultures, as is evident from various contemporary literary sources such as Plato (d. *ca.* 347 BC), Aristotle (d. 322 BC), Seneca (d. 65) and Pliny (d. 79). In the city-state of Sparta, for instance, only children expected to make good soldiers or healthy citizens were allowed to survive past infancy. In Ancient Egypt, in China, India and throughout the Orient, a similar approach was adopted toward 'defective' infants.[11]

The ancient Greeks apparently had few qualms about infanticide and would leave deformed or unwanted children exposed to the elements to perish. Such a cold act of exposure was perhaps less heinous, in their minds, than the hot act of forcefully murdering the child; it was a sin of omission that mitigated the savagery of a sin of commission. In Plato's *Republic*, Socrates, in describing how the guardians will be raised, tells Glaucon:

> Then the children as they are born will be taken in charge by the officers appointed for the purpose, whether these are men or women, or both … The children of good parents, I suppose, they will put into the rearing pen, handing them over to nurses who will live apart in a particular portion of the city; but the children of inferior parents and all defective children that are born to the others they will put out of sight in secrecy and mystery, as is befitting.[12]

---

[8] Ibn Taymiyya (d. 728/1328) said, 'To clarify the Way of Medina and its preference over other schools among the various other cities is among the most important of matters when the innovations of the ignorant and those who follow opinions, whims, and heresies of the egos become widespread, and God knows best.' See Ibn Taymiyya (2006), 163.

[9] Kilday is Dean and Professor of Criminal History in the Faculty of Humanities and Social Sciences at Oxford Brookes University. Her research and teaching focus on the history of violent crime and its punishment in Britain and America.

[10] Kilday (2013), 3.

[11] Ibid.

[12] Plato (1992), 142 (Book V, sec. 460b–460c).

In the *Politics*, Aristotle echoed a similar sentiment:

> As to the exposure and rearing of children, let there be a law that no deformed child shall live, but where there are too many (for in our state population has a limit), when couples have children in excess, and the state of feeling is averse to the exposure of offspring, let abortion be procured before sense and life have begun; what may or may not be lawfully done in these cases depends on the question of life and sensation.[13]

Classics scholar Jerry Toner, using a fictitious Roman nobleman speaking of the 'occupational hazard' of getting slave girls pregnant, writes:

> I like to treat these offspring with greater indulgence than I would normal slaves, and give them slightly better rations and easier work … Obviously I cannot be expected to treat all my illegitimate offspring in such a way. So if when born they look sickly, or if I already have enough in my household, I order the mothers to expose the infants by leaving them at the dump.[14]

Merciless as those views may seem, the 'right' to kill one's children can be found in Rome's earliest recorded law code, the Law of the Twelve Tables (*Leges Duodecim Tabularum*). Table VI legislated 'that terribly deformed children shall be killed quickly.' Roman law also permitted a father to kill any new-born female.[15] Among Stoic philosophers of Rome were those who did not consider a foetus human, thereby legitimizing abortion as an acceptable personal choice. It was only Christianity's powerful influence within Roman society that would eventually radically alter these views.[16]

As the religious traditions of the Axial Age penetrated large regions of the earth, they condemned infanticide as an affront to the sanctity of life. Abrahamic religious sentiment – and religious sentiment alone – shifted the attitudes of large numbers of peoples and inspired laws to prohibit infanticide and abortion. Child sacrifice, for instance, was thought to appease Molech, the god of the Ammonites, making infanticide a common practice in Phoenicia and other surrounding countries. But Leviticus 18:21 commands the Israelites, 'Do not give any of your children to be sacrificed to Molech.'[17] Due to the enormity of child sacrifice, the Mosaic law prescribed stoning as a suitable punishment.[18]

Genesis 9:6 further states, 'Whoever sheds the blood of man, by man shall his blood be shed; for in the image of God has God made man.'[19] An alternate reading of this text renders 'whoever sheds the blood of man in man,' which some rabbis argued referred to a foetus. For example, *Tractate Sanhedrin* of the Babylonian Talmud offers a rabbinical opinion concerning abortion:

---

[13] Aristotle (2005), 1999 (Book VII, sec. 1335b).

[14] Toner (2014), 70.

[15] See Barr (1966).

[16] Gorman (1982), 32.

[17] Barker et al. (2002), 225.

[18] Ibid., 225 and 228.

[19] Ibid., 24.

> In the name of Rabbi Yishmael[20] they said: '[A Noahide receives capital punishment] even for [destroying] a foetus.' What is the reason of Rabbi Yishmael? It is the verse 'he who sheds the blood of man in man (*adam bādam*) shall his blood be shed' (Genesis 9:6). What is the meaning of 'man in man?' This can be said to refer to a foetus in its mother's womb.[21]

Josephus (d. *ca.* 100),[22] a first-century Jewish historian, wrote, 'The law orders all the offspring to be brought up, and forbids women either to cause abortion or to make away with the foetus.'[23] Jewish rabbinical tradition prohibits abortion unless the pregnancy threatens the mother's life. Undeniably, Judaism's strong stance against both infanticide and abortion informed early Christianity and the doctrine of the Church that emerged. An early Christian handbook for Church doctrine, the *Didache* (*ca.* 85–110), states, 'Thou shalt not murder a child by abortion nor kill them when born.'[24] Some biblical scholars have even argued that the absence of abortion from the New Testament can be explained by its inconceivability to early Christians. In fact, according to C. Ben Mitchell:

> Early Christians did not just condemn abortion and infanticide; Christian communities were at the forefront of providing alternatives, including adopting children who were destined to be abandoned by their parents. Callistus (d. *ca.* 223) provided refuge to abandoned children by placing them in Christian homes. Benignus of Dijon (*fl.* 3rd cent.) offered nourishment and protection to abandoned children, including some with disabilities caused by failed abortions.[25]

Strong prohibitions against infanticide and abortion also exist in Hindu and Buddhist literature. India, despite Hinduism's condemnation of abortion, currently suffers from an epidemic of female feticide and even infanticide.[26] Buddhism, much to the chagrin of Western pro-choice advocates who view the faith as meshing with a progressive ethos, clearly condemns abortion in its earliest scriptures. The *Dhammapada*, an early collection of sayings of the Buddha, states, 'Considering others as yourself, do not kill or promote killing. Whoever hurts living beings ... will not attain felicity after death.'[27] Professor of religion and Zen teacher David R. Loy writes:

> Abortion [in Buddhist tradition] is killing. According to the Pali Canon, the Buddha said that it breaks the first precept to avoid killing or harming any sentient being. Any monastic who encourages a woman to have an abortion has committed a serious offense that requires expiation ... This absolute rule in early Buddhism is a source of discomfort and embarrassment to many Western Buddhists, and is often ignored by those who are aware of it.[28]

[20] Considered one of the most prominent 'fathers of Talmudic literature,' Rabbi Yishmael was a rabbinic sage of the second century.

[21] Schiff (2002), 52.

[22] A biographer from Jerusalem, Titus Flavius Josephus was also a Roman citizen. He recorded Jewish history and studied Jewish law with the Sadducees, Pharisees, and the Essenes.

[23] Mitchell (2013), 35.

[24] Ibid., 35.

[25] Ibid., 36.

[26] See Mohanty (2012).

[27] Cleary (1995), 47.

[28] Loy (2008), 67.

Concerning the sanctity of life, including the sanctity of life within the womb, tomes from the world's religious traditions could be written, but it remains safe to say that the normative pre-modern traditions of the world's religions have universally condemned abortion and infanticide. Islam, the last of the Abrahamic faiths, is no exception, for its primary source, the Qur'an, presents its teachings as an extension of previous dispensations.

## 6.3 The Qur'anic Ban on Infanticide

The great Prophets of Judaism and Christianity find constant mention as early Messengers in the Qur'an, and God reminds the Prophet Muhammad, 'Say, "I am not an innovator among the messengers"' (Qur'an 46:9, *al-Aḥqāf*). Pre-Islamic Arabs of the Arabian Peninsula practiced infanticide but employed a different, if no less brutal, method than the Greco-Roman culture's practice of death-by-exposure: the Arabs buried their children alive. They did it usually as a form of birth control, for reasons of poverty, or else out of shame at the birth of a girl. (The killing of male infants, driven by the scarcity of sustenance in the arid desert climate, was less common, though still practiced.) Commenting on the Qur'anic verse 'Do not kill your children from poverty,' (Qur'an 6:151, *al-An'ām*), Imam al-Qurṭubī (d. 671/1273)[29] states, 'Among [the Arabs] were those who also killed both their female and male children for fear of poverty.'[30]

Several verses in the Qur'an prohibit infanticide. The sixth chapter states, 'And thus their [belief in] false gods made the killing of their children appear good and led them to destruction while confusing them about true faith. If God willed, they would not have done that; so leave them and their lies' (Qur'an 6:137, *al-An'ām*). Shortly after those verses, the Qur'an lays out what are considered by Muslim scholars to be the first principles of Abrahamic morality:

> Say: Come, I will recite to you what your Lord has forbidden you. You should not associate anything with Him; and be good to your parents, and do not kill your children on account of poverty – We provide for you and for them – and do not approach sexual indecencies, open or secret, and do not kill the soul – which God has made sacred. (Qur'an 6:151, *al-An'ām*)

Another verse addresses this topic with the subtle nuance of *fear of poverty* as opposed to the previous verse, which prohibits killing the child *on account of poverty* – in other words, an actual impoverished state. The pronouns in the above verse (*for you and for them*) emphasize that God provides for the parents first and then the children in the case of actual poverty to alleviate their fears. In the following verse,

---

[29] A jurist and a scholar of Arabic, al-Qurṭubī is best known for his book on exegesis, *al-Jāmi' li-aḥkām al-Qur'ān* (*The General Judgments of the Qur'an*), also referred to as *Tafsīr al-jāmi'* or *Tafsīr al-Qurṭubī*. His commentary remains among the most important legal commentaries of the Qur'an.

[30] Al-Qurṭubī (1993), 7:86.

the pronouns are reversed (*them and you*), for the parents are afraid the addition of new children will reduce them to poverty despite their current well-being: 'And do not kill your children *out of fear of poverty* – We provide for *them and you.* Indeed, killing them is an enormous sin. And do not approach fornication: surely it is an obscenity and leads to an evil end. And kill not the soul which God has forbidden, except for just cause' (Qur'an 17:31–33, *al-Isrā'*). Commenting on this verse, Qāḍī Ibn al-ʿArabī (d. 543/1148)[31] relates a *ḥadīth* where the Prophet said killing a child from fear of poverty was the second gravest sin next to setting up 'partners with God.' Then Ibn al-ʿArabī mentions that infanticide 'is the greatest of sins because it is an assault on the entire species,' and also because it 'involves men taking on the qualities of predatory beasts.'[32]

Similarly, another verse also prohibits infanticide and pairs it with censure of sexual deviance: 'O Prophet, when believing women come to you to pledge allegiance to you that they will not associate anything with God, and will not steal, nor commit adultery, nor kill their children, nor bring a calumny which they have forged of themselves, nor disobey what is good, then accept their pledge and ask God to pardon them, for surely God is most forgiving, most merciful' (Qur'an 60:12, *al-Mumtaḥana*).

Regarding the practice of killing female infants, the Qur'an states, 'And when news of the birth of a daughter is given to one of them, his face darkens, and he grieves within. He hides himself from the people out of distress at the news he's given. Shall he keep it, in spite of ignominy, or shall he bury it (alive) in the dust? Oh, what an evil decision they make!' (Qur'an 16:58–59, *al-Naḥl*).

The Qur'an thus unequivocally prohibits infanticide; scholars, by consensus, hold this position based upon the Qur'an, the Prophetic tradition, and the consensus of the Companions. In the history of Islam, there has never been debate about this issue.

So what of abortion in Islam? In order to address that question, it will help to examine the surprisingly numerous verses in the Qur'anic discourse on embryology and the accompanying traditions attributed to the Prophet.

## 6.4 The Birth of Humans in the Qur'an and *Ḥadīth*

Ibn ʿAbbās (d. 67/687),[33] the Prophet's Companion and cousin, stated that the passage of time will continue to explain the Qur'an. We can appreciate the wisdom of that statement when we consider the Qur'anic verses and *ḥadīth* that relate to how and when human life begins, especially in light of what today's science has discov-

---

[31] Known mainly for his writings in exegesis and law, Qāḍī Abū Bakr ibn al-ʿArabī was a preeminent Mālikī jurist from Andalusia. He was the last student of Abū Ḥāmid al-Ghazālī (d. 505/1111).

[32] Ibn al-ʿArabī (2000), 3:149.

[33] A leading scholar and jurist of Islam as well as a narrator of *ḥadīth*, Ibn ʿAbbās was the son of the Prophet's uncle, ʿAbbās (d. 32/653).

ered about the process of birth. Scripture and science, taken together, can lead believers to rethink our understanding of when life begins, of the miracle of revelation, and most certainly of abortion.

However, commentaries on such Qur'anic verses and *ḥadīth* sometimes have mistakes, primarily because of difficulties in understanding the terms used. Those are not technical terms in the modern sense, despite often carrying quite precise meanings, and they are subject to the rhetorical demand for elegant variation. Moreover, of course, the commentators of those times simply lacked our present knowledge of scientific embryology and were dependent on the highly admirable but very insufficient information and procedures found in the Aristotelian and Galenic traditions.

### *6.4.1 More than a Clot*

Arabic words are notoriously difficult to translate due to the nuances involved in the root system of Arabic that cannot be replicated in other languages. In the first verses revealed to the Prophet Muhammad, the Qur'an declares, 'Read, in the name of your Lord, who created: created man from an *ʿalaq*' (Qur'an 96:1–2, *al-ʿAlaq*). The word *ʿalaq* was traditionally understood as simply a 'blood clot.' The root *ʿaliqa*, however, means 'to become pregnant'; according to Ibn Manẓūr's (d. 711/1311)[34] *Lisān al-ʿArab*, an authoritative Arabic dictionary, *ʿalaq* also means 'the desire of spouses for one another,' due to its root meaning 'to cling to.'[35] Other meanings are 'anything attached to something, something that imbeds itself into another, such as a mountain or earth, blood of any type, or a portion of it, the cord of a bucket, any cord that holds something, a leech, a clot.'[36] The most appropriate connotation is 'something that imbeds itself into something else,' as in the imbedding of an embryo, or blastocyst, into the woman's uterine wall. Another possible meaning is a clot, as in 'a small compact group of individuals,' given the blastocyst is a collection of rapidly dividing individual cells. The classical understanding and subsequent translation of *ʿalaq* as 'blood clot' is simply wrong, though understandable given that a miscarriage often reveals congealed lumps that appear to be blood clots from the prematurely formed foetus.

Also, regarding the creation of human beings, the Qur'an clearly states, in many verses, that we originate from the earth: 'God has caused you to grow as a growth from the earth, and afterwards, He will make you return there. He will bring you forth again anew' (Qur'an 20:55, *Ṭā-Ha*). 'God created you from the earth' (Qur'an 53:32, *al-Najm*). 'God created you from clay' (Qur'an 32:7, *al-Sajda*). 'We began

[34] A jurist and a judge, Ibn Manẓūr is the author of *Lisān al-ʿArab* (*The Tongue of the Arabs*), a twenty volume Arabic dictionary.

[35] Ibn Manẓūr (1993), 2:215.

[36] Ibid., 2:215–16.

the creation of the human being (*insān*) from clay' (Qur'an 37:11, *al-Ṣāffāt*). Another verse states that man was created from water: 'He is the One who created from water man and established bonds of kinship and marriage' (Qur'an 25:54, *al-Furqān*). These verses, according to exegetes, refer to the creation of Adam, peace be upon him, from earth and water, but they equally apply to all men, as earth and water are the sole components of our physical being.

Interestingly, the Qur'an also states that man was created from a *nuṭfa*: 'God fashioned man from a *nuṭfa*' (Qur'an 16:4, *al-Naḥl*). Again, we are confronted with the problem of translation. The meanings of *nuṭfa* are 'a minute quantity of fluid,' 'a drop,' 'a tiny drop left in a container,' 'a flowing drop,' 'drop of sperm,' 'female drop [ovum].'[37] What is striking about these Qur'anic verses is the accuracy with which they describe what we now know to be the male spermatozoon and the female ovum, both of which are shaped like a drop of water. The male reproductive cell, the spermatozoon, represents one of billions in the overall sperm ejected into a woman's womb. These tiny spermatozoa, each containing a unique genetic code, race to reach the released ovum, which also contains a unique code, but only a few complete the journey, and only one or two actually penetrate the female's ovum. The *ḥadīths* regarding this reproductive process reveal strikingly accurate details that pre-modern commentators misinterpreted due to their lack of the scientific knowledge necessary to understand them properly.

For instance, according to one *ḥadīth*, a Jewish man came to the Prophet and asked a question that, according to him, only a Prophet could answer: 'From what is a man created?' The Prophet replied, 'It's determined by both [the male and the female], from the *nuṭfa* of the man and from the *nuṭfa* of a woman.'[38]

In a different narration of the same *ḥadīth*, the man asked what determines the sex. He was told, 'A man's fluid is coarse white, and a woman's is translucent yellow (*aṣfar raqīq*). When they meet, if a male sperm (*maniyy*) (y chromosome) is dominant (*ʿalā*), then it is a boy. But if the female sperm (*maniyy*) (x chromosome) is dominant, then it is a girl.' The Prophet clearly distinguishes between the ovum (female *nuṭfa*) and the spermatozoon (male *nuṭfa*) and the sperm (*maniyy*), which he described as being both male and female (x and y chromosomes that a man receives from his mother and father).

An astonishing part of this *ḥadīth* is the description of the woman's contribution to conception: *aṣfar raqīq*, a precise translation of which is 'translucent yellow.' Only recently has technology enabled us to actually photograph, in colour, the release of an ovum from the ovaries; as it emerges, it is clearly a tiny egg in the shape of a drop, and its colour, due to the cumulus oocyte complex that surrounds the ovum, is described in the literature as 'translucent yellow.'[39] In short, the *nuṭfa* in the Qur'anic verses and the above *ḥadīth* refers to both the male 'drop' of sperm and the female 'drop' of the ovum, described elsewhere in the Qur'an and the

[37] Ibn Qayyim al-Jawziyya (1989), 220.

[38] Ibid., 220.

[39] Lousse and Donnez (2008): 833–4.

*ḥadīth*[40] as the woman's 'water' and the man's 'water,' both relatively accurate terms, given that more than seventy-five percent of the material is water.[41]

## 6.4.2 What Begins Life?

Another meaning of *nuṭfa* in modern technical terminology could be 'zygote' and the subsequent embryological stages during the first nine days. A zygote is formed by a fertilization of two gametes, male and female, before cleavage occurs. On the tenth day, embryogenesis results, and the *ʿalaq* phase begins in which the newly formed life imbeds (*taʿallaq*) in the uterine wall. The proof that *nuṭfa* also means zygote and embryo is in chapter seventy-six of the Qur'an, appropriately entitled 'The Human Being' (*al-Insān*). The first two verses state, 'Hasn't there been a time when man was nothing worth mention, for We made man from a mixed drop' (Qur'an 76:1–2, *al-Insān*).

The words 'mixed drop' are a translation of *nuṭfa amshāj*, an Arabic phrase that caused much confusion among commentators because the noun *nuṭfa* is in singular form while *amshāj*, its adjective, is plural; in Arabic grammar, the adjective, in a case like this, should agree with the noun in number. Al-Zamakhsharī (d. 538/1144),[42] in his attempt to solve this vexing grammatical dilemma, goes as far as saying *amshāj* is singular despite its clear plural form. It could also be an appositive of *nuṭfa*. The point, however, is the two *nuṭfa*s of the male and the female (i.e., the spermatozoon and ovum) become one *nuṭfa* mixed (*amshāj*) with the genetic material of the two parents. Setting aside whether it is an adjective or an appositive, the word *amshāj*, according to *Lisān al-ʿArab*, can mean 'the mixing of two colors' and 'the mixing of a man's water (spermatozoon) and a woman's water (ovum), then it goes from stage to stage.'[43] In modern Arabic, *mashīj*, the singular of *amshāj*, is 'gamete.'[44] This appears to be an excellent description, given that each human cell contains twenty-three pairs of chromosomes, and each chromosome is formed by the joining of two nucleotides, which make up the strand of DNA. Scientists have color-coded the strands of nucleotides to better visualize the DNA. The model of 'joining of two colours' in each strand is now universally used in teaching about the genetic code of life. In a well-known *ḥadīth* narrated by Ibn Masʿūd (d. 32/653),[45]

[40] In the case of the *ḥadīth*, which differs in the various narrations, oral transmission allows for the real possibility of mistakes in words or substitute words that convey a similar meaning, especially given the completely novel nature of the subject to the listeners.

[41] Cooper (2000), chap. 2.

[42] A scholar in exegesis, Arabic grammar, and rhetoric, al-Zamakhsharī is known for his major work, *al-Kashshāf ʿan ḥaqāʾiq al-tanzīl* (*The Discoverer of Revealed Truths*; also known as *Tafsīr al-Zamakhsharī*).

[43] Ibn Manẓūr (1993), 2:556.

[44] Wehr (1994), 1067.

[45] One of the earliest and closest Companions of the Prophet, Ibn Masʿūd was known for his erudition and knowledge of Sharīʿa.

the Prophet begins describing the process of human creation by saying, 'Verily, the creation of one of you is brought together in the mother's womb for forty days.'[46] Commenting on this *ḥadīth*, Mullā ʿAlī al-Qārī (d. 1014/1605)[47] states, 'The material of his creation (*māddat khalqihi*) is gathered and then protected.'[48] He then explains the meaning of the 'gathering' (*jamʿ*) using a tradition from al-Ṭabarī (d. 310/923)[49] and Ibn Mandah (d. 395/1005),[50] in which the Prophet was reported to have said:

> If God desires to create a servant, He does so through the man having intercourse with the woman in which his 'water' penetrates every root and part of her ['water'] (*ʿirq wa-ʿuḍw*), and on the seventh day, He gathers it, and then produces [a new life] from every 'genetic disposition' (*ʿirq*) back to Adam. [And then the Prophet recited the verse,] 'In whatever form He wishes to assemble you from various components (*rakkabak*)' (Qur'an 82:8, *al-Infiṭār*).[51]

The word the Qur'an uses for assemble (*rakkaba*) means 'to assemble from various parts' or 'put together,' 'to make, prepare out of several components or ingredients.'[52] Mullā ʿAlī then says, 'This meaning is confirmed by the Prophet's words when a light-skinned Arab woman gave birth to a black boy and her husband accused her of infidelity. The Prophet said, "Perhaps it is from a distant root (*nazʿahu ʿirq*)."'[53] Today we would call this a recessive gene. The *ḥadīth* implies the vast genetic variations that happen with each individual spermatozoon and ovum. Each contains a unique combination (*tarkība*) that will provide an entirely new individual never before existent.

### 6.4.3 Rethinking the Stage of Ensoulment

At what stage during the creation of the human being does ensoulment occur? Clearly, the Qur'an describes each stage of growth within the womb as one we passed through as a human being: 'Surely We created the human being from a quintessence of clay, and then We made him [man] a fertilized egg (*nuṭfa*) in a safe place, and then We made him [man] a clot, and then We made the clot an embryo, and then We made the embryo bones and clothed the bones in flesh, and then We originated another creation' (Qur'an 23:12–14, *al-Muʾminūn*). Commenting on this

---

[46] Al-Qārī (2014), 1:186.

[47] Mulla ʿAlī al-Qārī was a Ḥanafī jurist who authored many books on jurisprudence.

[48] Al-Qārī (2014), 1:186.

[49] Al-Ṭabarī is known as the Imam of the scholars of exegesis, and his Qur'anic exegesis is the most relied upon commentary in the Islamic tradition.

[50] Ibn Mandah was a Ḥanbalī jurist and well-known master of *ḥadīth*.

[51] Al-Qārī (2014), 1:187.

[52] Wehr (1994), 412–13.

[53] Al-Qārī (2014), 1:186.

verse, the eminent Malaysian scholar and metaphysician Syed Naquib al-Attas writes:

> From the fusion of the two gametes God created (*khalaqa*) a new individual organism; and from this organism He created (*khalaqa*) an embryo; and from the embryo He created (*khalaqa*) a foetus. Thus we see from this that the whole process in the various stages of the emergence of the animal being into definite shape and construction complete with organs is not something natural; i.e., it is not something due to the workings of nature, but that at every stage it is God's act of creation setting the created thing in conformity with its constitution in the womb (i.e., its *fiṭra*). Then from this final foetal stage, God originated (*ansha'a*) another creature. This refers to the introduction of the spirit (*al-rūḥ*) that God breathed into the animal being after He had fashioned it in due proportion.[54]

One of the derivations of the word 'originate' (*ansha'a*) in Arabic means 'to elevate.' It is the introduction of the immaterial aeviternal soul that elevates the new creation to a spiritual human being that exists as body and soul. The partially quoted aforementioned *ḥadīth* of Ibn Masʿūd says, 'Verily, the creation of one of you is brought together in the mother's womb for forty days in the form of a drop (*nuṭfa*), then he becomes a clot (*ʿalaqa*) for a like period, then a lump for a like period, then there is sent an angel who blows the soul into him.'[55] Based on this *ḥadīth*, the majority of scholars in the past claimed ensoulment was on the 120th day after conception.

A second interpretation argued that the words 'a like period' (*mithla dhālik*) refer back to the first forty, and thus all the stages occur during a forty-day period. Another *ḥadīth* in Imam Muslim's (d. 261/875)[56] collection (*Ṣaḥīḥ Muslim*) clarifies the ambiguity of the number of days in the above *ḥadīth* by saying the angel comes at six weeks.[57] Scholars have been in agreement that the ensoulment occurs immediately after the 'lump' (*muḍgha*) phase, when the foetus takes on a human form: modern science has confirmed this occurs around six weeks; the *ḥadīth* related by both Muslim and Abū Dāwūd (d. 275/889)[58] concurs with modern science.

The argument that ensoulment occurs soon after 40 days ultimately proves far stronger than the traditional majority view that it occurs after 120 days, given what we know of embryogenesis today. The basis for 120 days, if taken from the *ḥadīth* in its standard interpretation, would mean that the *ḥadīth* contradicts today's medical views that are based upon unshakeable evidence of embryonic organogenesis, where neuronal activity and heart tones are detected by the 6th week of

---

[54] Al-Attas (2015), 33–34.

[55] *Ḥadīth* no. 4 of al-Nawawī's *Forty Ḥadīths* (*al-Arbaʿīn*), found in Ibn Ḥajar al-Haytamī (2008), 197. Considered the master of the Shāfiʿī school of jurisprudence, al-Nawawī (d. 676/1277) was a *ḥadīth* scholar, linguist, and jurist.

[56] Imam Muslim is the author of *Ṣaḥīḥ Muslim*, the second most important book of *ḥadīth* and one of the six famous works on *ḥadīth*.

[57] Muslim (2013), 8:45 (*ḥadīth* no. 2644). Editor's note: Imam Muslim's version specifies a range for the arrival of the angel from 40 to 45 nights, i.e., around six weeks.

[58] A jurist and a *ḥadīth* scholar, Abū Dāwūd authored one of the six canonical works on *ḥadīth* (*Sunan Abī Dāwūd*). Editor's note: Abū Dāwūd's version of the *ḥadīth* of Ibn Masʿūd appears in Abū Dāwūd (2009), 7:93 (*ḥadīth* no. 4708).

gestation.[59] The well-known criterion among *ḥadīth* scholars is that a *ḥadīth* cannot contradict something known by reason with proofs beyond reasonable doubt. Thus, should a *ḥadīth* contradict agreed-upon factual knowledge, scholars either reject it or, if possible, reinterpret it if the language allows for other possibilities, as can be done in this case. As mentioned earlier, one alternate view among early scholars was that the three 40-day periods are not consequential but *concurrent*; the three stages occur in the same forty days based upon the ambiguity of the phrase 'a like period.' This interpretation, which the Arabic allows for, and given the soundness of its chain, remains the most plausible one.

## 6.5 Does Human Life Begin Before Ensoulment?

In the view of Imam Mālik ibn Anas (d. 179/795)[60] and the Mālikī scholars of the Way of Medina, a child (*walad*) is created at inception, when the exchange of genetic material occurs and the requisites for the formation of a unique human being exist. Were it not so, argue the jurists of this school, the Prophet would not have made blood compensation necessary if a person caused a woman to miscarry.

The *ḥadīth* related by Ibn Mājah (d. 273/887)[61] quotes the Prophet as saying, 'A miscarried foetus will fumble about the door of paradise saying, "I won't enter until my two parents enter."'[62] Khaṭīb al-Tabrīzī (d. 741/1340)[63] relates a similar version: 'Surely the miscarried foetus will dispute with its Lord if its parents end up in Hell, and it will be said, "O miscarried one, bring your parents to paradise."'[64] When a woman from the Hudhayl tribe struck another pregnant woman from her clan, causing her to miscarry, the Prophet told the woman's agnates that blood money was owed. When one of her clan members asked, 'Do we compensate for what never ate, nor drank, nor sighed, nor cried; can such a one be said to have been killed and died,' the Prophet replied, 'Are these the rhymes of the days of ignorance? Pay the blood money of the child.'[65]

---

[59] Allan and Kramer (2010), 12–31 and 32–164.

[60] Founder of the Mālikī school of jurisprudence, Imam Mālik is from the second generation, or Follower (*tābiʿīn*). A scholar of *ḥadīth* known for his major work, *al-Muwaṭṭaʾ*. After his death, his legal opinions and teachings in jurisprudence were written down in the book *al-Mudawwana al-kubrā* (*The Great Compilation*) by one of his students.

[61] A jurist and a scholar of *ḥadīth*, Ibn Mājah authored one of the six canonical works of *ḥadīth* (*Sunan Ibn Mājah*).

[62] Ibn al-ʿArabī (1992), 2:763. The *ḥadīth* has some weakness in its chain, but it is quoted by Mālikīs as one of their proofs that abortion is prohibited from inception. Editor's note: Ibn Mājah's version of the *ḥadīth* is no. 1608.

[63] A scholar of *ḥadīth*, Khaṭīb al-Tabrīzī authored the book *Mishkāt al-maṣābīḥ* (*The Niche of Lanterns*).

[64] Ibn al-ʿArabī (1992), 2:863.

[65] Al-Shawkānī (2005), 4:603. The *ḥadīth* is related by Ibn Ḥanbal, al-Bukhārī, and Muslim. Author of the well-known *Nayl al-awṭār* (*The Obtainment of the Objectives*), al-Shawkānī (d. 1250/1834) was one of the top scholars of Yemen in the twelfth and thirteenth century AH (eighteenth and nineteenth century CE).

The Mālikī scholars point out that the Prophet's ruling was not based on the stage of the pregnancy. They argue that the embryo is considered a child even at the earliest stages of pregnancy, and blood money would be owed. Moreover, the Prophet called the miscarried foetus 'a child' (*ṣabiyy*), and so the matter falls under the prohibition of the Qur'anic verses that prohibit killing children. Ibn Abī Zayd al-Qayrawānī (d. 386/996),[66] an authoritative voice in the Mālikī school and in the Islamic tradition, writes:

> Mālik says, 'If a pregnant woman is struck, causing her to lose her child, whether still in lump phase (*muḍgha*) or even an imbedded embryo (*'alaqa*), and nothing is discernible from its creation – neither eye nor finger nor anything else – if the women who know about such things determine that it was a child [i.e., that she was actually pregnant], then financial compensation is owed…' Ibn Shihāb (d. 124/742) said, 'Whether the foetus was formed or not [money is owed]. If there were twins or triplets, each demands compensation.'[67]

Imam al-Rajrājī (d. 633/1236),[68] in his commentary on Imam Mālik's position on abortion, also concurs, and adds that a foetus at any stage is considered a child.[69]

The term the Qur'an uses for a life within the womb is *janīn*, which means what is hidden from the eye or concealed; the greater the concealment, the more applicable the name. Thus, a zygote, embryo, blastocyst, and foetus are all called *janīn* in Arabic. Rāghib al-Iṣfahānī (d. 502/1108)[70] defines the *janīn* as 'a child (*walad*) as long as it is in the womb of its mother.'[71] Other Qur'anic verses affirm that God considers all stages of foetal development to be a human life: 'Does the human being think he'll be left for naught? Was he not an embryo from male and female fluid released?' (Qur'an 75:36–37, *al-Qiyāma*).[72] The verse could have said, 'Was he not created from an embryo,' but instead it states unambiguously, 'Was he not an embryo.' Another verse states, 'Surely We created the human being from a quintessence of clay, and then We made him into an embryo in a safe place' (Qur'an 23:12–13, *al-Mu'minūn*). Again, it says clearly that 'We made him into an embryo.' The Qur'anic narrative ineluctably defines our creation at each stage of our individual journeys within our respective wombs as a unique human being.

---

[66] Ibn Abī Zayd al-Qayrawānī is one of the most authoritative voices in the Mālikī school.

[67] Ibn Abī Zayd al-Qayrawānī (1999), 13:464.

[68] A jurist and scholar of *ḥadīth*, Abū al-Ḥasan 'Alī ibn Sa'īd al-Rajrājī wrote a seminal commentary on the Mālikī school's most important resource of Mālik's opinions, *al-Mudawwana*.

[69] Al-Rajrājī (2007), 10:222.

[70] A Persian scholar based in Baghdad, Rāghib al-Iṣfahānī was known for influencing his younger contemporary, Imam Abū Ḥāmid al-Ghazālī. His works on ethics, Qur'anic vocabulary, and Arabic literature are widely referenced.

[71] Rāghib al-Iṣfahānī (2014), 106.

[72] The Qur'an has ten variant recensions that contain different readings. Each is considered valid and transmitted by the Prophet to his Companions. They offer subtle nuances in meaning. In this verse, two readings, Nāfi' and 'Āsim, differ. One uses the masculine *yumnā*, and the other uses the feminine *tumnā*. This indicates that both the male and the female are releasing their respective *nuṭfa*s, which will commingle and become the *nuṭfa amshāj*. This appears to be a clear miracle of the Qur'an.

The ensoulment most likely relates to and initiates human brain activity that will eventually develop into the capacity for human thought, which, according to traditional Islamic metaphysics, is immaterial by nature and only occurs through the vehicle of, but is not synonymous with, the brain – hence, our distinction in English between mind and brain, and in Arabic between *ʿaql* and *dimāgh*. Michael Gazzaniga,[73] a leading researcher in cognitive neuroscience, writes that from the time of fertilization of the human sperm and egg, 'the embryo begins its mission: divide and differentiate.' Within hours, it develops layers of cells that then become the endoderm, mesoderm, and ectoderm, the layers that will give rise to every organ in the human body. Within weeks, the neural tube of the embryo spawns the central nervous system, the ventricles of the brain, and the central canal of the spinal cord. By the fourth week, he explains, the neural tube develops bulges that become the major divisions of the brain. He continues, 'Even though the foetus is now developing areas that will become specific sections of the brain, not until the end of week 5 and into week 6 (usually around 40–43 days) does the first electrical brain activity begin to occur.'[74]

This description of the development of the brain, and the timing of the start of brain activity, correspond quite precisely to the Prophetic tradition of ensoulment within six weeks. Still, the infusion of the soul (*nafkh al-rūḥ*), its nature, and its exact time remain a mystery. In Imam Muslim's collection, in a chapter entitled 'The Jew's Question to the Prophet about the Soul (*rūḥ*),' the Prophet was asked by a Jew about the nature of the soul. The Prophet was silent, and the narrator said, 'I knew something was being revealed to him.' When the revelation came, the Prophet replied from the Qur'an, 'They ask you about the soul. Say, "The soul is from the command of my Lord; and you are given but a little knowledge"' (Qur'an 17:85, *al-Isrāʾ*).[75]

## 6.6 Conclusion

The position of the scholars of the Way of Medina, that the foetus in all its stages is a living child, continues down to the present day without any dissenting voices. Qāḍī Ibn al-ʿArabī, a formidable Mālikī *mujtahid* (one who is capable of independent juridical reasoning, or *ijtihād*), says in his commentary of Mālik's *Muwaṭṭaʾ* (*The Well-Trodden Path*):

> Three states exist concerning child-bearing: the state before conception when *coitus interruptus* is used to prevent pregnancy, and that is permissible; the second state occurs once semen has been received by the womb, at which point it is impermissible for anyone to attempt to sever the process of procreation as is done by some of the contemptible mer-

[73] Gazzaniga is a distinguished Professor of Psychology at the University of California, Santa Barbara.

[74] Gazzaniga (2005), 4–5.

[75] Muslim (2013), 8:128 (*ḥadīth* no. 2794).

> chants who sell abortifacients to servant girls when their periods stop; the third situation is after the formation of the foetus and the ensoulment, and this third state is even more severe than the first two in its proscription and prohibition.[76]

This view is affirmed by other Mālikī scholars, with some minor dissensions. For instance, Qāḍī ʿIyāḍ (d. 544/1149)[77] says, 'Some opined that the embryo has no sanctity for the first forty days nor the legal stature of a child (*walad*); others argued that it is not permissible to disrupt conception or cause an abortion once conception has occurred in any way whatsoever! However, *coitus interruptus* differs in that it has not reached the womb.'[78] Most Mālikī scholars clearly believed in the sanctity of life from inception onward. Al-Kharashī (d. 1101/1690)[79] says, 'It is not permissible for a woman to do anything that would lead to an abortion causing the foetus to miscarry, nor is it permissible for the husband to do so, even if it is before forty days.'[80] Ibn Juzayy al-Kalbī (d. 741/1340)[81] says, 'If the womb receives the sperm, it is not permissible to attempt to thwart [conception] or harm it. Even worse involves an attempt once conception occurs, or worse yet after ensoulment, which, by consensus, is murder.'[82] Finally, in the authoritative collection of legal responsa of the Mālikī school, al-Wansharīsī (d. 914/1508)[83] writes, 'Our imams have prohibited using any drugs that cause infertility or that remove semen from the womb; this is the opinion of the masters and experts.'[84] Then, after quoting the statement above from *al-Qabas* (*The Firebrand*) of Qāḍī Ibn al-ʿArabī, he continues:

> If you have contemplated the conclusion of what was presented from the master jurist Qāḍī Abū Bakr [ibn al-ʿArabī], you should realize without any doubt that an agreement between the husband and the wife to abort their child or any attempt to do that is absolutely prohibited – forbidden! It is not permitted from any perspective. And if the mother should do so, she owes blood money and should be punished according to the discretion of the judge … Along the same lines, ʿIzz al-Dīn ibn ʿAbd al-Salām [d. 660/1262][85] was asked, 'Is it permissible to give a woman drugs that would prevent pregnancy?' He replied, 'It is not permitted for a woman to use medicine that would eliminate her capacity to become pregnant.'[86]

The references to induced abortion in early Islam are scarce and generally occur in books of jurisprudence, in sections on blood compensation (*diya*), which

---

[76] Ibn al-ʿArabī (1992), 2:763.

[77] A *ḥadīth* scholar from Morocco, Qāḍī ʿIyāḍ was a Mālikī jurist and a judge.

[78] ʿIyāḍ (1998), 8:127.

[79] A Mālikī jurist and Azharī scholar, al-Kharashī authored commentaries on Mālikī jurisprudence.

[80] Al-Kharashī (n.d.), 3:225.

[81] Ibn Juzayy al-Kalbī was a linguist, an exegete, Mālikī jurist, and formidable scholar of *uṣūl al-fiqh*.

[82] Ibn Juzayy al-Kalbī (1977), 141.

[83] Aḥmad al-Wansharīsī was a Mālikī jurist who compiled the most important work on legal responsa from the Mālikī school.

[84] Al-Wansharīsī (1981–1983), 3:370.

[85] Known as 'the Sultan of Scholars,' Ibn ʿAbd al-Salām was a leading Shāfiʿī scholar.

[86] Al-Wansharīsī (1981–1983), 3:370.

examine situations where someone caused a woman to lose her child. The permissibility of abortion was inconceivable to early Muslims even though abortifacients were readily available.

The Persian polymath Avicenna (Ar. Ibn Sīnā; d. 428/1037)[87] records more than forty abortifacients in his magisterial medical compendium *al-Qānūn fī al-ṭibb* (*The Canon of Medicine*). In the only section dealing with abortion entitled 'On Situations Requiring an Abortion,' he writes: 'There may be a situation in which you need to abort a foetus from the uterus in order to save the mother's life.'[88] He lists three conditions where a pregnancy threatens a woman's life and then lists several ways to induce an abortion in cases where those conditions exist. He gives no other reasons for aborting a foetus.[89]

The sole exception among Mālikī scholars regarding abortions was al-Lakhmī (d. 478/1085),[90] who permitted abortion of an 'embryo' (*nuṭfa*) before forty days. Arguably, he would recant his position if he knew what we know today about foetal development. Nevertheless, his position was never taken up for serious discussion by any Mālikī scholar and remains a mere mention as a sole dissenting voice in books of legal responsa.

Far too often today, the positions favouring the permissibility of abortions in other schools of jurisprudence are presented in articles and *fatwās* without the nuance that one finds in the original texts. This results from either disingenuousness or shoddy scholarship. For instance, Imam al-Ramlī (d. 1004/1596),[91] held in high esteem in the Shāfiʿī school, is invariably quoted as permitting abortion, but he clearly qualifies his position. He states, for instance, 'If the embryo results from fornication, [abortion's] permissibility could be conceivable (*yutakhayyal*) before ensoulment.'[92] He also believed that the stages of *nuṭfa*, *ʿalaqa*, and *muḍgha*, occurred during the first 120 days, but we now know they occur in the first 40 days; the question remains whether he would alter his position had he known this. Mistakenly, he also claims that al-Ghazālī (d. 505/1111),[93] perhaps the most important legal philosopher in the history of Islam, did not categorically prohibit abortion. In *The Revival of Religious Sciences*, al-Ghazālī discusses various positions of scholars on birth control and then states:

---

[87] A philosopher and a physician, Avicenna was known as the father of medicine in the Middle Ages. His book on medicine was used as a textbook in Europe until the seventeenth century.

[88] Avicenna (2014), 3:1262.

[89] Ibid., 3:1262.

[90] Al-Lakhmī, a formidable Mālikī jurist, was also knowledgeable in *ḥadīth* and Arabic literature.

[91] A late Shāfiʿī scholar, al-Ramlī is invariably quoted as permitting abortion, and along with Ibn ʿĀbidīn (d. 1252/1836) from the Ḥanafī school, he is the most quoted authority on abortion's permissibility. Nevertheless, a close reading of al-Ramlī's words leaves more doubt than certainty about the matter.

[92] Al-Ramlī (2003), 8:442.

[93] One of the most learned scholars of Islam and considered a renewer of the faith, Abū Ḥāmid al-Ghazālī was a theologian, philosopher, mystic, and Shāfiʿī jurist. His most famous work is the *Iḥyāʾ ʿulūm al-dīn* (*The Revival of Religious Sciences*).

> It should not be viewed like abortion or infanticide, because that involves a crime against something that already exists, although the creative process has degrees: the first degree of existence is the male sperm reaching the female egg in preparation for the beginning of life. To disrupt that is criminal (*jināya*). If it becomes a clot or a lump, the crime is even more heinous. And should ensoulment occur and the form completed, the crime is even more enormous; the most extreme crime, however, is to kill it once it has come out alive.[94]

Clearly in this passage, al-Ghazālī prohibits abortion, in no uncertain terms, during each stage of foetal development but opined that as the foetus developed within the womb, the severity of the crime increased by degrees. Even regarding *coitus interruptus*, according to a sound tradition from *Ṣaḥīḥ Muslim*, the Prophet stated, 'That is a hidden type of infanticide (*al-wa'd al-khafiyy*).'[95] Scholars interpret that to mean it is disliked, but the Prophet's strong language concerning birth control by likening it to a hidden form of infanticide indicates that aborting a foetus would surely be considered infanticide. And this is the position of the jurist Ibn Taymiyya (d. 728/1328),[96] who asserts that abortion is prohibited by consensus: 'To abort a pregnancy is prohibited (*ḥarām*) by consensus (*ijmā'*) of all the Muslims. It is a type of infanticide about which God said, "And when the buried alive is asked for what sin was she killed," (Qur'an 81:8, *al-Takwīr*) and God says, "Do not kill your children out of fear of poverty" (Qur'an 17:31, *al-Isrā'*).'[97]

The overwhelming majority of Muslim scholars have prohibited abortion unless the mother's life is at stake, in which case they all permitted it if the danger was imminent with some difference of opinion if the threat to the mother's life was only probable. A handful of later scholars permitted abortion without that condition; however, each voiced severe reservations. Moreover, none of them achieved the level of independent jurist (*mujtahid*). To present their opinions on this subject as representative of the normative Islamic ruling on abortion is a clear misrepresentation of the tradition. Those scholars permitted abortion only prior to ensoulment, which they thought occurred either within 40 days or 120 days. Further, these opinions were based on misinformation about embryology and a failure to understand the nuances of the Qur'anic verses and *ḥadīths* relating to embryogenesis. Modern genetics shows that the blueprint for the entire human being is fully present at inception, and thus we must conclude once the spermatozoon penetrates the ovum, the miracle of life clearly begins. Ensoulment occurs after the physical or animal life has begun. Given that at least twenty percent of fertilized eggs spontaneously abort in the first six weeks after inception,[98] the immaterial aspect of the human being,

---

[94] Al-Ghazālī (2010), 2:385–86.

[95] Muslim (2013), 4:161 (*ḥadīth* no. 141).

[96] The author of nearly three hundred works, Ibn Taymiyya was a theologian and a logician who was also highly regarded for his legal opinions.

[97] Ibn Taymiyya (1961–1967), 34:160.

[98] Jarvis (2017).

referred to as 'ensoulment' (*nafkh al-rūḥ*), would logically occur after that precarious period for the fertilized egg at around forty-two days; but God knows best.[99]

Abortions, especially those performed after forty days of foetal development, also violate a different teaching of the Islamic tradition: the prohibition of mutilation. A six-week-old foetus clearly has the form of a child, with budding arms and legs, a head, the beginning of eyes and ears. Imagery of actual abortions performed is pervasive in its depictions of ripped arms and legs from the bodies of foetuses. Ibn ʿAbd al-Barr (d. 463/1071)[100] said, 'There is no disagreement on the prohibition of mutilation.'[101]

The Qur'an states that God created us 'in stages' (Qur'an 71:14, *Nūḥ*). Each of these stages – the zygote, the embryo, the clot of cells, the lump formed and unformed, and finally the growing foetus – is a stage every human being experiences. The Prophet said, 'God says, "I derived the womb (*raḥim*) from My own Name, the Merciful (*al-Raḥmān*), so whoever severs the womb bond, I will sever him from My mercy."'[102] What constitutes a greater severance of the womb bond than aborting a foetus bonded to the womb? The act of abortion surely 'severs the womb bond,' and the womb is a place the Qur'an calls 'a protected space' (Qur'an 23:13, *al-Muʾminūn*), meaning God is its protector. Any act of aggression on that sacred space aggresses on a place made sacred by the Creator of life itself.

The Arabic word for 'womb' (*raḥim*) has an etymological relation to the word for 'sanctity' (*ḥurma*) in what Arabic linguists call 'the greater derivation.' The womb has a divine sanctity. God created it as the sacred space where the greatest creative act of the divine occurs: the creation of a sentient and sapiential being with the potential to know the divine. The miraculous inevitability of a fertilized egg occurs only by the providential care of its Creator. Each forebear – from the two parents to their four grandparents to their eight, exponentially back to a point where they eventually invert back to only two people – had to survive wars, famines, childhood sicknesses, natural disasters, accidents, and every other obstacle to the miracle that stands as the myriad number of people alive today. We are each a part of an unbroken chain back to the first parents.

Extreme poverty and the desire for independence from children in a world that has devalued motherhood through intense individualistic social pressures related to meritocracy, psychology, and even the misuse of praiseworthy gender egalitarianism are the primary reasons people in the West today choose abortions. No doubt, many women are genuinely challenged and feel inadequate and unprepared as mothers. The largest demographic among the poor in America remains single

[99] See elsewhere in this book for a neuroscientific argument of the 'ensoulment' as 'primary self-awareness' in Chap. 7, 'Where the Two Oceans Meet: The Theology of Islam and the Philosophy of Psychiatric Medicine in Exploring the Human Self,' by Asim Yusuf and Afifi al-Akiti.

[100] Ibn ʿAbd al-Barr is arguably the greatest *ḥadīth* scholar of Andalusia and a recognized master of Mālikī jurisprudence.

[101] Al-Būṣī (1999), 2:1036.

[102] Al-Tirmidhī (1937–1965), 4:315 (*ḥadīth* no. 1907).

mothers.[103] Abortions motivated by knowing, through the miracle of ultrasound technology, that the offspring will be female, as is the case in China and India, can be seen as an 'advanced' form of the infanticide that was practiced in ancient times after birth. Arguably, if the pre-Islamic Arabs had possessed ultrasound and modern methods of abortion, they would not have waited for the female child to come to term; rather, they would have aborted the infant in the early stages of pregnancy. Genetic testing can also now predict (not always reliably) any number of serious disabilities a child may be born with. Absent any religious injunctions on the sanctity of life, abortion is arguably a 'valid' way of dealing with unwanted pregnancies and overpopulation, not to mention the promotion of eugenics.

When the angels inquired as to why God would place in the earth 'those who shed blood and sow corruption,' God replied, 'I know what you do not' (Qur'an 2:30, *al-Baqara*). God knew there would be righteous people who would refuse to shed blood. Abortions are noted for the blood that flows during and after them. For anyone who believes in a merciful Creator who created the human being with purpose and providence, abortion, with rare exception, must be seen for what it is: an assault on a sanctified life, in a sacred space, by a profane hand.

## References

Abū Dāwūd Sulaymān ibn al-Ashʿath. 2009. *Sunan Abī Dāwūd*, eds. Shuʿayb al-Arnaʾūṭ, Muḥammad Kāmil Qarah Balilī, and ʿAbd al-Laṭīf Ḥirz Allāh. 7 vols. Beirut: Dār al-Risāla al-ʿĀlamiyya.

Allan, John, and Beverley Kramer. 2010. *Fundamentals of Human Embryology: Student Manual*. 2nd ed. Johannesburg: Wits University Press.

Aristotle. 2005. *Politics: Book VII*, trans. Benjamin Jowett. New York, NY: Barnes and Noble.

al-Attas, Syed Naquib. 2015. *On Justice and the Nature of Man*. Kuala Lumpur: IBFIM.

Avicenna. 2014. *The Canon of Medicine*, trans. Laleh Bakhtiar, O. Cameron Gruner, and Mazar H. Shah. 5 vols. Chicago, IL: Kazi Publications.

Barker, Kenneth L., et al., eds. 2002. *New International Version Study Bible*. Grand Rapids, MI: Zondervan.

Barnhart, Robert K., et al., eds. 1988. *Chambers Dictionary of Etymology*. New York, NY: H. W. Wilson.

Barr, Stringfellow. 1966. *The Mask of Jove: A History of Graeco-Roman Civilization from the Death of Alexander to the Death of Constantine*. Philadelphia, PA: Lippincott.

al-Būṣī, ʿAbd Allāh ibn Mubārak. 1999. *Ijmāʿāt Ibn ʿAbd al-Barr fī al-ʿibādāt: Jamʿan wa-dirāsa*. 2 vols. Riyadh: Dār Ṭayba.

Cleary, Thomas F. 1995. *Dhammapada: The Sayings of Buddha, Translated from the Original Pali*. New York, NY: Bantam Books.

Cooper, Geoffrey M. 2000. *The Cell: A Molecular Approach*. 2nd ed. Sunderland, MA: Sinauer Associates.

Gazzaniga, Michael S. 2005. *The Ethical Brain: The Science of Our Moral Dilemmas*. New York, NY: Harper Perennial.

[103] Semega et al. (2020), 3.

al-Ghazālī. 2010. *Iḥyā' 'ulūm al-dīn*, eds. 'Alī Muḥammad Muṣṭafá and Sa'īd al-Maḥāsinī. 6 vols. Damascus: Dār al-Fayḥā'.
Giubilini, Alberto, and Francesca Minerva. 2013. 'After-Birth Abortion: Why Should the Baby Live?' *Journal of Medical Ethics* 39 (5): 261–263.
Gorman, Michael J. 1982. *Abortion and the Early Church: Christian, Jewish and Pagan Attitudes in the Greco-Roman World*. Downers Grove, IL: InterVarsity Press.
Guttmacher Institute. 2020. 'Unintended Pregnancy and Abortion Worldwide: Fact Sheet.' Available at www.guttmacher.org/fact-sheet/induced-abortion-worldwide.
Herbermann, Charles G., et al., eds. 1907. *The Catholic Encyclopedia: An International Work of Reference on the Constitution, Doctrine, Discipline, and History of the Catholic Church*. 17 vols. New York, NY: Robert Appleton.
Ibn Abī Zayd al-Qayrawānī. 1999. *al-Nawādir wa-al-ziyādāt*, ed. 'Abd al-Fattāḥ Muḥammad al-Ḥulw. 15 vols. Beirut: Dār al-Gharb al-Islāmī.
Ibn al-'Arabī, Qāḍī Abū Bakr. 2000. *Aḥkām al-Qur'ān*. 4 vols. Beirut: Dār al-Kitāb al-'Arabī.
———. 1992. *al-Qabas fī sharḥ Muwaṭṭa' Mālik ibn Anas*, ed. Muḥammad 'Abd Allāh Wild Karīm. 3 vols. Beirut: Dār al-Gharb al-Islāmī.
Ibn Ḥajar al-Haytamī. 2008. *al-Fatḥ al-mubīn bi sharḥ al-arba'īn*, eds. Aḥmad Jāsim Muḥammad, Quṣayy Muḥammad Nawras Ḥallāq, and Abū Ḥamzah Anwar ibn Abī Bakr al-Shaykhī al-Dāghistānī. Beirut: Dār al-Minhāj.
Ibn Juzayy al-Kalbī. 1977. *al-Qawānīn al-fiqhiyya*. Beirut: Dār al-Qalam.
Ibn Manẓūr. 1993. *Lisān al-'Arab*, 18 vols. Beirut: Dār al-Kutub al-'Ilmiyya.
Ibn Qayyim al-Jawziyya. 1989. *Tuḥfat al-mawdūd bi-aḥkām al-mawlūd*, ed. Bassām 'Abd al-Wahhāb al-Jābī. Cyprus: Dār al-Bashā'ir al-Islāmiyya.
Ibn Taymiyya. 1961–1967. *Majmū'āt al-fatāwā*, ed. 'Abd al-Raḥmān ibn Muḥammad ibn Qāsim. 37 vols. Riyadh: Maṭābi' al-Riyāḍ.
———. 2006. *Tafḍīl madhhab al-Imām Mālik wa-ahl al-Madīna*, ed. Aḥmad Muṣṭafá Qasim al-Ṭaḥṭāwī. Cairo: Dār al-Faḍīla.
'Iyāḍ, Qāḍī. 1998. *Ikmāl al-mu'lim bi-fawā'id Muslim*, ed. Yaḥyá Ismā'īl. 9 vols. Mansoura: Dār al-Wafā'.
Jarvis, Gavin E. 2017. 'Early Embryo Mortality in Natural Human Reproduction: What the Data Say.' *F1000 Research* 5:2765.
Jaspers, Karl. 2003. *The Way to Wisdom: An Introduction to Philosophy*, trans. Ralph Manheim. 2nd ed. New Haven, CT: Yale Univerity Press.
al-Kharashī. n.d. *Sharḥ Mukhtaṣar Khalīl*. 8 vols in 4. Beirut: Dār al-Fikr.
Kilday, Anne-Marie. 2013. *A History of Infanticide in Britain: c. 1600 to the Present*. New York, NY: Palgrave.
Lousse, Jean-Christophe, and Jacques Donnez. 2008. 'Images in Reproductive Medicine: Laparoscopic Observation of Spontaneous Human Ovulation.' *Fertility and Sterility* 90 (3): 833–4.
Loy, David R. 2008. *Money, Sex, War, Karma: Notes for a Buddhist Revolution*. Boston, MA: Wisdom Publications.
Mitchell, C. Ben. 2013. *Ethics and Moral Reasoning: A Student's Guide*. Wheaton, IL: Crossway.
Mohanty, Ranjani Iyer. 25 May 2012. 'Trash Bin Babies: India's Female Infanticide Crisis.' *The Atlantic*. Available at www.theatlantic.com/international/archive/2012/05/trash-bin-babies-indiasfemale-infanticide-crisis/257672/.
Muslim ibn al-Ḥajjāj. 2013. *Ṣaḥīḥ Muslim*, ed. Muḥammad Zuhayr Nāṣir al-Nāṣir. 8 vols. Jeddah: Dār al-Minhāj.
Plato. 1992. *Republic*. New York: Everyman's Library.
al-Qārī, Mulla 'Alī. 2014. *al-Mubīn al-mu'īn*, ed. Sulaymān ibn 'Abd Allāh ibn Ḥammūd Abā al-Khayl. 2 vols. Riyadh: Dār al-'Āṣima.
al-Qurṭubī. 1993. *al-Jāmi' li-aḥkām al-Qur'ān*, ed. Sālim Muṣṭafā al-Badrī. 21 vols. Beirut: Dār al-Kutub al-'Ilmiyya.
Rāghib al-Iṣfahānī. 2014. *al-Mufradāt fī gharīb al-Qur'ān*. 7th ed. Beirut: Dār al-Ma'rifa.

al-Rajrājī, Abū al-Ḥasan. 2007. *Manāhij al-taḥṣīl fī sharḥ al-Mudawwana*, eds. Abū al-Faḍl al-Dimyāṭī and Aḥmad ibn ʿAlī. 10 vols. Beirut: Dār Ibn Ḥazm.

al-Ramlī, Shams al-Dīn. 2003. *Nihāyat al-muḥtāj ilā sharḥ al-Minhāj*. 3rd ed. 8 vols. Beirut: Dār al-Kutub al-ʿIlmiyya.

Saletan, William. 12 March 2012. 'After-Birth Abortion: The Pro-Choice Case for Infanticide.' *Slate*. Available at slate.com/articles/health_and_science/human_nature/2012/03.

Schiff, Daniel. 2002. *Abortion in Judaism*. Cambridge: Cambridge University Press.

Semega, Jessica, Melissa Kollar, Emily A. Shrider, and John F. Creamer. 2020. *Income and Poverty in the United States: 2019*. Washington, DC: US Government Publishing Office. Washington, DC, 2020.

al-Shawkānī. 2005. *Nayl al-awṭār min asrār Muntaqá al-akhbār*, eds. Aḥmad Muḥammad al-Sayyid, Maḥmūd Ibrāhīm Bazzāl, and Muḥammad Adīb al-Mawṣililī. 5 vols. Beirut: Dār al-Kalim al-Ṭayyib.

Thompson, Della, ed. 1996. *Oxford Modern English Dictionary*. 2nd ed. New York, NY: Oxford University Press.

al-Tirmidhī. 1937–1965. *Jāmiʿ al-Tirmidhī*, ed. Aḥmad Muḥammad Shākir. 5 vols. Cairo: Maṭbaʿat Muṣṭafā al-Bābī al-Ḥalabī.

Toner, Jerry P. 2014. *The Roman Guide to Slave Management: A Treatise by Nobleman Marcus Sidonious Falx*. New York, NY: The Overlook Press.

Yusuf, Hamza. 2018. 'When Does a Human Foetus Become Human?' *Renovatio: The Journal of Zaytuna College*. Available at https://renovatio.zaytuna.edu/article/when-does-a-human-fetus-become-human.

al-Wansharīsī. 1981–1983. *al-Miʿyār al-muʿrab wa-al-jāmiʿ al-mughrib ʿan fatāwá ahl Ifrīqīyah wa-al-Andalus wa-al-Maghrib*, ed. Muḥammad Ḥajjī. 13 vols. Beirut: Dār al-Gharb al-Islāmī.

Wehr, Hans. 1994. *Arabic-English Dictionary*, ed. J. Milton Cowan. 4th ed. Urbana, IL: Spoken Language Services.

**Dr Hamza Yusuf** is a leading proponent of classical learning in Islam. He is President of Zaytuna College and has taught courses on Islamic jurisprudence, ethics, astronomy, logic, theology, Prophetic biography, and *ḥadīth*, as well as other subjects. He has published numerous articles and translations, including *The Prayer of the Oppressed* and *Purification of the Heart*. He also serves as Vice President for the Forum for Promoting Peace in Muslim Societies, an international initiative that seeks to address the root causes that can lead to radicalism and militancy. He is listed in *The Muslim 500: The World's 500 Most Influential Muslims*.

# Chapter 7
# Where the Two Oceans Meet: The Theology of Islam and the Philosophy of Psychiatric Medicine in Exploring the Human Self

**Asim Yusuf and Afifi al-Akiti**

## 7.1 Introduction

At the nexus of metaphysics, psychology, health and ethics lies the same central conundrum: what is the human? In all of clinical practice, it is perhaps the concept of a 'mental illness' – the stock-in-trade of psychiatry and psychology – that raises this fundamental question most acutely. In the respective fields, this breaks down into a number of related questions.

- What is an illness? Is it possible to clearly define the border between the presence and absence of health? If so, what scales of measurement should be used to determine it: tissue damage, functional effectiveness or fulfilment of purpose?
- What is the 'mind' that psychiatrists and psychologists aim to heal and study? Is it merely an aspect of the brain – an illusory projection of a hundred trillion neural connections working in tandem – and thus reducible to the firing of neurons and chemical transmission across synaptic spaces? If so, is a highly complex concept like 'guilt' – the fuel of many a depression – reducible to mere physics and chemistry? Or is the 'person' something greater – a 'soul' that supervenes the body? If so, how precisely does it interact so intrinsically with the physical body, and is it possible to locate it either in brain or heart? And must these two perspectives be necessarily mutually exclusive, or can they be reconciled?

Questions such as these entail that the entire practice of medicine, especially in its sub-specialty of psychiatry, returns ultimately to critical philosophical concepts: personhood and identity, the origin, function and purpose of the human organism,

A. Yusuf (✉)
Royal College of Psychiatrists, British Board of Scholars and Imams, London, UK
e-mail: asimyusuf@nhs.net

A. al-Akiti
Oxford Centre for Islamic Studies, Oxford, UK
e-mail: afifi.al-akiti@worc.ox.ac.uk


A. al-Akiti, A. I. Padela (eds.), *Islam and Biomedicine*, Philosophy and Medicine 137, https://doi.org/10.1007/978-3-030-53801-9_7

and its place in the greater scheme of reality. It is also at this point that medicine tends to find itself at a loss. As a fully-fledged science, which the medical model has been throughout the twentieth century, it is – at minimum – epistemically reductionist in its approach, if not necessarily ontologically so. As such, it suffers from all the problems which beset scientific reductionism. This will be explored further on in the chapter in slightly more detail, though it bears noting that, across science as a whole, the great reductionist thesis – that all complex entities are ultimately reducible to more fundamental levels in nature – has experienced a number of significant set-backs.[1]

As such, given that these concepts – personhood, origin and purpose – are also the central themes of religious endeavour, it might be worthwhile exploring the answers that the great religions have provided. In answer to the obvious question – what does religion hope to offer that science cannot provide – one might argue that a holistic approach sometimes affords answers that a reductionist approach cannot.[2]

Indeed, this is the approach taken in this chapter. Sometimes, understanding requires a view of the whole picture; one needs to stand back, not squint ever yet closer. Medicine seeks to understand the integrative human from intracellular chemistry upwards, in order to sustain and preserve biological life. Religion seeks to understand the integrative human from Ultimate Reality (*al-Ḥaqq*) down, in order to sustain and preserve a greater life.

Equally, it may well be that, as has happened throughout Islamic history, the insights provided by the worldly sciences (*ʿulūm dunyawiyya*)[3] illuminate aspects of religious understanding about the nature of the human – if not her place in the scheme of reality – that were previously hidden in darkness. A good example of this was the incorporation of Hellenistic philosophy to provide a cosmological framework for the understanding of various aspects of scripture. Indeed, the Prophet Muhammad said, 'many of those who transmit understanding will do so to those who understand it better than they.'[4]

Enrichment works both ways.[5] Where the two oceans meet, one need not find an impassable barrier, nor a tempest of opposition, but perhaps a mingling of the waters

[1] Koperski (2015), 228–232. These range from the level of quantum mechanics in physics, through the apparent irreducibility of organic chemistry, to the irreducibility of phenotype to genotype in biology.

[2] It should also be noted at the outset that 'medicine' in this chapter refers to modern allopathic (or conventional) medicine. There are of course other theories of medicine, such as Chinese, Indian or Galenic traditional medicines which are far more holistic in their approach, but they will not be considered for the purposes of this chapter.

[3] Here 'worldly' entails both the Ghazālian meaning 'that which does not have an explicitly scriptural or revelatory basis' [al-Ghazālī (2011), 1:62], as well as the more common-place 'that which is concerned primarily with explaining observable phenomena on the basis of demonstrable laws.'

[4] Related by Abū Dāwūd (2009), 5:501 (*ḥadīth* no. 3660).

[5] A useful approach to this is the 'X' model: that is to say, each of the two fields (religion and science) have a view of the human in terms of origin, functioning and purpose, which are clearly distinct from one another. However, rather than being parallel approaches (II) with no point of conjunction, they instead cross over one another (X). Their very different ideas about origin (the 'past') and purpose (the 'future') of the human entity cross over each other at the point of human subjective experience (the 'present'). It is at these 'interfaces' that cross-fertilization of ideas and understanding is possible.

to the betterment of both. As God says in the Qur'an, 'soon shall we show them Our signs on the farthest horizons, and within their very selves, that it might become clear to them that this is the truth.'[6]

As with many scientific fields, the fundamental underlying assumptions of medicine almost invariably go unspoken and therefore largely unrecognized. Systems such as these tend to be rigorously internally coherent, and thus give the appearance of being totalizing explanations. However, despite appearances – and some clinicians' protestations to the contrary – this is not always the case. Every clinician has encountered situations and patients that have dumbfounded their expectations, where either the disease or response has not acted 'as it was supposed to,' for better or for worse. It is such situations that wrench clinicians out of their comfort zones, forcing them to either formulate a new explanation or hypothesis for what has happened, or (more usually) to accept that they do not understand the mechanisms of the human body as well as they thought they did. Both of these two can lead ultimately to an examination of the fundamental assumptions that underlie the discipline.

It is at the fringes of the various disciplines under discussion in this chapter that those fundamental assumptions begin to fray or even break down, inviting inquiry, challenge and critique. These are unlikely to destroy those respective disciplines, but careful questioning may indeed enrich and deepen the disciplines themselves. It is precisely these interfaces – specifically those between medicine and philosophy, psychiatry and medicine, and religion and these two clinical fields – that we wish to explore in this study, not necessarily to provide any answers, but hopefully to proffer some outline thoughts on the dilemmas raised.

The chapter, therefore, will address the light that the philosophies of medicine, psychiatry and religion can shed on the fundamental question of what it means to be human. It will do so by mining the interface of the philosophy and medicine to ask: *what is life/health?* And at the interface of the philosophy and psychiatry to ask: *what is mind/self?* At each stage, we will explore the possible contribution of Islamic philosophical theology[7] and spiritual cosmology[8] to the questions raised.

---

[6] Qur'an 41:53 (*Fuṣṣilat*).

[7] By 'Islamic philosophical theology' in this study is meant the strand – one of many – of Islamic theology, or *kalām*, represented by the Ghazālian-Rāzian synthesis of (Aristotelian and Neoplatonic) Hellenistic philosophy, as represented by Ibn Sīnā (d. 428/1037), with Islamic scriptural and dialectical approaches as represented by Ashʿarī and Māturīdī *kalām* schools. For an example of the Ghazālian synthesis, see Griffel (2009). See also n. 40 and n. 132 below.

[8] 'Spiritual cosmology' is a looser term, referring here primarily to the fusion of the above Islamic philosophical theology with a structured Ṣūfī experiential mysticism, to provide a basis for understanding the multi-layered relationship between Ultimate Reality and creation. It was hinted at in numerous places by al-Ghazālī (d. 505/1111) (as part of his '*ʿilm al-mukāshafa*' – unveiled metaphysical knowledge), but most definitively and influentially set out by the thirteenth-century Spanish mystic, Ibn al-ʿArabī (d. 638/1240), in his masterworks, *Fuṣūṣ al-ḥikam* (*Seals of Wisdom*) and *al-Futūḥāt al-Makkiyya* (*The Meccan Insights*). See also n. 152 below.

## 7.2 At the Interface of Medicine and Philosophy: What Is Health and Why Is It Sought?

At the heart of the relatively recent field of the philosophy of medicine, one finds the fundamental questions of what precisely health is, and why it is sought at all. This question is critical to our investigation, for the concepts of health and illness, when properly understood, can shed light on both what it means to be human, as well as the limitations of a purely naturalistic approach to our own intrinsic natures.

### *7.2.1 What Is Health?*

Few would question the idea that the guiding principle of medicine is beneficence; ultimately health professionals aim to relieve distress and suffering in their patients by restoring their health. The debate really begins around the question of what *constitutes* health and thus ill-health; the dividing line between them can be extremely both vague and highly subjective. Why, for example, does a blood pressure of 142/93 constitute illness, whilst one of 139/88 constitute health? This, then, is the primary issue addressed in the philosophy of medicine: what is health, and why is it sought?

The etymology of the word 'health' is itself fascinating, with roots tracing back to Proto-Indo-European, and encompassing meanings such as wholeness, soundness, freedom from injury, and holiness (on a similar note, 'ill' has etymological connotations denoting 'morally evil').[9] Two points should be noted here: firstly, each of these linguistic connotations of 'health' relate to debates that will be explored in this section, and secondly, the Arabic equivalent terms (*ṣāliḥ, ṣahiḥ)* have almost exactly the same spread of meanings.[10] This should be kept in mind as we proceed, as they relate to foundational concepts in this study moving forward.

### *7.2.2 Models of Health and Illness*

The DNA of the etymological ancestry of the word 'health' is echoed in modern attempts to more technically define the concept. These range from the narrowly naturalistic, by the philosopher Christopher Boorse: 'the absence of disease, where disease is an internal state which impairs normal functional ability …'[11], to the broad and amorphous, by the World Health Organization (WHO): 'a state of complete physical, mental and social well-being.'[12] They form the basis of two broad

[9] Klein (1966-67), 1:710. See also, Watkins (2011), s.v. '*kailo.*'

[10] Ibn Manẓūr (2003), 5:363.

[11] Boorse (1997), 1–134.

[12] *Constitution of the World Health Organization* (2006), 1 (Preamble).

trajectories of approaching the idea of wellness and illness: the 'medical' and 'biopsychosocial' models. Each of these, perhaps, raises more questions than they answer: about the subject-matter itself (health and disease), through the very *raison d'etre* of medicine, all the way to the nature and purpose of the human. The discussion also has a fascinating parallel with the approaches to Islamic law and spirituality, as will be addressed later on.

### 7.2.3 A Holist Perspective: The Biopsychosocial Model

From the perspective of the latter definition – health as a holistic sense of well-being – there is much to critique as well as to commend. Despite it being the preferred definition of the WHO, it stretches the very notion of health beyond what most clinicians would agree was their remit. Most clinicians would baulk at the idea that it was their responsibility to care for someone's social well-being, for example.

Anecdotally, such definitions are derided by most clinicians as being woolly, vague and unscientific, especially when held up to the precision science that is modern medicine. The complex – yet understandable – nature of the human being, as described below, is such that the narrower definition of health allows a much more effective investigation of illness and dysfunction, in turn allowing more effective management, in turn allowing concrete fulfilment of the goal of medicine: beneficence.

Despite this, it can be argued that the definition of health as a positive (well-being), rather than the absence of a negative (no disease), represents both the most intuitively appropriate formulation of the concept. Similarly, assisting others in achieving it fulfils the ideal of benevolence that lies at the very heart of medicine. It is also unitary, considering the entire human holistically, both in microcosm and macrocosm, rather than as merely a sum of their constituent parts.[13]

It crucially leaves the precise definition of 'well-being' open to individual interpretation, as it is ultimately a subjective lived experience rather than the imposition of an objective (normative or functional) standard. A Para-Olympian athlete objectively has a limitation on their functional ability, and statistically represents a deviation from the norm of the human species, but would bristle at the notion of being 'ill,' 'diseased' or in need of 'fixing.' Having a sense of well-being that exists despite external or internal limitations, living the best life one can in one's given circumstances, might be how most humans define being 'well.'

[13] On the Muslim theological discussion of the human microcosm and macrocosm, see for example, Chap. 4, 'The Concept of a Human Microcosm: Exploring Possibilities for a Synthesis of Traditional and Modern Biomedicine,' by Osman Bakar in this book.

### 7.2.4 Cosmic Holism: The Biopsychosocial Model Through an Islamic Lens

It is telling that, from an Islamic perspective, the ideal state one seeks in relation to this world is one of *ʿāfiya* – which is defined in very similar terms to the WHO definition of health: a state of well-being and absence of distress, which includes but is broader than the narrow biological notion of absence of physical disease or illness.[14] *ʿĀfiya* is considered both as an external reality – that the circumstances of one's life are amenable – but also as an internal, psychological one – the ability to cope with adverse life circumstances with equanimity.

Indeed, as opposed to the idea of ill-health being an undesirable state that impels the sufferer to rectify it, a great section of the classical works on Prophetic medicine (*ṭibb nabawī*) is about the 'piety of illness behaviour' – that is, how one reacts to, processes and deals with episodes of illness or injury with dignity, patience and fortitude. That is not to say that ill-health is sought – it is recognized as a harm, and seeking healing has a Prophetic precedent. At the same time, it is clearly considered to be part of the ebb and flow of human life, a trial sent by God to deepen one's consciousness and understanding, and thus a state of grace if passed appropriately. This is explored further in Ahmed Ragab's chapter of this book.[15]

The state of *ʿāfiya* thus parallels the holistic definition of health, but at the same time contains hints at the greater 'cosmic' relationships expressed in the linguistic sense of the word: *ʿāfiya* is near-synonymous with *ʿafw* (God-given exemption, forgiveness and kindness), God's name al-ʿAfuww (the Ever-Forbearing Possessor of Magnanimity), and also closely linked to the concept of *ʿiffa* (probity, integrity and moral continence). As such, holism itself is a relative term; depending on the cosmology in which it is utilized, it may or may not include spiritual and moral dimensions of human well-being.

Finally, it is important to note (for reasons that will be seen later) that *ʿāfiya* is sought as a means, rather than an end: a state of *ʿāfiya* is one which enables the human to meet their natural human needs, freeing them to fulfil the true purpose of their existence: to come to experiential knowledge of – and hence worship – their Lord.

### 7.2.5 A Reductionist Perspective: The Medical Model

Christopher Boorse's definition of health (in Sect. 7.2 above) would constitute the effective position of the vast majority of clinicians practising today: the state of health that is sought through treatment is the absence of disease. It is

[14] Al-Fīrūzābādī (2005), 1313 (s.v. '*ʿāfiya*').

[15] See Chap. 3, 'The Piety of Health: The Making of Health in Islamic Religious Narratives,' by Ahmed Ragab in this book.

(methodologically if not metaphysically) naturalistic, (epistemically if not ontologically) reductionist, and based ultimately upon the notion that the body is a machine that occasionally needs repairing to return it to proper functioning. The clinical examinations carried out by millions of practitioners every day are aimed at eliciting signs and symptoms of pathology, based on a clear assumption about what the proper functioning of each organ or system is. The diagnoses given (e.g., congestive cardiac failure) relate to damage or dysfunction of those parts, organs or systems, and the treatment plans are aimed at either restoring them to proper functioning or (more usually) mitigating their effects.

From the perspective of this naturalistic (or descriptivist)[16] approach to health and illness, therefore, the human is merely a collection of systems working in tandem, which are themselves comprised of organs and tissues, which are comprised of individual cells, which are comprised of intra-cellular components. Damage or dysfunction of the components – or disturbances of the delicate balance between them (homeostasis) – radiates outwards, affecting cells, tissues, organs, systems, and ultimately the human entity.

The principle underlying this is clearly reductionism: the human entity is composed of components (cells, organs, systems), themselves biological compounds bound together by their chemical properties, which in turn function according to the laws of physics. Health, then, is theoretically reducible to the smallest constituent molecules of the human organism, governed by the laws of quantum field physics, then chemistry (which is applied physics), then biology (which is applied chemistry).

Although, *prima facie*, this would appear to make perfect sense, it comes under severe strain when faced with the major objections – both philosophical and from scientific incoherence – raised against reductionism in the last few decades. Primary among these are the increasingly-recognized irregular and patchwork nature of fundamental physical laws, which appear 'not to talk to each other' at a base level,[17] the concept of emergence,[18] and – especially in relation to healthcare – the recent field of complexity sciences. This latter field seeks to understand natural processes in a non-reductive and non-linear way, recognizing that complex systems are dynamic and multi-dimensional, consisting of subtly interconnected relationships rather than a linear cause-effect one.[19]

There are three caveats to this (rather reductive!) account of medicine's reductive nature. Firstly, and critically, by-and-large, the system works. Medications aimed at, for example, regulating blood pressure by selective blockade of Beta receptors in the cardiac muscle (which themselves operate on the basis of the chemistry of attachment and bonding) would appear to do exactly that. Equally, a kidney damaged beyond repair can be 'swapped out' for another. The medical model allows for

---

[16] Fulford (2001): 80–85.

[17] Such that one cannot go from physics to chemistry, for example, without applying seemingly incoherent theories. See Koperski (2015), 168.

[18] This – simplistically – seeks to demonstrate via the scientific method that 'the whole is greater than the sum of its parts' – ibid., 232.

[19] Miles (2009): 409–410.

precision intervention; the body does indeed function as a well-oiled machine in many respects.

Secondly, the bewildering complexity of the human organism is in fact increasingly considered in medicine – the reductive simplicity of a piecemeal, building-block approach is balanced by recognition and partial understanding of the complex integrative systems of the body: the autonomic nervous system, lymph and blood circulation, immunological cascades and, above all, the intricate neuro-endocrinological feedback pathways that master-regulate human biological functioning.

Lastly and most prosaically, medicine is not infrequently functionally agnostic – interventions are instituted on the basis of outcomes, usually via large statistically significant trials, not because clinicians necessarily understand the precise mechanism by which the intervention is having an effect. The mantra is: if it works, use it today – understand its mechanisms tomorrow.

This is certainly the case for the most complex of all human systems: the higher-brain functions that regulate the activity of the 'mind': consciousness, perception, emotion, volition and rationality, which will be discussed in Sect. 7.3 below. The precise pathophysiology of everyday mental illnesses like depression and schizophrenia are poorly understood.[20] Research aside, clinical practice is almost entirely based on educated guesses retrospectively attained through observation of what interventions have worked. As will be explored in greater detail in the next section, the mind remains largely impenetrable to reductionist accounts. In short, as noted by Julian Reiss and Rachel A. Ankeny, 'philosophers of medicine continue to debate … whether more objective, biologically-based and generalisable accounts are preferable to those that incorporate social and experiential perspectives … none satisfy all of the desiderata of a complete and robust philosophical account that can also be useful for practitioners.'[21]

As an end-note, it is somewhat ironic that the very word for the absence of health – 'dis-ease,' and thus 'an absence of well-being' – is more closely related to the WHO definition than to the idea of organ dysfunction, yet the usage of the word itself is almost entirely naturalistic. The reductionist technical nomenclature appears to have eaten and digested the holism of the word itself.

---

[20] De Haan and Bakker (2004): 1–7. A search for 'the pathophysiology of schizophrenia' throws up papers covering neuronal transmission, synaptic problems, neuroanatomy, developmental and spectrum disorders, and a host of other possibilities.

[21] Reiss and Ankeny (2016).

### 7.2.6 Limitations of the Medical Model: Why Is Health Sought?

Despite the various advantages of the attempts to define health, there are two fundamental flaws at their very heart. Firstly, neither of them captures the essence of what appears to have been grasped by Neolithic nomads 7000 years ago in their usage of the term: health is greater than the internal human environment, greater even than the relationship between man and his immediate surroundings, but rather extends to the connection between the human entity and Ultimate Reality. This is something that appears not to have been addressed in critiques of the definitions of health within the philosophy of medicine, which is where the interface with the philosophy of religion might prove particularly useful. Secondly, closely linked to it and well-addressed in discussions around the medical model, is the idea that the definition of health and disease are premised on underlying assumptions about the nature and purpose of human life.

The primary critiques of the medical model (though it applies to more holistic accounts as well) are that it is predicated on the notions of norm and function. That is to say, it presupposes that there are norms for the human species, and (more importantly for our purposes) that the function of human life is to **survive and procreate**. This is clearly seen in the definition of health from perhaps the main figure in reductionist accounts of medicine, the philosopher Christopher Boorse: '[health is] the absence of … that which impedes normal functional ability,' where normal functioning is defined as 'making a contribution that is statistically typical to the survival and reproduction of the individual …'.[22] As pointed out by James G. Lennox, this makes the assumption that the goal of human life is the same as any other form of life, which is to survive and reproduce. Medicine, consequently, is concerned merely 'with biological fitness, rather than other human goals and values.'[23]

It is at this point that the ship of medicine runs aground on the shores of metaphysics. Medicine, in its daily practice, operates (effectively) on a principle of methodological naturalism: it assumes a purely empirical chain of cause and effect – perceivable by the senses, comprehensible to the intellect and thus predictable and objectively modifiable – and discounts any other factor. Medicine, in its fundamental definition of health and illness, however, assumes a *metaphysical* naturalism: the materialist philosophical outlook that nothing exists beyond the empirically perceivable. This is problematic for several reasons. Most prosaically, how does one deal with conditions that are universally considered states of ill-health, but have no identifiable pathology? The most obvious of these are the entire spectrum of mental illnesses, which would appear to be both largely undemonstrative of any observable pathology and also irreducible to the fundamental laws of cellular biology,

---

[22] Boorse (1997), 4.

[23] Lennox (1995): 499–511.

chemistry and physics. Questions raised by such illnesses of the 'mind' will be explored in Sect. 7.3.2 below.[24]

A deeper issue with the apparent metaphysical naturalism lurking at the heart of medicine is the conundrum that health, as an objectively verifiable marker of one's capacity to survive and fitness to reproduce, is the ultimate aim of medicine and is therefore sought as a means to that end. But why is health sought? Why is life the ultimate good?

Some, indeed, would argue the ultimate aim of medicine in less bluntly biological terms: that it is to preserve *quality* of life (or, in the WHO definition, 'a sense of [holistic] well-being'). Hybridizing definitions of health, that seek to bridge biological reductionism and experiential holism, provide examples of this, such those of as the philosopher Caroline Whitbeck, who defines health 'in terms of the physiological and psychological capacities of an individual that allow him or her to pursue a wide range of goals and projects,'[25] or Georges Canguilhem (d. 1995): 'that which confers a survival value … being able to fall sick and recover,'[26] although it can be argued that these fall more towards one or other definitional pole and subsequently suffer their respective drawbacks.

This, of course, largely eliminates the notion of a function or purpose to life, but invites a host of value judgments and assumptions about what precisely constitutes quality of life. It is differences about such assumptions that underlie ethical questions about, for example, interventions at the beginning and end of life, such as abortion and euthanasia. Notwithstanding this, preservation of quality of life manifestly ties in better with the more holistic definition of health, which – as shown above – is less practically useful for clinicians. Additionally, given the higher capacities of human functioning, the question of quality of life leads directly on to the discussion about the *nature* of the sentient self that perceives and appreciates that 'quality.'

Either way of course, life itself remains an essential precondition for its quality. As such, if one assumes that preservation of life itself is the ultimate aim of medicine, whether for its own sake or in pursuit of another objective, two questions are in turn inevitably raised: what is the purpose of life (and hence its nature)?, and why does its mere continuance in some form represent the ultimate good? These are obviously questions that clinicians would shy away from addressing as being outside their remit; yet – as has hopefully been demonstrated – they are begged by the very existence and enterprise of medicine itself. It is at this point that medicine interfaces with religion, which propounds answers to these very questions.

---

[24] Kinghorn et al. (2007): 40–45.

[25] Whitbeck (1977): 619–637.

[26] Canguilhem (1991), 105–119.

### 7.2.7 At the Interface of Medicine and Religion: What Is the Purpose of Life?

The definition of life is one of the great unanswered (and possibly unanswerable) questions of science; there is no single definition that has found broad acceptance.[27] There are literally hundreds of definitions of life, drawn from different sciences, each with its own drawbacks; many of which would appear to be largely descriptive within the context of their parent science, rather than in any way comprehensive. Given this, one might be tempted to mount an argument similar to that of the great intuitionist ethicist G. E. Moore (d. 1958) that, like 'goodness,' 'life' is a simple, non-analysable quality that can be apprehended, but not defined – you know it when you experience it.[28]

Minimally, however, it would appear that, scientifically, a living being might be defined as a unitary, complex, self-organizing entity with sensorimotor capacity – that is, the capacity to perceive and act.[29] Other aspects of life, such as growth and the ability to reproduce, are considered extensions of 'acting.' In terms of what is sensed and acted upon by living things, it is the perception of what is harmful and beneficial, and its avoidance/removal or acquisition/effecting. This characteristic is possessed by every living creature, from amoeba upwards, in as basic or sophisticated a manner as appropriate to its complexity.

Equally, the purpose (or *telos*) of life – as far as it is possible to discuss this from a scientific perspective – is merely to survive, and if this is impossible, then to perpetuate itself. This scientific reductionism is taken to its logical extension in Richard Dawkins' *The Selfish Gene*, whose hypothesis is that it is the very DNA (specifically, the gene unit) that 'seeks' to perpetuate itself, with the organism itself reduced to naught but a vehicle to effect this.[30] In this scenario, all of life is nothing more than the variably sophisticated reproduction of viruses.[31] This is not merely a reductive notion, but a profoundly depressing one, and still does not answer the question of why life – whether the sensing, capable organism itself or its DNA – would seek such perpetuation.

Although it is indisputable that every organism seeks to avoid harm, acquire benefit and perpetuate itself, it is a deeply unsatisfying thought that the purpose of organic life, in all its variation, beauty, and complexity, is merely this. This is especially so when one considers human life, with our rich interior worlds, our creative capacities and our emotional lives. This latter aspect, again, will be more thoroughly explored in Sect. 7.2.10 below.

---

[27] Cleland and Chyba (2002): 387–393.

[28] Moore (1922), 6–10.

[29] See Weber (2018): 'Something that is alive has organized, complex structures that carry out these [physiological] functions as well as sensing and responding to interior states and to the external environment and engaging in movement within that environment.'

[30] Dawkins (2016).

[31] A virus is considered a non-living entity; it is comprised of a strand of DNA with a protein capsule, invading cells in order to reproduce itself.

### 7.2.8 A Religious Account of the Nature and Purpose of Life

Sharīʿa, in its most commonly understood iteration of Islamic law,[32] operates along rather similar bases as modern biomedical ethics:[33] respect for autonomy,[34] beneficence,[35] non-maleficence[36] and social justice.[37] Its guiding principle is the avoidance of harm and acquisition of holistic benefit, and its ultimate aim is the making whole (*ṣalāḥ*) of man through reconciliation with the Divine.[38] This principle is operationalized in its five (or six, in different formulations) 'over-riding imperatives' (*maqāṣid*) – all of which are recognized to be part of the fundamental human impulse (*fiṭra*).[39] Foremost of the human goods that the Sharīʿa seeks to preserve – and above virtually all else – is worldly life; yet given the definitive Islamic belief in an eternal life-after-death, a very similar question could be posed: why is preservation of worldly life considered a good? And why, from a religious perspective, do humans seek it?

At the outset, the reader should note that there is no single 'Islamic perspective' on any given derivative theological question; there is a thousand-year legacy of rich intellectual discourse on most topics found in philosophy. Such topics might be addressed, therefore, via the prism of the dialectical theological schools of early and late classical *kalām*, the multiple Islamic philosophical approaches, or various strains of Ṣūfī or Shīʿī metaphysics. Doing so, however, would be far beyond the scope of this chapter; this and following sections should thus be considered nothing more than an inadequate overview. Our own particular preference tends to be the late Ghazālian[40] synthesis of Sunnī *kalām*, philosophy and Ṣūfī experiential knowledge, as framed by the twentieth century Turkish philosopher and theologian Bediüzzaman Said Nursi (d. 1379/1960).

---

[32] Sharīʿa in its broadest sense, as formulated by al-Ghazālī in his *Mīzān al-ʿamal* (*Balance of Action*) and much more fully in the *Iḥyāʾ ʿulūm al-dīn*, corresponds with a virtue-based approach to ethics; in its simplest sense it represents Divine-command ethics, whilst in its narrower sense resembles more the deontological natural moral law approach.

[33] Beauchamp and Childress (2012).

[34] As explicated in a number of legal maxims, most notably: 'actions are on the basis of intentions' (*innamā al-aʿmal bi-l-niyyāt*); and the Qur'anic dictum: 'there is no coercion in religion' (Qur'an 2:256, *al-Baqara*).

[35] The single overarching principle of Islamic law is 'avert harm and promote benefit' (*darʾ al-mafāsid wa-jalb al-manāfiʿ*). See Ibn ʿAbd al-Salām (2007), 1:6.

[36] As in the core legal maxim, 'harm is to be neither instigated nor reciprocated' (*lā ḍarar wa-lā ḍirār*).

[37] As per the implicit legal given that the law applies equally to all.

[38] Ibn ʿAbd al-Salām (2007), 1:5–32.

[39] Ibn Ashur (2006), 71–84.

[40] Abū Ḥāmid al-Ghazālī (Lat. Algazel) is arguably the most influential Islamic thinker of all time: a twelfth century Persian polymath renowned for his unrivalled mastery in various fields of the traditional Islamic sciences like theology, jurisprudence and its principles, but also, unusually for his time, the 'rival' fields of philosophy and logic. He was also a Ṣūfī master deeply informed by his own mystical experiences, which he incorporated into his oeuvre in subtle (some might say sneaky) ways.

Notwithstanding this, Islam, as one might expect, provides a radically different perspective on the purpose of life, but – somewhat more unexpectedly, perhaps – proffers a comprehensive alternative explanation that both incorporates and transcends the naturalistic perspective on the nature of *all* (not merely *human*) life.

### *7.2.9 An Islamic Account of the Nature of Life*

Muslim theologians have had much the same struggle that others approaching this most fundamental of concepts have encountered, with the added (and intriguingly modern) difficulty that their definition must necessarily encompass non-biological life (like angels and *jinn*) as well.

Nonetheless, they tended to define life in very similar terms to those employed by modern scientists – sensorimotor capacity – though of course on the basis of a very different cosmological system.[41] It should be noted that Islamic theologians tended to discuss the nature of life insofar as it is a pre-eternal attribute of God, the Necessary Existent. As such, this definition of life is explicitly adduced for *created* animate beings, thus excluding the Divine. For traditional theologians such as al-Bājūrī (d. 1276/1860), then, the nature of life is minimally the ability to perceive (*idrāk*), and more expansively, the ability to perceive, choose and act.[42]

Again, the sophistication with which this is done is commensurate with the sophistication of the organism, but all life is defined by this quality or attribute. In Islamic cosmology, this extends beyond organic life to angels, other sentient beings and even God Himself, though in a manner befitting His divinity and entirely beyond creation's capacity to understand.[43]

In terms of created living beings, what is perceived, chosen and acted upon is precisely the same as in naturalistic accounts: 'the avoidance of the harmful and the acquisition of the beneficial' (*darʾ al-mafāsid wa-jalb al-manāfiʿ*). All living beings thus are – to the extent commensurate with the order of their creation – possessed of a form of knowledge, will and power: the attributes that demarcate life. Thus far, the Islamic account largely matches the previous naturalistic one. Lest it be thought that this is a case of religious borrowing, it should be borne in mind that Islamic theologians and thinkers, though undoubtedly owing something to the Greek philosophers

---

[41] Most Sunnī Muslim theologians adopt an occasionalist, atomistic approach to cosmology, where material reality has no necessary spatial or temporal connection, and permanence is an additional but not logically necessary feature. The basic unit of matter is the indivisible particle or *jawhar*, within which attributes (or accidents) subsist.

[42] Al-Bājūrī (1423/2002), 175. A more inclusive classical definition, also by al-Bājūrī, is 'the attribute that allows knowledge, will and power to subsist within a being' (ibid., 176). Ibrāhīm al-Bājūrī was a Cairene Shāfiʿī jurist and Ashʿarī theologian who occupied the post of Shaykh al-Azhar from 1847–1860.

[43] For a glimpse of this supra/trans-organic cosmology, see Chap. 4, 'The Concept of a Human Microcosm: Exploring Possibilities for a Synthesis of Traditional and Modern Biomedicine,' by Osman Bakar in this book.

that came before and whose 'Sharīʿa-compliant' teachings were eventually inherited and incorporated into Islamic discourse, were engaged in these discussions hundreds of years before they were taken up by biologists.[44]

### 7.2.10 An Islamic Account of the Purpose of Life

Where the religious account truly passes beyond the naturalistic one, however, is not in its discussion of the *nature* of life, but of its *telos*. Islam provides two intertwined perspectives on the purpose of life, both of which intimately relate to its nature: one human (*ego*centric), the other profoundly *theo*centric. In brief, the former is that the purpose of life is to come to recognize, know and hence worship one's Creator; the latter is that the purpose of life (and more broadly, existence itself) is to manifest the perfect attributes of God. Religion has been described as the movement from a self-centred view of existence to one centred on Ultimate Reality.[45] This is perhaps most marked in the writings of Ṣūfī theologians and philosophers, who provide an entirely God-centred explanation for existence itself, and life in particular.

They explain that creation itself is naught but a manifestation of the attributes of God, a conscious witness to those attributes, and itself witnessed by God. Here it is crucial to note that, in Islamic scripture and theology, God's perfection encompasses His attributes of both absolute gentleness and absolute rigour (*ṣifat al-jamāl wa-l-jalāl*). As He is the Exalter, He is the Abaser; as He is the Giver of Life, He is the Bringer of Death. Transcendent beyond the mere principle of moral goodness, God is the principle of Existence itself.[46]

In like vein, the act of creation – the original and the continuously-occurring – is itself an expression of both loving kindness (*jamāl*) and absolute dominion (*jalāl*) on the part of the Creator. He is described in the very beginning of the Qur'an as 'the Creator, Sustainer and Nurturer of the Universes, All-Beneficent, All-Compassionate, Absolute Sovereign of the Day of Judgment,' (Qur'an 1:2–4, *al-Fātiḥa*) and His creative act is repeatedly linked to these qualities.[47] The true blessing of existence is merely to exist – hence to be observed by God. Of all the hypothetically possible versions of an entity, all of which exist in the knowledge of God, only one was chosen by Him to exist, and it is this one is witnessed by Him.

From a creation-centric perspective, in several places in the Qur'an, we are told that 'everything in the heavens and the earth glorifies God,' and, more explicitly,

---

[44] Prior to the Islamic philosophers, many of whose views were not accepted by theologians anyway, the prevailing definition of life had been Aristotle's principle of 'animation' – see Weber (2018).

[45] Hick (1989), 240.

[46] Sachiko Murata (1992), 55. For more on the ontological reflection of God being the principle of Existence itself, see also, Chap. 4, 'The Concept of a Human Microcosm: Exploring Possibilities for a Synthesis of Traditional and Modern Biomedicine,' by Osman Bakar in this book.

[47] Nursi (2010), 120.

that 'the seven heavens, the earth and all within them glorify Him; there is not a single thing save that it sings His praise, but you are not given to understand their praise.'[48] Glorification of God is not a one-way monologue; it is heard and responded to by Him. To exist is thus to be in dialogue with God. Theologians further explain that the glorification of God by each object in creation is 'by the tongue of its state.'[49] For inanimate objects, therefore, this 'glorification' occurs by the mere fact of the existence of the object – Islam can be seen, from this perspective, to advocate a form of panpsychism.

Living beings – specifically but not exclusive to animals by the very word of scripture[50] – are considered to be a step above this, both in their ability to glorify God and their manifestation of His attributes. The theologians explain that 'the deer glorifies God by its fleeing from the lion; the lion glorifies God by its pursuit of the deer.'[51] Animate beings glorify God via expression of the instinctual faculties afforded by being alive: seeking out benefit and avoiding harm. Put another way, the ultimate metaphysical purpose of a living being is fulfilled through its own nature.

Living beings also consciously manifest attributes of God: in a famous *ḥadīth*, the Prophet explained that 'God diffused one hundredth part of His attribute of mercy throughout existence; by virtue of that does the mother camel raise her hoof to shelter her cub; by virtue of that is compassion manifested between themselves.'[52] Though God is possessed of attributes of gentleness and rigour, to bowdlerize the words of Martin Luther King Jr. (d. 1968), 'the arc of God's justice is long, but it bends towards mercy.'[53]

Human life is yet a quantum leap beyond this, both in terms of worship and its manifestation. Possessed of the same instinctual drives as other living beings, humans have the additional faculty of sentience, intellect and conscious volition: they may make a moral choice to come to know God or not. Additionally, human beings have the unique ability, by means of their rich, complex interior lives and ratio-emotional states, to manifest the attributes of God more fully and perfectly than anything else in existence. Hence Allāh declared that 'We have honoured the children of Adam,'[54] and the famous (but disputed) Prophetic declaration, 'imbue yourselves with the attributes of God.'[55]

This entails the notion that the 'order' of creation – from least sophisticated to most – is actually related to the increasing capacity to fulfil the purpose of creation. More about the nature of the human, and its relationship to its ultimate purpose, is

48 Qur'an 57:1 (*al-Ḥadīd*) and 17:44 (*al-Isrā*ʾ).

49 Al-Ālūsī (2005), 27:221.

50 For example, trees and foliage are described as 'falling prostrate before God' – Qur'an 55:6 (*al-Raḥmān*).

51 Al-Ālūsī, 27:221.

52 Al-Bukhārī (2012), 8:8 (*ḥadīth* no. 6000).

53 Martin Luther King Jr. originally said: 'The arc of the moral universe is long, but it bends towards justice.' See King Jr. (1965).

54 Qur'an 17:70 (*al-Isrā*ʾ).

55 Al-Ghazālī (1985), 15.

dependent upon understanding the nature of self, and so will be left for a later section (7.3.16). However, it is sufficient for our current purposes to conclude that, from the Islamic perspective, the purpose of life may be approached from two perspectives: to glorify God and to manifest His attributes, and this purpose finds fulfilment in the very nature of the living being.

### 7.2.11 *Why Is Health Sought?*

To return to the original discussion, why does the ultimate purpose of medicine appear to be the restoration of health and preservation of either life or its quality? The religious contribution to this fundamental question – unanswered and perhaps unanswerable from a naturalistic or medical frame of reference – may be stated as follows: given that the **purpose** of life is fulfilment of the ultimate creational good (the recognition and adoration of God), and that the **nature** of life is such that it allows this, life is an instrumental good and ought to be preserved.

It is also natural for mortal beings to seek a form of immortality, given that they 'seek' (with varying degrees of consciousness of it) to manifest the attributes of an eternal and transcendent God. This is the fundamental survival instinct, which drives the pursuit of benefit and avoidance of harm, but can only be done via procreation. It is the nature of living beings to be finite, whilst seeking an infinity beyond themselves. For the human, however, given their greater capacity to manifest these attributes, there is another path, necessitated by the acquisition of moral choice: immortality of the conscious self that endures beyond the death of the physical body.

It is thus the nature of humans, as the most sophisticated of sentient living beings, to pursue immortality via one means or the other – survival/procreation as the instinctual mechanisms, but conscious immortality as the higher one. The more effective their ability to survive and thrive, the greater is their opportunity to seek out God and fulfil the purpose of their lives. Additionally, the better their quality of life – their state of *ʿāfiya* – the better they are able to manifest God's divine attributes in creation and fulfil their moral responsibilities to the rest of creation as God's vicegerents. One of the major aspects of *ʿāfiya* is physical and mental health, and hence the medicine that brings it about is a human good – a manifestation of not only human, but Divine benevolence in creation. Life and health are thus necessary means to the ultimate purpose of human existence, while death and illness detracts from it.

## 7.3 Mind and Soul: At the Interface of Psychiatry, Medicine and Philosophy

As noted in the introduction, the concept of a 'mental illness' raises fundamental questions about the nature of the human and, by extension, of the cosmos. As the concept of illness, when pursued to its utterest ends, leads on to investigations about the nature and purpose of life, the concept of a 'mental' illness raises bedrock questions about the nature and purpose of the sentient, conscious unitary self.[56]

This section will thus explore the nature of consciousness in terms of mental and brain states, examine the relationship between psychiatry and medicine, provide an overview of what the minimalist and strong variants of the medical model, as well as cognitive neuroscience, can contribute to the understanding of 'self,' before discussing the Islamic theological approach to this most fundamental of questions.

### *7.3.1 Self, Soul and Mind*

The term 'psychiatry' is a nineteenth century one, deriving from the Medieval Latin *psychiatria*, which in turn is derived from the Greek words *psyche* (soul/self) and *iatreia* (healing); the meaning conveyed is thus: 'healing the soul/self,' Similar terminology – *ʿilm/muʿālajat al-nafs* (the study/healing of the soul/self) – is found in al-Ghazālī's *magnum opus*, the *Iḥyāʾ ʿulūm al-dīn* (*Revival of the Religious Sciences*),[57] and has been utilized throughout Muslim history.[58]

Clinically, of course, very few psychiatrists would characterize themselves as 'soul doctors,' but most would be content to be referred to as 'mind doctors.' The concepts of 'mind' and 'soul' are closely interlinked, both referring to the subjective, thinking, self-aware *self.* The fundamental difference between them is the metaphysical systems they connote: naturalist versus idealist, reductionist or emergent versus holistic.[59] It might be pithily stated thus: the mind is self *qua* self; the soul is self *qua* God. Within their respective systems, therefore, these close cognates assume very different meanings: the soul is usually considered a distinct entity that supervenes onto and interacts in some way with the physical body; the mind is usually considered a function that arises in some way from that physical body.

Thus when pressed further on what precisely they treat, most psychiatrists would argue that 'mind' is in fact an aspect of brain function. This brings us to the heart of the issue: the mind/brain dichotomy. What in fact is the mind, and if it is a function of the brain, how does the concept of 'mind' arise from it? Are brain states identical with mental states, or are the latter fundamentally different, yet ontologically dependent upon the former?[60]

---

[56] It should be noted at the outset of this section that we will utilize what appears to us to be the most appropriate terms for concepts such as consciousness and sentience. This is done in full cognizance of the fact that different fields have differing technical terms for them, such as primary consciousness for self-awareness and percept for sentience in the neurosciences. An agreed translational framework across philosophy, science, psychology – and theology – is sorely required.

[57] Gilʿadi (1989): 81–92.

[58] ʿAbd al-Ḥamīd, Najāti, and al-Sayyid (2008).

[59] Koperski (2015), 282.

[60] Yalowitz (2014).

The concept of the unitary, sentient self is, perhaps, most *a priori* of truths that we have – the ultimate ontological given.[61] As such, and as seen with the concept of 'life' (Sect. 7.2.7 above), it might be best described as one of those simple, unanalysable concepts that is simply apprehended but impossible to satisfactorily define. At its root lies the conundrum of the nature of consciousness, which in reality returns to three questions: *what* is it?, *how* does it arise?, and *why* does it exist? These are known as the descriptive, explanatory and functional problems of consciousness.[62]

For most of human history, 'self' would have been synonymous with the idea of the soul – a notion so commonplace throughout human history that it might be considered one of the great human universals. The dualist notion of 'soul' being separate in some way from, and transcendent beyond, the material body – to say nothing of enduring after physical death – is less universal, but still highly prevalent.[63]

Yet it was precisely the concept of 'soul' (or essence) that became the primary target of the Humean logical positivist, materialistic ontology that developed from the nineteenth century onwards. As a metaphysical construct, it cannot be directly demonstrated empirically.[64] The closest parallel, however, is precisely the notion of the self-aware, subjective self – the 'I.' It was this that became understood as the 'mind.' An understanding of how primary self-awareness – an *a priori* truth – arises from the substance of the human body is thus the conundrum at the very root of any physicalist ontology: what is 'I'?

Approaches to 'mind' in science and philosophy are multifarious and far too extensive to go into in this chapter. Suffice to say that they encompass substance and property dualist, monist, reductive and non-reductive physicalist, functionalist, supervenience and quantum mechanical theories.[65] The more developed theories include:

- *Reductionist Physicalist* approaches that would type-identify molecular brain states with mental constructs (e.g., a particular change in neuronal activity is exactly the same as the decision to lift up one hand);[66]
- *Emergence* approaches that utilize complexity sciences to posit mind as arising from, dependent upon, but not identical with, brain states (e.g., the decision to

---

[61] As seen in Descartes famous *cogito ergo sum*, but also six centuries before in Ibn Sīnā's *al-Shifāʾ* (*The Healing*): '[the unperceiving soul] is unaware of anything except the fixedness of its own individual existence (*thubūt annaʾiyyatihā*).' Cited in Marmura (1986): 383–395.

[62] Van Gulick (2018).

[63] This does necessarily entail a belief in a next life, of course. One of the notable exceptions to the idea of an immortal soul, interestingly, would seem to have been the Arab pagans at the time of the Prophet Muhammad, who did not appear to have any real belief in a hereafter, saying, 'who will revive these dry bones when they have crumbled to dust?' Qur'an 36:87 (*Yā Sīn*).

[64] As in, in terms of substance or tissue – though proponents would argue that its indirect effects encompass every process within the body, or at least, the conscious, voluntary aspect of human perception and behaviour.

[65] Van Gulick (2018), 44–52.

[66] Papineau (2002).

lift up one hand is different from the neuronal activity, but cannot exist without it);[67]

- *Anomalous Monist* approaches, that would token-identify mental and brain states in various ways (lifting up one's hand is a particular instantiation of specific neuronal activity, but there is no one-to-one relationship between them);[68]
- *Quantum Mechanical* approaches, that would consider the mind as a supervenience phenomenon similar to a Bose-Einstein condensate,[69] or arising from quantum effects on microtubules within neurons.[70]

At the root of this question lies a potentially unsolvable issue: the gap between the objective and subjective known as the hard problem of consciousness.[71] As first so-labelled by David Chalmers in 1995,[72] it examines the explanatory gap between descriptions of objective occurrences, such as the firing of a neuron or release of a synaptic transmitter, and subjective experiences (or qualia), such as the taste of chocolate. In other words, is the relationship between objective reality and our experience of it even possible to explain? It is called a 'hard' problem because, rather than not yet having the answer because of an epistemic gap, it may be rationally impossible to *ever* construct an answer to the question from within a naturalistic framework.[73] The philosophical position that it is impossible to solve the problem of consciousness is known as mysterianism, and its adherents include significant philosophers and scientists such as Colin McGinn,[74] Steven Pinker and the neuroscientist Sam Harris.

This leaves us with the notion – deeply unsettling to metaphysical naturalists and logical positivists – that the most fundamental intuitive fact of human existence is impossible to empirically prove or falsify.[75] Put another way, consciousness is a metaphysical truth. The following sections will look at this issue in more detail, examining whether psychiatry or cognitive neuroscience can shed more light on the question of the *what*, *how* and *why* of the conscious self.

[67] Hasker (2001), 27.

[68] Yalowitz (2014), 5–6.

[69] Zohar and Marshall (1990).

[70] Penrose (1994).

[71] Howell and Alter (2009): 4948.

[72] Chalmers (1995): 200–19.

[73] From a theological point of view, of course, consciousness is a function of the soul: the subjective experience of the external world that is objectively processed via demonstrable changes in neural substrates.

[74] McGinn (1989): 349–66.

[75] Howell and Alter (2009).

### 7.3.2 Psychiatry and Medicine

The objective-subjective distinction is mirrored in the fields of cognitive neuroscience and psychology/psychiatry. A significant subset of the former is about determining the neural correlates of consciousness, whilst the primary focus of the latter is about investigating the subjective human experience.

Psychiatry has historically had an uneasy relationship with medicine. Although it is a medical specialty, and all psychiatrists are fully trained doctors, the extent to which it gels with the modern medical model has always aroused uncertainty and suspicion in the minds of other clinicians. A recent discussion, for example, is whether the treatment of mental disorders should be removed entirely from the domain of medicine and be studied and managed under the field of cognitive neuropathology.

All these discussions return ultimately to the question of how precisely a mental disorder – and thus the conscious human mind experiencing it – is to be fundamentally conceptualized: is it an objective malfunction of neuronal processes or a subjective experience of psychic distress and disorder? Is the sentient human self, by extension, merely an illusory construct, the sum of all the brain's inputted data, systematized and processed by the mind-bogglingly complex structures of the neural connectome, or something greater than the sum of its parts? Is the brain – or perhaps the nervous system more generally – where soul and body co-mingle?[76] Are any of these necessarily mutually exclusive?

Medical questions about mental health and disorder are thus intimately connected to philosophical questions about the nature of the human self. This is borne out in the recent and developing discipline of the philosophy of psychiatry, where discussions fall into three primary groupings: (1) those that approach psychiatry as a specialist science using the methods of the philosophy of science; (2) those that examine the conceptual issues that arise with the very idea of a mental illness; and (3) those that explore issues relating to psychopathology and the philosophy of mind.[77] Each of these relate in some way or another to the fundamental question posed by this chapter: what is the nature and purpose of the conscious human self?

### 7.3.3 Psychiatry and the Medical Model

It is unquestionable that most mental health professionals, in actual clinical practice, lean much more towards the holistic biopsychosocial model of health than that of the medical model: they will explicitly consider factors beyond the merely

[76] Rafaqat Rashid's discussion of the nature of death, in this book, demonstrates another practically relevant example of this philosophical dilemma. See Chap. 9, 'The Intersection between Science and Sunnī Theological and Legal Discourse in Defining Medical Death.'

[77] Murphy (2017).

biological in terms of pathogenesis and management, and tend to aim for precisely the sense of patient-led subjective 'well-being' (in terms of relief of symptoms and their consequences, if nothing else) than repair of tissue or even sometimes restoration of 'proper' functionality. The brain of a grieving old widow, experiencing comforting audio-visual hallucinations of her deceased husband that keep her company but who is otherwise getting on with her life, is unquestionably objectively dysfunctional, but would be judged by most practitioners to need nothing more than observation, because treatment would probably increase her distress.

This leaning towards the biopsychosocial model is, quite simply, because the concept of the mind itself is holistic rather than reductive. One might in fact argue that it makes little clinical sense to think of the 'mind' in terms of the sum of its neurobiological processes, but rather in terms of the subjective sense of a unitary self, as that is both more intuitive and more accurate in terms of human self-perception. The precise difference between mind and brain might even be summed up as: mind = subject (or 'I'), brain = object (or 'it').

Nonetheless, there has been a general agreement over the last several decades that psychiatry specifically, as a branch of medicine, must (and does) adopt an evidence-based medical model – that is: 'the consistent application of modern medical thinking and methods.'[78] This is because psychopathology (the symptoms of mental illness) is understood to 'represent the manifestation of disturbed functioning within a part of the body (the brain),'[79] which is the very core of the medical model as noted in the previous section. However, given the complexity of the questions thrown up by the very idea of a mental illness, some of which will be explored below, it has become necessary to distinguish between two different interpretations of the medical model.

### 7.3.4 *The Minimalist Medical Model*

The first of these, a minimalist model, employs a syndromic approach to health and illness. In it, the concept of disease is merely the 'unfolding of a suite of symptoms,'[80] and bears no necessary connection to aetiology or pathophysiology. The second, the 'strong' interpretation of the medical model, necessitates specific causal hypotheses about mental illnesses.[81] In other words, in the minimal model, diagnosis is made on the basis of symptoms and course of illness; in the strong model, it is made on the basis of demonstrable or strongly inferable brain pathology. Both, of course, are empirical in nature, but the latter demands explanations that cite pathogenic

78 Black (2005), 3–15.

79 Guze (1992), 44.

80 Ibid.

81 Murphy (2017), 4.

processes in the brain[82] (this does not have to be reductive, as it can include emergent approaches such as system dysregulation).

The minimalist model is the default in clinical psychiatry – the Diagnostic and Statistical Manual (DSM) and the International Classification of Diseases (ICD)[83] list diagnoses and categories primarily on the basis of symptoms rather than aetiology or pathophysiology.[84] Because of this, they have come in for heavy criticism from advocates of the strong medical model, who will sometimes cite them as 'Exhibit A' for why psychiatry is not a true medical sub-speciality. This is not an unjustified criticism – diagnosing someone as having major depression on the basis of them having five out of nine symptoms for a certain length of time is a bit like a doctor diagnosing 'chest pain.' Is a refugee of war, forced to flee their home, traumatized by the loss of family, friends, home and income, who feels sad, hopeless and helpless, the same as a socially and psychologically untroubled person who wakes up one morning with the same set of symptoms?

Either way, the aetiological agnosticism of this model makes it entirely unhelpful in answering our primary question – if it does not comment on the nature of any specific disorder, it most certainly will not shed any light on the nature of the unitary self that is experiencing that disorder.

### *7.3.5 The Strong Medical Model*

This leaves us with the strong medical model, which unlike the minimalist variant, explicitly focuses on elicitable pathology. Simply put, if an asthma attack – defined as disturbed bronchial constriction and relaxation – can be traced back to the neurochemical relationship between cell receptors in the bronchial walls, the parasympathetic nervous system, and the calcium channels in the smooth muscle of the bronchi, then psychopathology such as a hallucination or depressed mood should be equally traceable back to the neural substrate of certain areas of the brain. This is the model that most working psychiatrists would profess to adopt (albeit with a lot of hand-waving about it being 'more complicated than this, obviously'): schizophrenia is ultimately about excess striatal dopamine, and depression is about a depletion of serotonin levels in the hippocampal synaptic space.[85]

This model – the default upon which most of medicine operates – has its own problems. When it comes to the strong model, even the term 'mental illness' can be viewed as problematic unless specifically referent to disorders in higher functioning that ultimately arise from brain pathology. The *extenso ad absurdum* of this is that,

[82] Andreasen (2001), 172–176.

[83] The RDoC model, a very different approach to determining pathology, will be discussed later on (see Sect. 7.3.8 below).

[84] World Health Organization (1992), 5.

[85] It is a *lot* more complicated: see Harvard Health Publishing (2019).

in the absence of demonstrable tissue pathology, it becomes impossible to diagnose (and thus justify treatment for) any mental illness at all. Indeed, Emil Kraepelin (d. 1926), one of the forefathers of psychiatry and the effective originator of the minimalist interpretation, himself viewed it as a stop-gap measure until a true picture of pathology emerged.[86] A century later, we are little further on.[87]

In practice, both models are employed. Clinicians will diagnose largely on the basis of symptomatology (guided by their clinical *nous* in terms of adherence to or departure from the diagnostic schemes), but propose to accept ideas about pathogenesis in terms of suggested treatment plans. In other words, a person may be diagnosed as having OCD on the basis of their symptoms and degree of behavioural and functional disturbance, but be treated with a combination of SSRIs and psychotherapy on the basis of a presumed pathogenesis.

### 7.3.6 Reductionism and Strong Model Psychiatry

In general, but especially for our purposes, the primary issue with the strong model is its reductionism. As explained earlier, this is the idea that all complex entities are ultimately reducible to more fundamental levels in nature. It takes two forms: ontological and epistemic reductionism – respectively, the idea that all matter is merely the sum of its smallest constituents, and the idea that the laws governing all matter are reducible to the most fundamental laws of physics.[88] This, combined with naturalism – the belief that only matter exists – entails that all of existence is no more than subatomic particles governed by the laws of particle or quantum state physics.

In this model, therefore, mental states such as beliefs, emotions and intentions[89] (and disturbances in them) can only be understood as expressions of cellular biology, which itself is merely the chemistry of organic molecules, which in turn are governed by the physics of the atoms of which they comprise. As such, a depressed person's conscious decision to jump off a building is at root no different from the effect of gravity on their falling body. This is not only intuitively fallacious, but entails a hard scientific determinism: there is demonstrably no such thing as choice.[90]

It is critical to note here that the principle of reductionism itself, the basis of much of modern science during the twentieth century, is not directly scientifically demonstrable. It is a meta-theoretic shaping principle: a paradigm assumption made

---

[86] Kraepelin (1991), 1:4.

[87] Murphy (2017).

[88] Koperski (2015), 226–7.

[89] Or *ʿilm*, *ḥāl* and *ʿamal al-qalb*, to use the Islamic terms.

[90] The first proponent of this idea was Pierre-Simon Laplace (d. 1827) and what became known as 'Laplace's demon.' See Saunders (2000): 517–44.

about the way reality operates – that causality operates uni-directionally from part to whole.[91] This principle itself has been strongly challenged, as will be seen later.

### 7.3.7 The Limitations of the Strong Medical Model

Modern psychiatry, therefore, as with the rest of medicine, is considered to arise from a reductive, physicalist understanding of reality. This is the position that there is only one 'substance' of reality – that which is measurable and observable – and nothing that cannot be empirically demonstrated can be deemed to exist. This idea is closely connected to logical positivism, the epistemological position that any proposition is meaningless unless it is based either on empiricism or necessary logical truth.[92] This would include every metaphysical proposition, of course. Any statement about the soul, therefore, is *prima facie* a meaningless utterance.[93] Unfortunately for devotees of this approach, the same might very well be said for consciousness itself – not only does one's own consciousness not actually exist from a reductive perspective, even talking about it is meaningless.

Setting this aside, there remain major problems with this approach, which relate to two primary concepts. One of these is potentially solvable – the lack of granular knowledge about brain anatomy and physiology; the other is almost by definition insoluble within the paradigm of materialism – reductionism and the hard problem of consciousness.

To look at some of exemplar problems in more detail: firstly, there is no solid, one-to-one evidence of primary tissue pathology in the regions referred to by the 'dopamine' and 'serotonin' hypotheses of schizophrenia[94] and depression[95] – the conditions are significantly more complicated. These hypotheses operate on the basis of a manipulationist model of causation[96] (we know that if we make change 'x,' then 'y' is prevented, therefore 'x' must be causally related to 'y'). As such, if reducing dopamine delivery to a particular area reduces psychosis, then psychosis must have something to do with excess dopamine. As mentioned in the previous section, quite a lot of medicine starts out with this type of approach, and it can be statistically shown to be generally effective. However, with other domains of medi-

---

[91] Koperski (2015), 26–29.

[92] Ayer (1936).

[93] The pros and cons of logical positivism are beyond the scope of this study, but it is probably worthwhile noting that its own founding proposition: 'every proposition not based on empirical fact or necessary truth is meaningless' is itself not based on empirical fact or necessary truth, and so by its own logic is meaningless! A metaphysical statement refuting metaphysics is a snake consuming its own tail. This is one reason why its originator, Ludwig Wittgenstein (d. 1951), eventually moved away from it.

[94] Toda and Abi-Dargham (2007): 329–336.

[95] Krishnan and Nestler (2008): 894–902.

[96] Whitbeck (1977): 627–8.

cine, this is usually a preface to discovering the *actual* pathological process at play; in psychiatry, we appear to be little closer to discovering this, largely due to the sheer complexity of the mind/brain. Equally problematic and probably related, this blunt manipulationist approach tends to yield significantly less effective results than similar approaches in other fields of medicine.

Secondly, is it possible to explain the effectiveness of psychotherapy within a reductionist paradigm? How can a conscious thought in the 'mind' have an impact on neural operations at granular level? If, as appears to be the case, CBT can be as effective at treating depression as an SSRI medication – not just in terms of relief of symptoms, but also in bringing about actual neural rewiring[97] – then can a conscious thought trigger a release of serotonin or remodel the brain? It has been demonstrated that long term meditation can alter brain structure and function, as well as create powerful feelings of well-being and peacefulness.[98] But how does an abstract subjective concept like 'a positive thought' relate to the nuts and bolts of brain chemistry? Both these demonstrable findings would appear to necessitate the consideration of a form of supervenience: the idea that higher-level processes, whilst ontologically dependent on lower-level substrata, can supervene on them, leading to a form of reverse-directional causality.[99]

Thirdly and perhaps most fundamentally, we return to the hard problem of consciousness. There is a significant category shift to be made between the paradigms of objective granular neural functioning and those of subjective experience. How does electro-chemical activity become a subjective experience? Equally, is it not simply a category error to try to reduce a sophisticated depressogenic idea like guilt to a specific neural substrate?[100] Nancy C. Andreasen, an advocate of the strong interpretation of the medical model, nonetheless argues against reductionism in psychiatry on this basis,[101] and the reductionist endeavour is increasingly being challenged in neuroscience.[102]

This 'experiential barrier' is one that it may be conceptually impossible to cross from a physicalist or reductionist perspective. As seen previously, peering closer and closer does not necessarily make the picture clearer. Philosophically, one might question whether it is even logically conceivable for humans to transcend the limitations of their own brain structures and functions to understand them in true holistic fashion. To take another example, the Special Theory of Relativity strongly postulates eternalism: the idea that time, as merely a dimension of existence, is as mathematically constrained as space, and that the future, therefore, is 'written.'[103] From the perspective of the human, however, this is simply impossible to apprehend – the

---

[97] Linden (2006): 528–538.

[98] Jeeves and Brown (2009).

[99] Koperski (2015), 232.

[100] This is not to say that there *aren't* neural correlates, just that guilt being *merely* a neurotransmitter is unsupportable.

[101] Andreasen (1997): 1586–93.

[102] Krakauer et al. (2017): 480–490.

[103] Petkov (2009), 172.

'flow of time' is simply wired in to the structures of our brains.[104] Similarly, can the brain, as the neural substrate of the mind, ever be a tool to understand the mind – to say nothing of reality itself (material or metaphysical)?

In terms of determining an answer to our prime question, therefore, the strong medical model is hamstrung by both its epistemic shortcomings and its reductionism. Despite the fact that the stock-in-trade of psychiatry is mental illness, it cannot satisfactorily explain what the nature of the conscious being experiencing it might be.

### *7.3.8 Psychiatry, Emergence and Cognitive Neuroscience*

As we have seen, analysing the concept of a mental disorder throws up fundamental philosophical questions about consciousness: what it is, how it arises, and why it is present at all. It is particularly in answer to these questions that the pitfalls of a reductive approach to mental states become clearly manifest. It is then ironic, perhaps, that in search of an answer, we should briefly turn to perhaps the most ostensibly reductive of all disciplines dealing with the mind: cognitive neuroscience, particularly its sub-discipline of neuro-philosophy.

This field is concerned with the study of the biological processes that underlie cognition, with a specific focus on the neural connections in the brain that are involved with mental processes, and identifying the neural correlates of consciousness.[105] From it has emerged the RDoC model, a research framework for new approaches to investigating mental disorders which integrates many levels of information (from genomics and circuits to behaviour and self-reports) in order to explore basic dimensions of functioning that span the full range of human behaviour.[106] In the course of this, a large number of neural substrates, action loops and functional pathways have been determined.

To make some sense of this, some have proposed a model comprising different levels of neural functioning, within which a particular causal or explanatory mechanism can be validly applied – despite this being nonsensical when applied to a different level. David Marr distinguished between three levels of explanation of neural functioning in cognitive science:

- the highest specifies the 'computational task' being undertaken (e.g., communicating effectively);
- the middle describes the representations and algorithms that carry out the goal (the necessary circuits and pathways between different areas of the brain, including memory, language, motor, sensory, association, etc.);

[104] Lockwood (2005), 69.

[105] Gazzaniga, Ivry and Mangun (2019).

[106] See the website of 'Research Domain Criteria (RDoC)' hosted by the National Institute of Mental Health (USA): https://www.nimh.nih.gov/research/research-funded-by-nimh/rdoc/index.shtml.

- the lowest describes the actual neural substrate and electro-chemical processes that occur to bring it about (which neurons fire, which neurotransmitters are released into the synaptic space between them).[107]

When applied to a concept like vision, the model works relatively well: seeing is explicable at each of the three levels utilizing different explanatory tools. However, when applied to psychological explananda, this trifold model is subjected to significant stress. The three levels are not three variant explanations of the same process, but three different *representations* of (or ways of talking about) the same process.

In this schema, whilst cognitive neuroscience is primarily concerned with the middle and lowest levels of neural functioning, clinical psychiatry is concerned with disorder at the highest. However, it is also patently multifactorial in its approach: epidemiologically, it considers factors ranging from strictly biological, like genetics, through complex interactional mediating ones like the concept of guilt, to social ones like bereavement or loss of status. As hard as it may be to reduce the concept of guilt to a specific neurobiological substrate, it is even more difficult to contemplate doing so with something like bereavement. And while it is possible to model psychiatric psychopathology (as dysfunction) using the highest cognitive level, and also equally useful to understand something of the neurobiology at cellular or synaptic level (in terms of psychoactive agents), connecting the two to demonstrate how the former arises from the latter is deeply problematic: one is merely explaining experiences like distress in subjective terms, but neural activity in chemical terms. The hard problem yet remains.

Underlying all of this is a more fundamental issue still – the (possibly *a priori*) inability to explain the 'fourth' level of brain functioning: the conscious self. Even the highest level of modelling of brain functioning – explaining computational tasks or goals – assumes the obvious: that they are all subsumed to a unitary, living entity working towards the ultimate goal (whether that be survival or something greater, as discussed above). The explanatory leap from explaining specific tasks undertaken by the brain to its logical and necessary extension of the sentient self is even more opaque to reason than the jump from neurobiology to task-based functions. And just as explanatory models at one level are inapplicable outside of that level, so too there is no plausible neuroscientific explanatory model within a reductionist framework for the subjective experience of personhood.

### 7.3.9 Cognitive Neuroscience and Emergence

It is cognizant of this latter objective – the search for an explanation for consciousness – that the limitations of reductionism were first demonstrated, and the need for a radically different approach recognized.[108] This inverse-reductionist theory is

[107] Marr (1982), 24–25.

[108] Hasker (2001), 45–58.

known as emergence: the whole is ontologically greater than the sum of its parts. It is characterized by three premises: the higher level (A) is irreducible to the lower level (B); the behaviour of A cannot be predicted by B; and what is observed of A is novel and unexpected given its base.[109] It has found applications across the sciences, from chaotic dynamics in quantum physics to the hermaphroditic change of clown-fish in biology,[110] but is particularly applicable to the question of consciousness.

Emergence has given rise to an experimentally supported model of consciousness: the dynamic core hypothesis of neuroscientists Gerald Edelman and Giulio Tononi.[111] They propose that it has a dual nature, distinguishing between lower-order (volitional) and higher-order (sentient) consciousness possessed of animals and humans respectively, on the basis of the relative complexities of their cerebral cortices. They further posit what they consider to be a likely neurophysiological basis for conscious awareness: a widespread functional interconnectedness across the brain comprised of two-way neural interactions, which is a complex, highly differentiated and ever-changing neural state known as the reticular activating system. This is an oft-cited example of emergence: conscious awareness is not reducible to two-way neuronal firing, cannot be explained by it, and is an unexpected consequence of it.

The reticular activating system, however, is primarily associated with awareness and arousal – it modulates the difference between wakefulness and sleep, for example, in both animals and humans.[112] The extension of the hypothesis to account for sentient consciousness – the full subjective experience of 'I' – entails the additional involvement of the symbolic representation, memory and linguistic centres of the brain. This has far less experimental support and a much more tenuous neurophysiological basis; it is more of a positing by analogy. As such, though it goes some way towards doing so, the dynamic core hypothesis cannot resolve the explanatory gap of subjective experience versus objective occurrence.

### *7.3.10 The Interface Between Cognitive Neuroscience and Psychiatry*

Another way to look at this question is to ask what mental disorder can teach us about the mind. As we have seen, in terms of understanding the complexities of the brain's functioning, it is worthwhile to explore it by means of levels. Clinical psychiatry examines disorders at the highest level of brain functioning, namely that of functional processes. As such, examining dysfunction in these processes can be useful in more clearly explicating their functions and purposes.

---

[109] Batterman (2009).

[110] Koperski (2015), 233.

[111] Edelman and Tononi (2000), 103.

[112] Garcia-Rill (2009), 8:137–143.

By proper understanding of the concept of a delusion, for example, one can seek to map out the cognitive process of belief – how from a computational perspective, information becomes knowledge that might be swayed or amended by further information, which in turn becomes a firm conviction that is unshakeable no matter what other information is presented.[113] Neuropsychological work done on this has helped to clarify two-factor theories of belief formation: the first step is an impairment in one's reception of external information (my wife appears odd…), the second is an impairment in one's ability to evaluate that belief (… so she must have been replaced by a robot).[114] It is the impairment in the evaluative component of knowledge formation that truly sets apart a delusion.[115]

Some of the psychopathology encountered in clinical psychiatry can also throw up philosophical conundrums. If 'mental' is referent to primary consciousness (self-awareness) and intentionality (conscious purpose), how does one explain something arising 'in the mind' but not 'of the mind'? Consider, for example, the difference between three internal thoughts: a person recalling a fond memory, an annoying tune stuck in their head, and the psychiatric phenomenon of a thought insertion.[116] The first is both self-attributed and intentional (my thought that I chose to recall); the second is self-attributed but unintentional (my thought, but I didn't choose to recall it and can't get rid of it). The third, however, is something entirely different: an entirely introspective awareness of an episode in my mind that is, nonetheless, experienced as someone else's thought. This may be explained as alienated self-consciousness,[117] but it is also instructive about the limitations of a purely materialistic philosophy of mind.[118]

Most intriguing, from a philosophical perspective, is the question: why psychiatry? The very idea of dysfunction in higher cognitive processes, the 'spanner in the works' of mental processing, begs the deeper question of why such an elaborate system exists in the first place. After all, the more complex a system, the more likely it is that errors will occur – and there is perhaps nothing in the universe more complex than the human brain. Why, then, have human beings evolved (or been endowed) these higher cognitive faculties in the first place? Is this enormously complicated

---

[113] This is what the Qur'an describes as 'placing a lock upon the heart' (Qur'an 47:24, *Muḥammad*) and 'the stamping of the soul' (Qur'an 47:16, *Muḥammad*).

[114] Davies and Coltheart (2000): 1–46.

[115] Much of al-Ghazālī's work in moral psychology – in fact, one might argue, the *raison d'etre* of the *Iḥyāʾ* as a whole – is to determine subconscious factors that impair the soul's ability to properly evaluate external information about the nature of the world and the hereafter in relation to God, and thus to take correct moral decisions and increase one's knowledge of God.

[116] The deeply discomfiting experience of a thought that one recognizes as not being one's own, but that an external agency has inserted into one's mind.

[117] Stephens and Graham (2000).

[118] Islamic thought, on the other hand, would allow for such experiences to be explained, as it would fold into notions of the 'multifarious self,' which include ideas about the 'internal or accompanying devil' (*nafs al-shayṭān* or *al-qarīn al-sūʾ*). This is experienced much more commonly as the unbidden, negative automatic thought that arises within the mind, from which both mental and ethical disorders are born. The thought insertion phenomenon would be a heightened version of this – a dissociative experience brought via the mechanism of dislocation of the conscious self.

machine not an overly complex tool by which to ensure mere survival, or does it have another function? This question relates directly back to the question posed in the previous section – posed but unanswerable from a materialist perspective – about the nature and purpose of not life, but the self.

No matter how partial or unsatisfying, then, cognitive neuroscience has at least attempted to address some of our core questions: consciousness is a complex mental state of heightened awareness and focus; it emerges functionally from highly differentiated neural activation across wide areas of the cortex. As to why it is present, the best answer is that the complexity of the cerebral cortex simply engenders it, which of course begs the question above: why is the human cortex so complex? Science is still unable to ultimately explain the brute fact of the self. The 'I' would appear to be a metaphysical given.

### *7.3.11 The Mind in Religious Metaphysics*

At this point, once again, a materialist ontology runs aground on the shores of metaphysics. For all the detail provided about how the higher processes of the brain work and why they might become dysfunctional, it does not satisfactorily answer the question about the nature and purpose of the subjective self.

Given the methodological constraints of a purely empirical scientific approach to the question of 'what is the self,' it is certainly worthwhile investigating a religious approach, bearing in mind that the explanatory toolkit of Islamic philosophical theology, whilst internally robust and coherent, is not the same as the scientific one. It is also a given that, in order to accept the answers proffered by a religious approach to these most fundamental metaphysical questions,[119] one must accept its underlying assumptions about the nature of reality: that it is metaphysical, not merely material, there actually exists that which cannot be proven empirically, and self cannot be understood divorced from Ultimate Reality. However, it is submitted that equally, rejection of these assumptions is equally empirically unprovable: ignorance is not evidence, after all. This is especially when one considers that naturalism does not provide answers to the questions that undergird the entire enterprise of medicine.

### *7.3.12 Islam and the Nature of the Soul*

Given the above, what then does Islam have to say about the nature, origin and purpose of the self? Before answering, I refer the reader back to the caveat noted above (Sect. 7.2.8) – there are several nuanced approaches to this question that are beyond the

---

[119] That are nonetheless, as has hopefully been shown, necessary ones to answer in order for the entire superstructure of materialism and medicine to exist and operate in the first place.

scope of this study to explore in the detail they deserve. Though the unitary self (*nafs*)[120] is mentioned repeatedly in scripture, the most fascinating aspect of discussion within the 'house of Islam' on its nature, however, is perhaps the most fundamental and authoritative one – the brief but brutal Qur'anic summation of the question: 'They ask you, [O' Muhammad] about the soul (*rūḥ*). Tell them: it is the affair of my Lord, and you have been given but little knowledge of it.'[121] This echoes the contention made earlier about the conceptual impossibility of the mind being able to understand its own nature.

Nonetheless, discussion about the nature of the soul and selfhood – partly inherited from classical Greek enquiries into the same question, yet largely fuelled by frequent but gnomic insights from scripture – is a recurring feature of early Islamic psycho-theological discourse. The *kalām* theologians and philosophers approached the question from a metaphysical and scriptural standpoint, whilst Ṣūfī theoreticians added an ethico-spiritual dimension.[122] In other words, theologians tend to ask: 'what is the soul?', whilst mystics tend to ask: 'what is it for?'[123] As with the question of life, the discussion around the soul centres on fundamental investigations about its nature and purpose. This parallels the descriptive and functional problems of consciousness in modern philosophy of science; though while science focuses on the explanatory problem (how does consciousness arise?), religion tends to focus more on the functional problem (what is the purpose of the conscious soul?).

One might expect that Muslims, as committed theists, plumped for a thoroughly Cartesian dualist approach – that the human is comprised of body and soul. However, one finds that historical theological discussions about the nature of the soul were significantly more nuanced than this. As ably summarized by Ayman Shihadeh,[124] one finds a broad spread of opinion across Muslim scholarship that reflects in many ways modern discussions around the topic of selfhood. In brief, they range from the monist – even strictly physicalist – approaches of the early Ashʿarī theological tradition through to virtually Neoplatonic dualist formulations from the classical philosophical tradition. A middle theological ground – of sorts – was developed by major later theological figures such as al-Ghazālī (d. 505/1111) and Fakhr al-Dīn al-Rāzī (d. 606/1210),[125] who set the course for later classical Islam and the *madrasa* syl-

---

[120] The need for a consistent lexicon and translational framework applies particularly to the terms *nafs* (self or soul, etc.), *ʿaql* (intellect or mind, etc.), *rūḥ* (spirit or soul, etc.) and *qalb* (lit. heart), which have been utilized to denote different aspects of self in classical and contemporary Islamic literature.

[121] Qur'an 17:85 (*al-Isrāʾ*). It should be noted that this is not necessarily a reference to the *human* soul, as discussed in the exegetical literature in some detail.

[122] It should be noted that the categories 'theologian and Ṣūfī mystic' are far from exclusionary; especially in the later period, many occupied both roles simultaneously though, like al-Ghazālī, they might 'wear different turbans' depending on which field they were speaking from.

[123] The most interesting parallel to this is actually the discussions about the Names of God in Islamic literature: the primary concern of the theologians was how to define them, whilst the critical additional concern of the Ṣūfīs was how to embody them within oneself.

[124] Shihadeh (2012b): 413–416.

[125] Fakhr al-Dīn al-Rāzī was one of the most important figures in the later development of Islamic theology, most famous for his master-work *al-Tafsīr al-kabīr* (*The Great Exegesis*), one of the most important reference-works in all exegetical literature. A twelfth century Persian, he was one of the major proponents of Islamic philosophical theology, deeply influenced by Ibn Sīnā and al-Ghazālī, while still being critical of both of them.

labus itself. They promulgated a thoroughgoing interactionist substance dualist approach to the notion of body and soul that owed as much to the pioneering cognitive theories of the philosophical giant Ibn Sīnā (d. 428/1037) as it did to the early Ashʿarī theology and Ṣūfī metaphysics.

### 7.3.13 Monist Physicalist Perspectives on the Soul

From the perspective of Ashʿarī theology, luminaries of early orthodox Sunnī Islam such as al-Ashʿarī[126] (d. 324/936) and ʿAbd al-Qāhir al-Baghdādī (d. 429/1038) viewed man as a purely physical entity, comprised of atoms (substance) and the accidents (attributes) that inhered in them. It was the structure of the atoms within man (i.e., his *binya*) that properly classified him as 'human,' rather than any metaphysical aspect. His inherent accidents included a special class (*ṣifat al-ḥayy*) unique to living beings, such as perception and movement, that were conditional upon the central attribute of life.[127] There was no need to theoretically postulate anything beyond the purely corporeal, no extrinsic 'animating force' that was required. The notion of the soul itself was only admitted – with not inconsiderable theoretical difficulty – as a concession to the explicit word of scripture, and even then, viewed as a strictly material entity residing within the human.[128]

In more modern language,[129] the early Ashʿarīs adopted a reductive physicalist approach to the notion of the human that would be comprehensible to biologists: comprised of cells, each one 'generative' of its own life-force, operating together. The individual atoms of the heart (or brain, for some) had the additional attribute (here, read: function) of intellect (*ʿaql*), through which conscious thought, reflection

---

[126] Abū al-Ḥasan al-Ashʿarī was the founder one of the two Sunnī 'Orthodox' schools of Islamic theology or *kalām*. A tenth century scholar, he was deeply influenced firstly by the Muʿtazilī rationalist school of al-Jubbāʾī (d. *ca.* 915), and then by the luminaries of the traditionalist *ḥadīth* movement such as Ibn Ḥanbal (d. 241/855), eventually developing a synthesis that became mainstream Sunnī orthodoxy.

[127] Shihadeh (2012a): 445.

[128] Ibid.: 465.

[129] For ease of understanding, Ashʿarī notions of occasionalism (and hence strict material noncausality) will be excluded from this discussion. In short, the doctrine is that metaphysically (and possibly methodologically as well) one does not admit any form of necessary causality except the independent Will of God. Nothing other than God causes anything to occur, and there is no such thing as natural law. All apparent cause and effect is merely that – empirical observation of correlation that is (at best) regular enough to be considered 'effective causality,' but which cannot ever be proven. This is a remarkably Humean notion that has been modified somewhat by various thinkers, but operates best at a metaphysical (or quantum) level rather than at a methodological one. Indeed, even in the general word-usage of the Ashʿarī theologians, 'normal' causal efficacy is taken for granted; for example, the description of the soul as 'that which imparts life to the body.'

and contemplation could occur. Additionally, the notion of human exceptionalism as being a consequence of his '*binya*' (particular and unique bodily structure), rather than the soul per se, would appear, at first glance, to dovetail well into similar modern notions about human genetics and epigenetics as being that which sets them apart from other living organisms.

The primary problem identified with this approach historically, however, was exactly the same as noted earlier with the materialist reductive approach: where does the notion of the subjective, unitary, sentient self fit into this picture? The nature of man, in this Ashʿarī framework, is ontologically fragmentary,[130] and its conceptualization of the spirit as 'just another bit somewhere' exacerbates rather than ameliorates this fragmentation.

As is the case with a number of central Ashʿarī doctrines, the focus on elucidating and promulgating a cohesive and totalizing approach to the Divine nature tends to leave the nature of man somewhat stuck epistemically. In other words, because both the Divine and human nature were being discussed within the same ontological framework, a theocentric explanatory system would always give priority to Divine unity, even if it rendered the account of man's nature somewhat unsatisfactory.[131] This became such a fundamental problem that the notion appears to have effectively been discarded during the sixth/twelfth century in favour of the Ghazālian or Rāzian synergistic approach.[132]

### 7.3.14 *Ibn Sīnā's Dualist Perspective of the Soul*

The most influential and far-reaching contribution to the question of the human self in Islamic theology was undoubtedly that of the tenth century polymath and philosopher *par excellence*, Ibn Sīnā,[133] who was also one of the most influential medical theorists in history. His writings on the subject are wide-ranging and well documented elsewhere; nonetheless a relatively (compared to other theoreticians) detailed view will be presented here, primarily because his account was so influential for later Islamic thought.[134]

---

[130] Indeed, neither man nor anything other than God is considered to be 'one' in a metaphysical sense, but only in a conventional one. See al-Qushayrī (1968), 78.

[131] Shihadeh (2012a): 475.

[132] The reasons for and mechanisms behind this momentous and stark fundamental shift in theological anthropology are poorly understood, but may have something to do with the emergence – via celebrated orthodox scholars like al-Ghazālī and (even more so) Fakhr al-Dīn al-Rāzī – of a cogent alternative that preserved the unitary nature of man without compromising the necessarily unitary nature of God. See also, al-Akiti (2009), 51–100.

[133] Unquestionably the most famous Islamic philosopher, Abū ʿAlī ibn Sīnā (Lat. Avicenna) was perhaps the most influential philosopher of the pre-modern age. He was also a peerless physician whose *al-Qānūn fī al-ṭibb* (*The Canon of Medicine*) was taught for centuries. His unique philosophical system was anthropocentric within a theological context.

[134] Ivry (2012), 12.

He not only developed earlier Platonic theories about the nature of the soul and its relationship to the body, but also made the understanding of the human the lynchpin of his entire philosophical system – this in direct contrast to the previous system, in which the nature of man was an after-thought. By focusing on anthropology – specifically the 'rational soul,' which derives its ability to contemplate abstract intelligibles from the atemporal Active Intellect (*ʿaql al-faʿʿāl*) [135] – he was not only able to systematize a comprehensive, internally coherent explanatory system that incorporated all the classical philosophical sciences as well as traditionally theological topics like revelation, miracles, theodicy and eschatology, but also to expound on the fundamental questions of the origin, nature and purpose of man.

In his well-known thought experiment to illustrate the idea of the self, known as 'the flying/suspended man,' he argued that a person totally deprived of any form of sensory input from the beginning of his existence would still know that he exists. This is because of the rational soul is *a priori* self-aware,[136] requiring nothing external to have this most basic knowledge. This thought experiment prefaced the famous meditation of René Descartes (d. 1650), '*cogito ergo sum*' (I think, therefore I am), by 600 years, and arguably bettered it, because it was used to rationally prove the existence of the self, rather than the existence of God.[137]

From the Avicennan perspective, the rational soul – as possessed uniquely by man – is the ultimate purpose of the creation. It is created by God via the celestial intellects as an immortal, immaterial, 'simple' substance that individuates upon its instantiation (or ensoulment) into a particular body. It is a self-subsistent, immaterial entity that is thus associated with the human body and which comes into existence along with it, but is neither imprinted in nor dependent upon it. It is pure consciousness, attributed primarily with direct unmediated knowledge of itself (*ʿilm al-ḥuḍūrī*).[138]

Crucially, this intellect is entirely distinct from the 'lower' aspects of the soul, such as the life-force enabling growth, movement and basic perception that – as noted earlier – is common to all living beings, but also from the imaginative faculty shared by animals and humans. The crucial distinction, for Ibn Sīnā, with the rational soul was in its origin (from the metaphysical rather than material), its nature (a simple rather than material substance, deriving knowledge not from sense experience but directly from the Active Intellect), and its purpose (to perceive, *in imitatio Dei*, universals and abstract intelligibles: the pure atemporal theoretical sciences of mathematics and metaphysics).[139]

By doing so, it would achieve the classical Aristotelian goal of *eudaimonia* – human flourishing, or moral and spiritual contentment. The rational soul has two functions: one primary – the fulfilment of theoretical wisdom through

[135] The lowest of the ten emanations of the celestial spheres. Latin scholastics translated this as *intellectus agens*. Apart from 'Active Intellect,' it can also be translated as: agent intellect, active intelligence, active reason, or even productive intellect.

[136] That is, it is its very nature to be aware of itself, this is not something it learns after the fact.

[137] Marmura (1986): 383.

[138] Aminrazavi (2003).

[139] Gutas (2012): 417–8.

contemplation of the intelligibles, and one secondary – the fulfilment of practical wisdom through making moral, rational choices. As such, the rational soul serves as the conduit between the material world, navigated via the practical philosophies such as ethics, and the metaphysical world, navigated via the theoretical philosophies such as ontology. From here, Ibn Sīnā develops a thoroughly rationalistic account of the human soul and its place in the cosmos, delivering a powerful integrated vision of the nature of the universe and man's place within it.[140]

Compellingly, and perhaps understandably given his medical background, he also promulgates an account of developmental psychology through the development of human physiology. The entirety of the human soul, then, is the animating life-force, which is divided into vegetative, animal and rational aspects. The vegetative relates to tasks such as growth, digestion, and so forth, whilst the animal aspect accounts for the mechanism of volition: external sense perception, volition, and the five 'inner senses': common sense (*ḥiss mushtarak*),[141] imagination (*khayāl*),[142] the imaginative/cogitative power (*quwwa mufakkira*),[143] estimation (*wahm*),[144] and memory (*ḥāfiẓa*).[145]

The theory of the five internal senses (*al-ḥawāss al-bāṭina*) mark a major development of the psychology espoused by Aristotle (d. 322 BC), specifically his concept of *phantasia*, and strongly influenced later philosophers.[146] This aspect of living beings is shared to a certain extent by other animals, and is physically located by Ibn Sīnā – following Aristotle and Galen (d. 216) – in the subsequent ventricles of the brain.[147] It is, as noted, with the rational, transcendent aspect of the soul that the human is truly distinguished from other orders of creation. In this, Ibn Sīnā intriguingly prefaces modern discussions in neuroscience, which distinguish between 'lower-order consciousness' – the ability to construct a mental scene with limited semantic or symbolic content, and higher-order consciousness, which is accompanied by a sense of the self and the ability to construct the past and future, as well as developed language.[148]

Ibn Sīnā's account, unifying, powerful and rational, provides a truly thoroughgoing disquisition of the nature of the human entity. It explicates the origin, nature

[140] Hall (2004), 62–86; cf. Gutas (2012), 425.

[141] The internal combination of the information from the external senses to create subjective perception.

[142] The faculty allowing retention of the perceptions of the common sense once their object is no longer perceptible – hence an aspect of memory and recall.

[143] The ability to compare and modify the stored forms, hence the cogitative faculty, which Ibn Sīnā considered to be possessed of by animals as well, though functioning only imaginatively in them, rather than rationally, as in humans.

[144] The ability to give salience to one or other, hence to discriminate the harmful from the beneficial. Both Ibn Sīnā and al-Ghazālī link this to the affective component of the human.

[145] The storing of the conclusions of the estimative judgments of the *wahm* ready for recall.

[146] Black (1993): 219–258.

[147] Ivry (2012), 14–15.

[148] Edelman and Tononi (2000), 110.

and purpose of the subjective human self – further making it the centrepiece of a totalizing 'theory of everything' – as well as clearly locating the perceptive, volitional and motor aspects of living beings within the brain. It not only connects the subjective, unitary aspect of the human entity to its bodily form as well as the world around it, via the mechanisms of the vegetative and animal aspects of the soul respectively, but to metaphysical reality via the rational soul.

Ibn Sīnā also wrote relatively extensively about the neurological basis of mental illnesses such as anxiety, mania, melancholia and psychosis on the basis of his widely-accepted medical theories. Although some of his ideas would naturally require modern updates, he provides ample scope for overlap between the medical approach to the mind and a religiously informed one.

There would appear to be two major issues with his approach. The first is his separation of the imaginative faculties and the intellectual ones – necessitated by the rather Platonic need to keep the immaterial soul purified from the 'corruption' of bodily form. The second is his overarching account of metaphysical reality; if the purpose of the soul is merely to perceive the realities of mathematics and metaphysics – that is to say: the universe – the Divine fits into the picture only indirectly and tangentially. From a unitary perspective as well as a religious one, this is somewhat unsatisfying – why should the soul find beatitude in the perception of abstractions?

### *7.3.15 A Ghazālian Compromise and the 'Orthodoxification' of Dualism*

Despite its clear precedence in classical Greek thought, Ibn Sīnā's powerful account deeply influenced Muslim understandings of the nature of the human afterwards. This is primarily manifested in al-Ghazālī and Fakhr al-Dīn al-Rāzī, notwithstanding their severe critiques of Ibn Sīnā and the latter's differences with the former.[149] These two widely-accepted orthodox scholars of Sunnī Islam are generally considered to be Ashʿarī theologians; both of them, however, are more accurately identified as founders of the tradition of philosophical theology in Islam.[150] For the purposes of this chapter, only al-Ghazālī's additional contributions – directed primarily towards the second critique of Ibn Sīnā above, will be addressed.

Al-Ghazālī is perhaps the paragon syncretic Muslim thinker: widely read across intellectual disciplines, careful and critical in his approach, but willing to fully understand ideas from outside his technical purview and incorporate those which were not entirely contradictory of traditional approaches to scripture and religious teachings. He was, however, not merely a transmitter of sciences; al-Ghazālī was

---

[149] Shihadeh (2005): 141–179. For al-Ghazālī, in particular, see al-Akiti (2009), 60–83.

[150] That is, primarily traditional theologians, but deeply influenced by Muslim Peripatetic philosophy. This is as opposed to Ibn Rushd (Lat. Averroes; d. 595/1198), for example, who was a theologically-influenced philosopher. See al-Akiti (2009), 91–6.

highly creative not simply when it came to original ideas or theories, but in terms of improving the approaches of others and synthesizing them into a greater theological venture. As Tzvi Langermann puts it in his succinct account of our earlier study of al-Ghazālī's technique of borrowing from the Greek-inspired Avicennan scientific tradition: 'al-Akiti detects, uncovers, and displays three levels of writing in al-Ghazālī's approach to *falsafa* (Hellenistic philosophy), particularly as formulated for the Muslim public by Ibn Sīnā. He presents this philosophy as ugly in his *Maqāṣid* (*Intentions of the Philosophers*): it appears ugly because he includes without comment teachings that are clearly unacceptable. However, in his *Tahāfut* (*Incoherence of the Philosophers*), this same philosophy is presented as merely bad: specific faults are identified and criticized. Finally, in the corpus of texts known as the *Maḍnūn* (*Restricted*), philosophy is seen to be good; sound philosophical doctrines are exploited in order to formulate key Muslim beliefs. Al-Ghazālī's project allows him to present a coherent explanation of the world, expressed in traditional terms, whose rationale derives from Avicennan science and philosophy; but he is also able to articulate the traditional, orthodox faith in philosophical terms. The differences in presentation between the good, the bad, and the ugly often amount, as al-Akiti amply demonstrates, to nothing more than the addition or excision of a single word or phrase. In doing so, al-Ghazālī puts into practice a dictum attributed to ʿAlī (d. 40/661), the Prophet's nephew, which states that the true and the false can be very similar indeed, just like the venom of a snake so closely resembles its antidote.'[151]

Additionally, however, al-Ghazālī very clearly wrote over an extended period of time during which his views on a number of discussions shifted, but also for different audiences.[152] All this has led to understandable complaints that al-Ghazālī's actual position on a number of matters is difficult to pin down.[153]

A paradigm case for this is al-Ghazālī's treatment of Ibn Sīnā's anthropology,[154] and subsequent addressing of our primary question: what is the self, and what is its purpose? This, one might argue, was the primary focus of most of al-Ghazālī's later oeuvre, though he dealt with it from the highly pragmatic perspective of a spiritual master rather than the abstract approach of a philosopher.[155] Rather frustratingly, however, he does not in any work openly attributed to him provide a thorough-going

[151] Langermann (2009), viii–ix.

[152] A major philosophical collection of written texts attributed to him is literally entitled 'That Which Should Be Restricted from Those Incapable of Understanding It,' (*al-Maḍnūn bi-hi ʿalā ghayr ahli-hi*), or simply, the *Restricted Corpus*, which al-Akiti identifies as al-Ghazālī's authentic work and basis for the allusions (*talwīḥāt*) and references to *ʿilm al-mukāshafa* – the unveiling of metaphysical reality – found scattered throughout his *magnum opus*, the *Iḥyāʾ*. See al-Akiti (2009), 52 and 84–90. For a description and catalogue of the *Maḍnūn* corpus itself, see al-Akiti (2008).

[153] Marmura (2005), 273–99.

[154] Shihadeh (2016), 2:126.

[155] Karamustafa (2007).

account of the nature and purpose of the human soul.[156] Instead, more or less fragmentary discussions are scattered throughout his works, including the *Iḥyāʾ* (most thoroughly in Book XXI of the *Iḥyāʾ*, entitled, *Sharḥ ajāʾib al-qalb* [Explaining the Wonders of the Heart], which Richard J. McCarthy calls 'peak Ghazālī'),[157] the *Munqidh min al-ḍalāl* (*The Deliverance from Error*; where much insight can be found in his entirely original 'spectrum-theory' of *ilhām*),[158] and his oft-overlooked *Maqṣad al-asnā fī sharḥ asmāʾ Allāh al-ḥusnā* (*The Best Means in Explaining God's Beautiful Names*), where one finds the seeds of a comprehensive explanation of existence by means of the Divine Names, such as is later more fully developed by the famous Ṣūfī, Ibn al-ʿArabī (d. 638/1240), and the modern Turkish thinker, Said Nursi.

Despite not-inconsiderable controversy, largely due to his allusive (and even evasive) style of writing on this issue, it seems clear to most that al-Ghazālī appropriated the Avicennan theory of selfhood virtually in its entirety.[159] This, of course, would entail a decisive break with Ashʿarī monist notions of the soul and a strictly physicalist view of reality. The points at which al-Ghazālī differs from Ibn Sīnā, however, are absolutely fundamental. According to Taneli Kukkonen, al-Ghazālī categorically rejects Ibn Sīnā's '*mabdaʾ wa-l-maʿād*' (beginning and end point) – that is to say, his views on the Divine nature, the underlying metaphysical structure of reality, and soteriology.[160] From al-Ghazālī's much more orthodoxy-grounded perspective, Ibn Sīnā's ideas about aspects of these are not merely incompatible with Muslim belief but also logically incoherent, and it is on these three points that he charges his predecessor with disbelief.

A potted summary of the Ghazālian perspective, which eventually became the foundation for Muslim theology thenceforth, might run as follows. Creation exists in hierarchical form: the sensible world or the material dimension (*mulk*) being the lowest and corresponding with the three-dimensional material reality accessible to the senses; beyond that is the immaterial dimension (*malakūt*); and beyond that is the atemporal

[156] Gianotti (2001). There is, however, one dedicated manual on the soul attributed to al-Ghazālī, namely the *Maʿārij al-quds fī madārij maʿrifat al-nafs* (*The Ascent to the Divine Through the Degrees of Knowing the Soul*), which certainly deserves further study. Al-Akiti identifies this as a work belonging to al-Ghazālī's *Restricted Corpus*, see al-Akiti (2009), 55 n. 13. For a flavour of the discussion of the soul in the *Maʿārij*, see al-Akiti (2004), 189–212.

[157] Al-Ghazālī (1999), 309.

[158] For an analysis of *ilhām* as found in the *Munqidh* and its apparent provenance from the *Maʿārij*, see al-Akiti (2004), 197–200.

[159] Al-Akiti (2009) observes: 'One reason why al-Ghazālī finds Ibn Sīnā so attractive that he ends up becoming his favourite *falsafī* author is that Ibn Sīnā's writings did present the best unified general system of scientific thought that included psychology … Indeed, al-Ghazālī was himself one such systematizer, and probably the first from the religious community to recognize and attend to this successful synthesis. He, in turn, did what his predecessor did, but this time integrated Avicennan psychological theory fully into a religious framework and, indeed, crowned it there. It is thus not surprising that we find that the *De Anima* tradition [of Aristotle] is transmitted effectively through *kitāb* [Book] XXI of the *Iḥyāʾ*… which in turn, not only prefaces the *akhlāq* [ethical] books of the *Iḥyāʾ*, but forms the theoretical basis for the philosophical ethics embedded in those books' (56-5 n. 15). On the subsequent controversy arising from this Ghazālian synthesis, see, for example, ibid., 90–1.

[160] Kukkonen (2012): 542.

dimension or the plane of the Divine attributes (*jabarūt*).[161] These latter two are effectively higher-dimensional realities, so to speak, as they overlay the material dimension. The act of creation (*al-khalq wa-l-amr*) 'commences' in the atemporal dimension, which instantiates a particular manifestation of God's attributes in the immaterial dimension, which in turn instantiates (or mirrors) a manifestation in the material dimension.

The *qalb* (heart), which in (often-misunderstood) Ghazālian parlance signifies not the muscular pump but the true reality of the human self (*ḥaqīqat rūḥi-hi*) and which is the locus for knowledge of the Divine, is from the immaterial dimension.[162] Ensoulment, or *nafkh al-rūḥ*, is not necessarily about 'becoming alive,' but about the instantiation of this true human reality within the body, with the accompanying individuation.

This human reality is intrinsically connected to the body, through which it develops in stages (*aṭwār*): first vegetative, then animal aspects, culminating in discernment and then intellection. The former allows it to interact with the world, and the latter with abstract realities. However, neither of these are its primary purpose. Al-Ghazālī coins a neologism: *quwwa qudsiyya*, the (largely passive) divine, holy or spiritual faculty,[163] which is a level of perception and understanding beyond that of the intellect, and relates to the immaterial and atemporal dimensions. It is through this divine faculty that the human achieves their ultimate purpose: to know, contemplate and – most crucially – perceive their Lord.

This human spirituo-intellectual reality, as a mirror impressed with the innate capacity to understand universals but more so the potential to discern the ineffable Creator, may be freely gifted the awakening of this divine faculty. However, in order to acquire this, it is required to polish the mirror to preserve it from the rust of the lower, instinctual self (possibly the result of the soul's encounter with bodily needs and carnal desires of this world). This is accomplished through *jihād al-nafs* as well as contemplation of the external world.[164]

Through this approach, al-Ghazālī adopts the vast majority of Ibn Sīnā's systematic theory of the soul, whilst stripping it of its overtly Hellenistic terminology and synthesizing it thoroughly with Islamic scriptural theology and the nascent field of Ṣūfī experiential metaphysics.[165] The mechanics of the interplay between body and soul remain largely Avicennan; what is dramatically altered is the idea of a multidimensional view of reality and the nature and purpose of the human self within it.

As the soul relates to the higher levels of existence via the higher cognitive functioning of the brain, it both perceives (consciously or not) specific instantiations of

[161] In some works, al-Ghazālī cites the *jabarūt* as being the intermediary between the *mulk* and the *malakūt*, see Kukkonen (2012), 558. The original order is generally the approach taken in post-classical Ṣūfī works, though.

[162] Al-Ghazālī (2013), 126.

[163] Kukkonen (2012): 544.

[164] Ibid., 557.

[165] This two-stage Ghazālian editorial process, one of 'appropriation' – critically adopting scientific materials from Ibn Sīnā – and the subsequent 'naturalization' stage – adapting them to suit his own theological project, by employing religious idioms and allusions (*talwīḥāt*), is described in al-Akiti (2009), 62 n. 25.

the Divine attributes and can develop so as to more perfectly perceive those same instantiations in higher dimensions of existence, ultimately attaining perfect perception of the Ultimate Reality that is God,[166] which may be apprehended as joy, dread, awe or reverence.[167]

Inherent within the soul are the tools with which to do so: an active rational faculty (*quwwa ʿaqliyya*), and a passive divine or spiritually perceptive faculty (*quwwa qudsiyya*) – though this may only be awakened by an act of Divine grace – to the extent that God permits. The ultimate life-purpose of the reflective, self-aware human soul (the *ʿaql/qalb/nafs/rūḥ*), therefore, is to make the only true moral choice: the conscious decision to remove potential barriers to this perception. It achieves this by cultivation of the virtue ethic approach, as most systematically promulgated through the *Iḥyāʾ*, in order to remove qualities that muddy clear spiritual perception and acquire ones that clarify it.

This, in turn, is perception and acquisition of true (metaphysical) benefit and harm, thus instantiating the most fundamental markers of life itself, but in the highest and most perfect form. This is to sense, choose and act on that which is truly destructive (because it leads to non-fulfilment of the purpose of the immortal soul) and salvific (because it facilitates its fulfilment).

Further, the *Iḥyāʾ* is neatly divided into a first-half section that deals with human action in the external world, and the last-half section that deals directly with these harmful and beneficial qualities themselves. This is because, by virtue of the embodiment of the human self, mental dispositions manifest as action. They are operative relationally, both in respect to the human interaction with God, and their interaction with the created universe – hence the first half of the *Iḥyāʾ* is itself divided into two halves: the first dealing with the human self's relationship with God, and the second dealing with their relationship with creation. Key to understanding the body-soul construct in Islam is to recognize that each is affected by the other: harmful actions are not just manifestations of a polluted soul, but themselves pollute the mirror of the soul. Those actions reflective of (or engendering) harmful qualities which hinder the human capacity to know God are deemed blameworthy (*madhmūma*); their opposites are deemed praiseworthy (*maḥmūda*).

The relationship between external action and internal state is thus a mutual feedback loop – which is strongly reflective of the relationship between the neuroplastic brain and words/actions. The human soul needs to be embodied, because without this, it can neither acquire nor reflect those salvific qualities required to fulfil its purpose of perceiving God.

---

[166] Kukkonen (2012): 558.

[167] Al-Ghazālī (2003), 199.

## *7.3.16 What is the Nature and Purpose of the Self?*

Drawing together both scientific and classical Islamic theories of the subjective self, then, we believe it is possible to attempt a non-contradictory and satisfactory answer to the descriptive, explanatory and functional questions of consciousness. The scientific approach finds accounting for the nature of the self problematic, and is largely silent on its purpose; the religious approach is largely silent or out-of-date on the mechanics of mind-body interactivity. It is at the mingling of the waters of science and religion, then, that the answer may be found, provided one abandons an *a priori* commitment to metaphysical naturalism.

The **soul** (*rūḥ*) is the primordial human reality, or pure consciousness: a metaphysical instantiation of the *amr Allāh* – a Divine charge designed for no less a purpose than knowing its Creator. Given what we now know of the neuroscientific theories of self, we believe that one can validly argue, within an Islamic context, that the soul-as-consciousness instantiates at ensoulment[168] via emergence upon the brain of the human as **mind** (*ʿaql*), initially as primary self-awareness. This soul-as-mind is a functional rather than substantive entity (an attribute rather than a substance), arising possibly as per the dynamic core hypothesis (discussed above in Sect. 7.3.9). Soul, mind and body (more specificially, the nervous system) together comprise the integrative **self** (*nafs*). As it receives sensory inputs, it develops both lower-order and higher-order self-consciousness, as well as reflexive consciousness of that which is other than itself: external creation.

As expressed in the previous section, that creation is itself the manifesting of God's perfection: it is the effect of the Divine act of creating, which arises from the Names of God, which point to His entity. The entirety of the material dimension or, the sensible world, is thus the expression of God's attributes of absolute rigor (*jalāl*) and absolute beauty (*jamāl*), which together combine to make immanent (*tashbīh*) God's transcendence (*tanzīh*). To perceive the material, then metaphysical, levels of creation is thus to perceive God's *jalāl* and *jamāl* with increasing *tanzīh* as one filters out the material substrate of the material dimension, then the immaterial dimension, then the atemporal dimension. This filtration is an ethico-spiritual endeavour – the act of purifying the soul of the qualities that hinder clear perception, so as to arrive ultimately at *mukāshafa* – the unveiling of metaphysical reality.

In order to facilitate this perception of God's perfection, the subjective human self has thus been afforded a number of faculties according to the Muslim tradition:

- First, by mere virtue of the soul being embodied and possessed of a nervous system (i.e., being alive), it is possessed of the capacity to instinctually perceive benefit and harm.

168 The famous *ḥadīth* of Ibn Masʿūd (d. 32/653) concerning the foetus can be read to temporally locate ensoulment at around 40 days or 6 weeks – the exact time that both the nervous and circulatory systems begin to function. For the Muslim theological argument of this position, see Chap. 6, 'When Does a Human Foetus Become Human?' by Hamza Yusuf in this book.

- Next, by virtue of the complex neuroendocrine feedback pathways of the mid-brain, this instinctual perception is experienced as emotions: primarily 'fear' and 'desire,'[169] but also every other 'secondary' emotion that arises from them.[170]
- Then next, by virtue of the rational capability,[171] mediated through the higher cognitive structures and functions of the brain, the soul is capable of perceiving this benefit and harm through the prism of space and time, and so to abstract their universal meanings beyond particular instantiations, including but not limited to ethical abstractions (so here, benefit as 'good' and harm as 'evil').
- And finally, by virtue of the awakened divine or spiritual faculty,[172] the highest instantiations of human contemplative emotion – themselves products of the benefit/harm instinct – are manifested in response to the highest abstractions of true, unitary, metaphysical benefit and harm: the attributes of both absolute gentleness and absolute rigour of God.

The highest manifestation of fear, then, is **awe**: the response to God's *jalāl*. The highest manifestation of desire is **love**: the response to God's *jamāl*. The highest manifestation of abstract thought, found at the utterest limits of its capacity, is **bewilderment**: the response to God's *tanzīh*. The highest and most transcendent experience of awe, love and bewilderment is precisely the spiritual experience of the utterly overwhelming Divine presence. It is witnessed by means of fear and desire (at its most basic, instinctual level of the self) and reason (at its most highest, sublime level of the self), but mediated through the divine or spiritual faculty, either directly or through the prism of God's instantiation in creation.

This is the true purpose of the self: to be alive, and to be human, is to have the unique capacity to experience Ultimate Reality. All this, in turn, is summarized in the *shahāda* of Islam: an acceptance of absolute metaphysical reality (*there is none truly worshipped but God*) and an acceptance of the means by which it may be perceived and attained (*Muhammad is the Messenger of God*).

### *7.3.17 Mind, Soul and Brain*

The reason, then, for the (seemingly excessive) complexity of the brain is precisely in order to permit this 'higher order' intellectuo-spiritual functioning. As the purpose of all life is fundamentally theocentric – to recognize and adore God – rather

[169] This is the *quwwat al-shahwa* (desire) and the *quwwat al-ghaḍab* (irascible) at its most basic, instinctual level of the *nafs*.

[170] The concept of altruism – the perception of 'fear' and 'desire' on behalf of others and acting upon them – thus the emotional capacity of the human to experience and instantiate 'mercy,' is absolutely critical to a full understanding of human nature, experience and potential, but unfortunately beyond the scope of this chapter.

[171] The *quwwat al-ʿaql*.

[172] The *quwwat al-qudsiyya*.

than merely survive and reproduce, the purpose of the subjective human self is to accomplish this in the most perfect way possible. The human being needs everything that an animal requires to maintain life (hence all the lower-order cognitive functions of the 'inner senses' as described above in Sect. 7.3.14), as well as to be capable of intellection, in order to contemplate abstractions, which in turn can proceed to the 'spiritual' contemplation of the highest metaphysical realities.

In this way, the materialist theory of the self is thus turned on its head. Rather than the brain requiring – and thus creating – the illusion of selfhood in order to make sense of its innate complexity, the unitary self is provided with a brain precisely as complex as it needs to be in order to permit perception. In other words, the soul, in order to fulfil its primary purpose of knowing and perceiving Ultimate Reality (God), requires both embodiment and the capacity to intellect. The whole of human physiology is thus effectively to support life whilst this purpose is being fulfilled. The complexity of the neural connectome – way beyond what is required to merely sustain biological life – is a requirement for the human entity because its purpose is not merely to survive and reproduce. Rather, to fulfil its true purpose of metaphysical perception, the brain's structure and neural functioning need to be capable of processing both abstract intellection and to have the potential of unlocking transcendent spiritual and religious experiences (which also appear to be mediated through neural centres).

## 7.4 Conclusion

A mental disorder may be defined variously in the field of psychiatry as the absence of health, the presence of suffering, a pathological process, or disturbance of functioning.[173] From a holistic Islamic perspective, however, we would venture to define it thusly: a disorder of perception, consciousness and intentionality – understood as that which impedes any of the primary, secondary and tertiary purposes of the self: to perceive and know God (spiritual experience), to recognize and adopt those stable mental dispositions (or traits) which facilitate that experience, and to navigate the material world in such a way as to engender and encourage – via ethical action – development of those traits, and to remain safe whilst this is being undertaken. In other words, preservation and facilitation of religion, intellect and life/health: three of the primary purposes of Divine Law (*maqāṣid al-sharīʿa*).

An integrative Islamic approach to psychology, therefore, cannot be divorced either from metaphysics or ethics, and it would be most accurately designated as metaphysical psycho-ethics. Mental illnesses such as psychosis, within this framework, would be viewed as invariably harmful disorders, because they hinder the necessary mental function of accurate perception, and may effect actions harmful to the self, either directly (through harm to self) or indirectly (through harm to others),[174] materially or metaphysically. Conditions such as depression or anxiety, on the other hand, might either be construed as disorders of brain functioning (i.e., damage to the apparatus of perception/volition) or disorders of 'soul' functioning

[173] Gelder, Mayou, and Cowen (2001), 87–88.

[174] From an Islamic theological perspective, therefore, harming others is considered metaphysically harming the self.

(instantiations of mental dispositions that hinder the soul's capacity to experience God). Both of these manifest or crystallize in the subjective human experience (i.e., the mind).

This, however, would need to be carefully ascertained within a clear framework. An apparently negative emotion like sorrow is not necessarily a spiritually harmful experience: a person's sorrow might actually be positive – a means for them to have an experience of God's rigour followed by the feeling of relief that is an experience of God's kindness. This is where the Islamic psychotherapist (traditionally the Ṣūfī master) would come to the fore: diagnosing the precise nature and consequence of an episode in a person's interior life, distinguishing between a biological malfunction and the higher order spiritual one.

In sum, examining the concept of a 'mental illness' – the stock-in-trade of the naturalistic sciences of medicine and psychiatry – brings to the fore the fundamental underpinnings of not only health, but the very nature of life and self. Yet it is through religion, not science, that these most fundamental questions find an answer. Yes, one needs to choose whether to accept the underlying assumptions of either religion or science – metaphysical idealism or naturalism – but one must also accept that the latter leads to an explanatory dead-end, whilst the former provides a way forward. At the same time, religionists need to recognize that the sciences of medicine, cognitive neuroscience and even psychiatry provide essential understandings of the mechanistic processes through which body and soul might interact and find fulfilment in each other.

In dogged pursuit of the conceptual bases of psychiatry, then, the traveller invariably arrives at the shores of metaphysics, calling out: what is reality, what is life, and what does it mean to be human? And in answer, Islam replies: reality is the manifestation of the Divine splendour, life is the opportunity to experience it, and the purified human soul is the locus of its ultimate fulfilment.

> *He released the two oceans. They meet. Yet there is a barrier between them they do not cross. Which, then, of your Lord's blessings do you both deny? Pearls and corals come forth from them. Which, then, of your Lord's blessings do you both deny?*[175]

## References


Abū Dā'ūd Sulaymān ibn al-Ash'ath. 2009. *Sunan Abī Dāwūd*, eds. Shu'ayb al-Arna'ūṭ, Muḥammad Kāmil Qarah Balilī, and 'Abd al-Laṭīf Ḥirz Allāh. 7 vols. Beirut: Dār al-Risāla al-'Ālamiyya

'Abd al-Ḥamīd, Ibrāhīm Shawqī, Muḥammad 'Uthmān Najātī, and 'Abd al-Ḥalīm Maḥmūd al-Sayyid. *'Ilm al-nafs fī al-turāth al-Islāmī*. 3 vols. Cairo: Dār al-Salām, 2008.

al-Akiti, Afifi. 2004. 'The Three Properties of Prophethood in Certain Works of Avicenna and al-Ġazālī.' In *Interpreting Avicenna: Science and Philosophy in Medieval Islam*, eds. Jon


[175] Qur'an 55:19–23 (*al-Raḥmān*).

McGinnis and David C. Reisman. Islamic Philosophy, Theology and Science: Texts and Studies, eds. Hans Daiber and David Pingree, no. 56. Leiden: Brill.

———. 2008. 'The *Maḍnūn* of al-Ghazālī: A Critical Edition of the Unpublished *Major Maḍnūn* with Discussion of His Restricted, Philosophical Corpus.' 3 vols. DPhil diss., University of Oxford.

———. 2009. 'The Good, the Bad, and the Ugly of *Falsafa*: Al-Ghazālī's *Maḍnūn*, *Tahāfut*, and *Maqāṣid*, with Particular Attention to Their *Falsafī* Treatments of God's Knowledge of Temporal Events.' In *Avicenna and His Legacy: A Golden Age of Science and Philosophy*, ed. Y. Tzvi Langermann. Cultural Encounters in Late Antiquity and the Middle Ages, no. 8. Turnhout: Brepols.

al-Ālūsī. 2005. *Rūḥ al-maʿānī fī tafsīr al-Qurʾān al-ʿAẓīm wa-al-sabʿ al-mathānī*, eds. al-Sayyid Muḥammad Sayyid and Sayyid ʿUmrān. 30 vols. Cairo: Dār al-Hadīth.

Aminrazavi, Mehdi. 2003. 'Avicenna's (Ibn Sīnā) Phenomenological Analysis of How the Soul (*Nafs*) Knows Itself (*ʿIlm Al-Ḥuḍūrī*).' In *The Passions of the Soul in the Metamorphosis of Becoming*, ed. Anna-Teresa Tymieniecka. Islamic Philosophy and Occidental Phenomenology in Dialogue, no. 1. Dordrecht: Kluwer.

Andreasen, Nancy C. 1997. 'Linking Mind and Brain in the Study of Mental Illnesses: A Project for a Scientific Psychopathology.' *Science* 275 (5306): 1586–1593.

———. 2001. *Brave New Brain: Conquering Mental Illness in the Era of the Genome*. New York, NY: Oxford University Press.

Ayer, A. J. 1936. *Language, Truth and Logic*. London: Victor Gollancz.

al-Bājūrī, Ibrāhīm. 1423/2002. *Tuḥfat al-murīd ʿalā Jawhar al-tawḥīd.* Damascus: Dār al-Bayrūtī.

Batterman, Robert W. 2009. 'Emergence in Physics.' In *Routledge Encyclopedia of Philosophy Online*, ed. Edward Craig. Available at https://www.rep.routledge.com/articles/thematic/emergence-in-physics/v-1

Beauchamp, Tom L., and James F. Childress. 2012. *Principles of Biomedical Ethics*. 7th ed. Oxford: Oxford University Press.

Black, Deborah L. 1993. 'Estimation (*Wahm*) in Avicenna: The Logical and Psychological Dimensions.' *Dialogue* 32 (2): 219–258.

Black, Kevin J. 2005. 'Psychiatry and the Medical Model.' In *Adult Psychiatry*, eds. Eugene H. Rubin and Charles F. Zorumski. 2nd ed. Blackwell's Neurology and Psychiatry Access Series, ed. Ronald B. David. Malden, MA: Blackwell.

Boorse, Christopher. 1997. 'A Rebuttal on Health.' In *What Is Disease?*, eds. James M. Humber and Robert F. Almeder. Totowa, NJ: Humana Press.

al-Bukhārī. 1422/2001. *Ṣaḥīḥ al-Imām al-Bukhārī al-musammá al-Jāmiʿ al-musnad al-ṣaḥīḥ al-mukhtaṣar min umūr Rasūl Allāh wa-sunanihi wa-ayyāmih*, ed. Muḥammad Zuhayr ibn Nāṣir al-Nāṣir (the Sulṭāniyya edition). 9 vols. Beirut: Dār Ṭawq al-Najāh.

Canguilhem, Georges. 1991. *The Normal and the Pathological*, trans. Carolyn R. Fawcett. New York, NY: Zone Books.

Chalmers, David J. 1995. 'Facing Up to the Problem of Consciousness.' *Journal of Consciousness Studies* 2 (3): 200–219.

Cleland, Carol E., and Christopher F. Chyba. 2002. 'Defining Life.' *Origins of Life and Evolution of the Biosphere* 32 (4): 387–393.

Davies, Martin, and Max Coltheart. 2000. 'Pathologies of Belief.' *Mind and Language* 15 (1): 1–46.

Dawkins, Richard. 2016. *The Selfish Gene: 40th Anniversary Edition*. Oxford: Oxford University Press.

de Haan, L., and J. M. Bakker. 2004. 'Overview of Neuropathological Theories of Schizophrenia: From Degeneration to Progressive Developmental Disorder.' *Psychopathology* 37 (1): 1–7.

Edelman, Gerald M., and Giulio Tononi. 2000. *A Universe of Consciousness: How Matter Becomes Imagination*. New York, NY: Basic Books.

al-Fīrūzābādī. 2005. *al-Qāmus al-muḥīṭ*, ed. Muḥammad Naʿīm al-ʿIrqsūsī. Beirut: Muʾassasat al-Risāla.

Fulford, Kenneth W. M. 2001. 'What is (Mental) Disease?: An Open Letter to Christopher Boorse.' *Journal of Medical Ethics* 27 (2): 80–85.

Garcia-Rill, E. 2009. 'Reticular Activating System.' In *Encyclopedia of Neuroscience*, ed. Larry R. Squire. 10 vols. Amsterdam: Elsevier.

Gazzaniga, Michael S., Richard B. Ivry, and George R. Mangun. 2019. *Cognitive Neuroscience: The Biology of the Mind*. 5th ed. London: W. W. Norton.

Gelder, Michael G., Richard Mayou, and Philip Cowen. 2001. *Shorter Oxford Textbook of Psychiatry*. Oxford: Oxford University Press.

al-Ghazālī. 1985. *al-Maqṣad al-asnā fī maʿrifat al-asmāʾ Allāh al-ḥusnā*, ed. Muḥammad ʿUthmān al-Khusht. Cairo: Maktabat al-Qur'ān.

———. 1999. *Deliverance from Error: An Annotated Translation of al-Munqidh min al-Ḍalāl and other relevant works of al-Ghazālī*, trans. Richard Joseph McCarthy. Louisville, KY: Fons Vitae.

———. 2003. *Kitāb al-Arbaʿīn fī uṣūl al-dīn*, eds. ʿAbd Allāh ʿAbd al-Ḥamīd ʿIrwānī and Muḥammad Bashīr al-Shaqafa. Damascus: Dār al-Qalam.

———. 2011. *Iḥyāʾ ʿulūm al-dīn*. 10 vols. Jeddah: Dār al-Minhāj.

———. 2013. *al-Munqidh min al-ḍalāl wa-l-mufṣiḥ bi-l-aḥwāl*. Jeddah: Dār al-Minhāj.

Gianotti, Timothy J. 2001. *Al-Ghazālī's Unspeakable Doctrine of the Soul: Unveiling the Esoteric Psychology and Eschatology of the Iḥyāʾ*. Brill's Studies in Intellectual History, no. 104. Leiden: Brill.

Gilʿadi, Avner. 1989. 'On the Origin of Two Key-Terms in al-Ġazzālī's *Iḥyāʾ ʿUlūm al-Dīn*.' *Arabica* 36 (1): 81–92.

Griffel, Frank. 2009. *Al-Ghazālī's Philosophical Theology*. New York, NY: Oxford University Press.

Gutas, Dimitri. 2012. 'Avicenna: The Metaphysics of the Rational Soul.' *The Muslim World* 102 (3): 417–425.

Guze, Samuel B. 1992. *Why Psychiatry Is a Branch of Medicine*. New York, NY: Oxford University Press.

Hall, Robert E. 2004. 'Intellect, Soul and Body in Ibn Sīnā: Systematic Synthesis and Development of the Aristotelian, Neoplatonic and Galenic Theories.' In *Interpreting Avicenna: Science and Philosophy in Medieval Islam*, eds. Jon McGinnis and David C. Reisman. Islamic Philosophy, Theology and Science: Texts and Studies, eds. Hans Daiber and David Pingree, no. 56. Leiden: Brill.

Harvard Health Publishing. 24 June 2019. 'What Causes Depression?: Onset of Depression More Complex Than a Brain Chemical Imbalance.' Available at https://www.health.harvard.edu/mind-and-mood/what-causes-depression

Hasker, William. 2001. *The Emergent Self*. Ithaca, NY: Cornell University Press.

Hick, John. 1989. *An Interpretation of Religion: Human Responses to the Transcendent*. New Haven, CT: Yale University Press.

Howell, Robert J., and Torin Alter. 2009. 'The Hard Problem of Consciousness.' *Scholarpedia* 4 (6): 4948.

Ibn ʿĀshūr, Muḥammad al-Ṭāhir. 2006. *Treatise on Maqasid al-Shari'ah*, trans. Mohammed El-Tahir El-Mesawi. Washington, DC: International Institute of Islamic Thought.

Ibn Manẓūr. 2003. *Lisān al-ʿĀrab*. 9 vols. Cairo: Dār al-Ḥadīth.

Ivry, Alfred L. 2012. 'Arabic and Islamic Psychology and Philosophy of Mind.' In *The Stanford Encyclopedia of Philosophy*, ed. Edward N. Zalta. Summer 2012 ed. Available at https://plato.stanford.edu/entries/arabic-islamic-mind/

Jeeves, Malcolm, and Warren S. Brown. 2009. *Neuroscience, Psychology and Religion: Illusions, Delusions, and Realities about Human Nature*. Templeton Science and Religion Series. West Conshohocken, PA: Templeton Foundation Press.

Karamustafa, Ahmet T. 2007. *Sufism: The Formative Period*, The New Edinburgh Islamic Surveys, ed. Carole Hillenbrand. Edinburgh: Edinburgh University Press.

King Jr., Martin Luther. 1965. 'The Arc of the Moral Universe Is Long, but It Bends Towards Justice," Our God Is Marching On (How Long, Not Long): 25 March 1965, Montgomery

Alabama, USA.' In *Speekola: All Speeches Great and Small.* Available at: https://speakola.com/ideas/martin-luther-king-jr-how-long-not-long-1965.

Kinghorn, Warren A., Matthew D McEvoy, Andrew Michel, and Michael Balboni. 2007. 'Professionalism in Modern Medicine: Does the Emperor Have Any Clothes?' *Academic Medicine* 82 (1): 40–45.

Klein, Ernest. 1966–67. *A Comprehensive Etymological Dictionary of the English Language: Dealing with the Origins of Words and Their Sense Development Thus Illustrating the History of Civilization and Culture.* 2 vols. Amsterdam: Elsevier.

Koperski, Jeffry. 2015. *The Physics of Theism: God, Physics and the Philosophy of Science.* Oxford: Wiley-Blackwell.

Kraepelin, Emil. 1991. *Psychiatry: A Textbook for Students and Physicians*, ed. Jacques M. Quen, and trans. Helga Metoui and Sabine Ayed. 2 vols. Canton, MA: Science History Publications.

Krakauer, John W., Asif A Ghazanfar, Alex Gomez-Marin, Malcolm A. MacIver, and David Poeppel. 2017. 'Neuroscience Needs Behaviour: Correcting a Reductionist Bias.' *Neuron* 93 (3): 480–490.

Krishnan, Vaishnav, and Eric J. Nestler. 2008. 'The Molecular Neurobiology of Depression.' *Nature* 455 (7215): 894–902.

Kukkonen, Taneli. 2012. 'Receptive to Reality: Al-Ghazālī on the Structure of the Soul.' *The Muslim World* 102 (4): 541–561.

Langermann, Y. Tzvi. 2009. 'Foreword.' In *Avicenna and His Legacy: A Golden Age of Science and Philosophy*, ed. Y. Tzvi Langermann. Cultural Encounters in Late Antiquity and the Middle Ages, no. 8. Turnhout: Brepols.

Lennox, James G. 1995. 'Health as an Objective Value.' *Philosophy of Medicine* 20 (5): 499–511.

Linden, David E. J. 2006. 'How Psychotherapy Changes the Brain: The Contribution of Functional Neuroimaging.' *Molecular Psychiatry* 11 (6): 528–538.

Lockwood, Michael. 2005. *The Labyrinth of Time: Introducing the Universe.* Oxford: Oxford University Press.

Marmura, Michael E. 1986. 'Avicenna's 'Flying Man' in Context.' *The Monist* 69 (3): 383–395.

———. 2005. 'Al-Ghazālī on Bodily Resurrection and Causality in the *Tahāfut* and the *Iqtiṣād*.' In *Probing in Islamic Philosophy: Studies in the Philosophies of Ibn Sīnā, al-Ghazālī and Other Major Muslim Thinkers*, ed. Michael E. Marmura. Binghamton, NY: Global Academic Publishing.

Marr, David. 1982. *Vision: A Computational Investigation into the Human Representation and Processing of Visual Information.* San Francisco, CA: W. H. Freeman.

McGinn, Colin. 1989. 'Can We Solve the Mind-body Problem?' *Mind*, New Series 98 (391): 349–366.

Miles, Andrew. 2009. 'Complexity in Medicine and Healthcare: People and Systems, Theory and Practice.' *Journal of Evaluation in Clinical Practice* 15 (3): 409–410.

Moore, G. E. 1922. *Principia Ethica.* Cambridge: Cambridge University Press.

Murata, Sachiko. 1992. *The Tao of Islam: A Sourcebook of Gender Relationships in Islamic Thought.* Albany, NY: SUNY Press.

Murphy, Dominic 2017. 'Philosophy of Psychiatry.' In *The Stanford Encyclopedia of Philosophy*, ed. Edward N. Zalta. Spring 2017 ed. Available at https://plato.stanford.edu/entries/psychiatry/

National Institute of Mental Health. 'Research Domain Criteria (RDoC).' Available at https://www.nimh.nih.gov/research/research-funded-by-nimh/rdoc/index.shtml.

Nursi, Bediüzzaman Said. 2010. *The Rays: Reflections on Islamic Belief, Thought, Worship and Action*, trans. Hüseyin Akarsu. The Risale-i Nur Collection. Somerset: Tughra Books.

Papineau, David. 2002. *Thinking About Consciousness.* Oxford: Clarendon Press.

Penrose, Roger. 1994. *Shadows of the Mind: A Search for the Missing Science of Consciousness.* Oxford: Oxford University Press.

Petkov, Vesselin. 2009. *Relativity and the Nature of Space time.* 2nd ed. The Frontiers Collection. Dordrecht: Springer.

al-Qushayrī. 1968. *al-Taḥbīr fī al-Tadhkīr*, ed. Ibrāhīm Basyūnī. Cairo: Dār al-Kātib al-ʿArabī.

Reiss, Julian, and Rachel A. Ankeny. 2016. 'Philosophy of Medicine.' In *The Stanford Encyclopedia of Philosophy*, ed. Edward N. Zalta. Summer 2016 ed. Available at https://plato.stanford.edu/archives/sum2016/entries/medicine/

Ibn ʿAbd al-Salām, ʿIzz al-Dīn. 2007. *al-Qawāʿid al-kubrā al-mausūm bi-Qawāʿid al-aḥkām fī iṣlāḥ al-anām*, eds. Nazīh Kamāl Ḥammād and ʿUthmān Jumʿa Ḍumayriyya. 2 vols. Damascus: Dār al-Qalam.

Saunders, Nicholas T. 2000. 'Does God Cheat at Dice?: Divine Action and Quantum Possibilities.' *Zygon* 35 (3): 517–544.

Shihadeh, Ayman. 2005. 'From al-Ghazālī to al-Rāzī: 6th/12th Century Developments in Muslim Philosophical Theology.' *Arabic Sciences and Philosophy* 15 (1): 141–179.

———. 2012a. 'Classical Ashʿarī Anthropology: Body, Life and Spirit.' *The Muslim World* 102 (3): 433–477.

———. 2012b. 'Introduction: The Ontology of the Soul in Medieval Arabic Thought.' *The Muslim World* 102 (3): 413–416.

———. 2016. 'Al-Ghazālī and *Kalām*: The Conundrum of His Body-Soul Dualism.' In *Islam and Rationality: The Impact of al-Ghazālī*, ed. Georges Tamer. 2 vols. Islamic Philosophy, Theology and Science: Texts and Studies, no. 96. Leiden: Brill.

Stephens, Lynn G., and George Graham. 2000. *When Self-Consciousness Breaks: Alien Voices and Inserted Thoughts*. A Bradford Book. Cambridge, MA: MIT Press.

Toda, Mitsuru, and Anissa Abi-Dargham. 2007. 'Dopamine Hypothesis in Schizophrenia: Making Sense of It All.' *Current Psychiatry Reports* 9 (4): 329–336.

van Gulick, Robert. 2018. 'Consciousness.' In *The Stanford Encyclopedia of Philosophy*, ed. Edward N. Zalta. Spring 2018 ed. Available at https://plato.stanford.edu/entries/consciousness/

Watkins, Calvert, ed. 2011. *The American Heritage Dictionary of Indo-European Roots*. 3rd ed. Boston, MA: Houghton Mifflin.

Weber, Bruce. 2018. 'Life.' In *The Stanford Encyclopedia of Philosophy*, ed. Edward N. Zalta. Summer 2018 ed. Available at https://plato.stanford.edu/archives/sum2018/entries/life/

Whitbeck, Caroline. 1977. 'Causation in Medicine: The Disease Entity Model.' *Philosophy of Science* 44 (4): 619–637.

World Health Organization (WHO). 1992. *The ICD-10 Classification of Mental and Behavioural Disorders: Clinical descriptions and Diagnostic Guidelines*. Geneva: World Health Organization.

———. 2006. *Constitution of the World Health Organization*. 45th ed. Geneva: World Health Organization.

Yalowitz, Steven. 2014. 'Anomalous Monism.' In *The Stanford Encyclopedia of Philosophy*, ed. Edward N. Zalta. Winter 2014 ed. Available at https://plato.stanford.edu/entries/anomalous-monism/

Zohar, Danah, and I. N. Marshall. 1990. *The Quantum Self: Human Nature and Consciousness Defined by the New Physics*. New York, NY: Morrow.

**Dr Asim Yusuf OBE** is a Fellow of the Royal College of Psychiatrists and a practising clinician with a special interest in Mental Health and Spirituality. He is acknowledged as one of the leading figures in western Islamic psychological studies. He has been granted an *ijāza* (formal religious authorization) to instruct students in the art and science of Islamic thought by a number of scholars, and is the founder and Director of the Nur al-Habib Foundation and sits on the British Board of Scholars and Imams.

**Dato' Dr Afifi al-Akiti** is the Kuwait Fellow in Islamic Studies at the Oxford Centre for Islamic Studies, and teaches in the Faculty of Theology, University of Oxford. He is a Fellow of Worcester College, Oxford. Dato' Afifi is trained as a theologian in both the Islamic and Western traditions. His areas of expertise are Islamic theology, law, and science. He has worked on several BBC documentaries, including the award-winning *Science and Islam* (2009). Since 2010, Dato' Dr Afifi has been listed in *The Muslim 500: The World's 500 Most Influential Muslims*.

# Chapter 8
# Muslim Values and End-of-Life Healthcare Decision-Making: Values, Norms and Ontologies in Conflict?

**Mehrunisha Suleman**

## 8.1 Introduction

Biomedicine predominates globally as a theoretical system of understanding health and disease. Practically, that means the application of scientific data from bench to bedside, through population-based studies; and informing on a sound basis the systematic design and delivery of efficient and effective models of care to prevent and/or counter disease and to promote health. Traditionally, the biomedical model of health and disease has focused on physical systems often diagnosed quantitatively through biochemical, electrical and other empirical modes of measurement. George L. Engel's (d. 1999) pioneering paper emphasising a 'biopsychosocial' model of health and disease, stressed the importance of social, psychological, and physical dimensions of illness.[1] It offered a revolutionary framework for education, training and research. The wider perspective offered by Engel's model in the understanding of illness coincided with transitions in models of care.

Historically, doctors were the principle decision makers within the clinical context. This authority was often linked to their superior knowledge, training and experience of disease pathologies, management, and prognosis. Despite rapid biomedical advancement in recent decades, healthcare innovation and a shift in focus towards technologically driven healthcare, has been paradoxically coupled with a decline in

[1] Engel (1977): 129–136. 'Biopsychosocial': 'bio' here refers to biological components, such as age, gender or genetics. 'Psycho' refers to psychological components, such as thoughts, emotions, or beliefs. 'Social' refers to factors such as family circumstances, cultural influences or environmental factors.

M. Suleman (✉)
University of Cambridge, Cambridge, UK
e-mail: ms520@cam.ac.uk


A. al-Akiti, A. I. Padela (eds.), *Islam and Biomedicine*, Philosophy and Medicine 137, https://doi.org/10.1007/978-3-030-53801-9_8

the authority of health services and health service personnel, particularly doctors.[2] Patients, families and communities have been experiencing a diminished trust in health services[3] that have been gearing more towards a 'commodity centric' model of care.[4] The response to this has been recent calls for patient-centred care, shared decision-making and kindling shared partnerships between healthcare users and providers.[5]

In addition to changes in models of care, there has been a transformation in the generation, organization, and use of medical knowledge. The advent of evidence-based medicine[6] has marked the importance of integrating robust empirical evidence with individual clinical expertise, to ensure effective and efficient care. Both research and practice within biomedicine are conducted through normative processes that are approved through the systematization of biomedical research through collaborations such as Cochrane[7] and the establishment of randomized controlled trials[8] as the panacea of biomedical enquiry. The latter and former have also demarcated the epistemological framework of biomedical knowledge and practice as largely empirical.

The systematization of research in ensuring evidence-based practice has been welcomed, yet such processes and frameworks deal only with biomedical *gnosis* and *praxis*. The healthcare context is rarely a sterile and controlled environment; commonly it consists of plurality, diversity and often fragmentation and uncertainty. Healthcare providers, patients and families, who interact within such a context, be that within an institution or in the community, carry with them not only biomedical *gnosis* and *praxis*, but also individual and socio-cultural histories, languages, values and beliefs. In the United Kingdom, in particular, a demographically diverse, increasing multi-ethnic and multi-faith population, interlocutors within the healthcare context will encounter myriad sources of *gnosis* and *praxis*. End-of-life care (EOLC) is a key area of clinical research and practice where such interfaces and interactions are acute. Ensuring patient-centered care and shared decision-making whilst relying on empirical biomedical systems of *gnosis* and *praxis* can raise challenges for practitioners and patients alike within end-of-life care. For example,

[2] Stange (2010): 100–107.

[3] O'Neill (2002).

[4] Heath (2006): 846–847.

[5] Frosch and Kaplan (1999): 285–294.

[6] Sackett (2005), 2:3.

[7] See: www.cochrane.org. The charity was formed in 1993, in the UK, to facilitate systematic reviews of randomized control trials in healthcare.

[8] The National Institute for Health and Care Excellence (UK) defines 'randomised controlled trial' as: 'A study in which a number of similar people are randomly assigned to 2 (or more) groups to test a specific drug, treatment or other intervention. One group (the experimental group) has the intervention being tested, the other (the comparison or control group) has an alternative intervention, a dummy intervention (placebo) or no intervention at all. The groups are followed up to see how effective the experimental intervention was. Outcomes are measured at specific times and any difference in response between the groups is assessed statistically. This method is also used to reduce bias.' See: https://www.nice.org.uk/glossary?letter=r.

studies about hydration, at the end-of-life, reveal equivocal evidence, from empirical research, for clinical practice.[9]

The UK's multi-faith and multi-ethnic population comprises a growing population of Muslims,[10] many of whom either access or provide healthcare services within the National Health Service. Yet, very little is known about the beliefs, processes and practices they rely on when deliberating decisions within end-of-life care, such as those associated with death, dying and remembrance. This chapter will investigate the role and extent to which religious views and values influence end-of-life care decision-making when juxtaposed with biomedical *gnosis* and *praxis*. There is a need to understand better the values and perspectives of Muslim patients and families as well as Muslim healthcare providers and those of another and no faith who have experience of caring for or working with Muslims. Although studies have been conducted investigating the role of Muslim physicians' faith in decision-making,[11] and others have assessed the views of the Muslim community,[12] few such studies have been conducted in the UK. There are also a limited number of studies[13] carried out in the UK looking in particular at the qualitative decision-making between different stakeholders in end-of-life care, involving Muslim patients and families. This study seeks to assess not only the individual views, values and practices of different stakeholders but also the layers of complexity that co-exist when decision-making involves the juxtaposition of biomedical and religious sources of deliberations within end-of-life care.

This chapter will provide an analysis of the experiences, practices, and moral deliberations of healthcare users and providers within the context of end-of-life care. The latter offers a lens through which the collocation of Islam and biomedicine can be researched. The chapter findings point to a synchronicity between Islam and biomedicine in end-of-life care decision-making. Normatively, for Islam and Muslims, such synchronicity emphasizes a growing need for experts who are able to adequately navigate the two spheres of knowledge, understanding and practice.

## 8.2 Methodology

To assess the role and extent to which Islam and the beliefs, values and practices of Muslims influence decision-making within end-of-life care in the UK, an empirical qualitative study was carried out.

---

[9] Good et al. (2014): 2–16.

[10] Kettani (2010), 1387–1390.

[11] Mahdi et al. (2016): 403–421.

[12] Padela et al. (2012): 708–715.

[13] Gaveras et al. (2014): 1–11.

## 8.3 Sampling

Sampling was carried out in London and Birmingham, to maximize the opportunity to evaluate the influence of Islam in end-of-life care decision-making, as these two cities have the highest population of Muslims in the UK.[14] Sampling was also carried out in Cambridge, despite the small population of Muslims, to include narratives of stakeholders in a varied socio-demographic profile.

Given the aim of the study, the following types of key stakeholders were identified as important and included in recruitment:

1. Muslim patients and family members;
2. Healthcare professionals (doctors, nurses, physiotherapists, psychologists, etc.) – Muslim and non-Muslim;
3. Bereavement staff, funeral service staff, mortuary staff and coroners – Muslim and non-Muslim;
4. Chaplains (multi-faith and/or Muslim);
5. Imams and/or Islamic scholars involved in end-of-life care decision-making.

The rationale for sampling these five types of interviewees was because they constitute the five groups most likely to be able to provide insight into the role of Islam and the beliefs, values and practices of Muslims as pertaining to decision-making within end-of-life care. The reason for interviewing diverse actors, at multiple levels and throughout the pathway of patient and family care, was to allow for an assessment of the multiple relevant perspectives within end-of-life care in different contexts. A purposive sampling method was employed to capture a range of experiences.

Emails were sent systematically to all hospices, in London, Birmingham and Cambridge, listed on the Hospice UK website[15] to recruit hospices and individual participants into the study. An email including a brief of the study was sent via the Hospice UK mailing list. Emails were also sent to chaplaincy offices at hospital trusts in the three cities. Once interviews began, further recruitment was carried out via Internet searches (purposive sampling) and emailing of suitable participants as well as recruitment based on the advice of interviewees (snowballing).

A total of 74 interviews were conducted. This number was based on my being able to interview a sufficient number of suitable individuals within each of the participant categories such that data saturation was reached, i.e., until a point was reached beyond which it was judged the addition of new themes was unlikely.

---

[14] Ali (2015), 26.

[15] See: https://www.hospiceuk.org/about-hospice-care/find-a-hospice.

## 8.4 Ethical Review

As the study involves direct participation involving human subjects, it has undergone review by the University of Cambridge School of Humanities and Social Sciences Ethics Committee as well as the NHS Health Research Authority (IRAS number: 220682).

## 8.5 Semi-structured Interviews

As one of the objectives of the study was to investigate whether and how Islam and the beliefs, values and practices of Muslims influence their understanding and approaches to end-of-life care, the semi-structured interview presented the ideal means of probing and also challenging participants' views to better understand their reasoning and experiences. Green and Thorogood describe the interview as 'a conversation that is directed, more or less, towards the researcher's particular needs for data.'[16]

For in-depth interviews with participants, an open-ended thematic topic guide was developed (see Appendix 1) to ensure that the same themes were covered in each of the five interview tiers. The guide, however, provided flexibility to ensure that questioning could occur freely and to allow the interviewer to choose the questions appropriate to the context and to enable suitable probing of topics and issues that were pertinent and arose within the interview.

## 8.6 Framework Analysis

A framework approach has been used to analyse the data, as it has been described as a flexible method of analysis in allowing for both inductive and deductive contributions to analysis. Concepts and themes from the literature were used as pre-existing theoretical constructs during the analysis of the data (deductive analysis), alongside an inductive approach, whereby themes were identified directly from the qualitative data before re-visiting the literature.[17] This method also has the advantage that although in-depth analysis can take place across the entire data set, the process of coding and charting ensure that the views of each participant remain connected within a matrix.[18] The data analysis in this study employs the thematic framework analysis method that was devised by Ritchie and Lewis.[19]

---

[16] Green and Thorogood (2009), 95.

[17] Gale et al. (2013): 1–8.

[18] Ibid.

[19] Ritchie and Lewis (2003).

Semi-structured interviews were audio recorded and transcribed. Using data from notes taken at the interviews, and transcriptions of the audio recordings a framework analysis approach was employed.[20] The method I used reflects the framework analysis requirements described first by Ritchie and Lewis who suggest that the framework should ensure the investigator:[21]

1. Remains grounded in the data;
2. Permits captured synthesis – this is reflected in the charting process where verbatim text is reduced from its raw form;
3. Facilitates and displays ordering – again this is reflected in the charting process;
4. Permits within and between case searches – the charting process allows for searching and comparisons to be made within and between data sets.

Such a method ensures that the data analysis process is systematic, comprehensive and flexible to enable new ideas to be generated. It also enables refinements and ensures transparency to others. Ritchie and Lewis's method of analysis is one that involves an 'analytical hierarchy' which begins with familiarization of the data or data management followed by the generation of descriptive accounts and finally abstraction through the development of explanatory accounts.[22] The following describes how I carried out these steps of analysis:

1. Familiarization with the data – this first step was employed to ensure, as primary investigator, I remained close to the data and this involved immersion in the data with repeated reading of field notes, summaries and transcripts, in order to list key ideas, recurrent themes and patterns. I did not code at this stage and instead summarized the key points participants made via a summary sheet for each interview. A selection of the transcripts was discussed with my research team at the Centre of Islamic Studies (Cambridge), during the early stages of the interview period, to enable me to develop an initial systematic reflection of the data.
2. Generating themes – a coding scheme was developed by identifying all the key issues, concepts and themes. This was carried out by drawing on *a priori* issues and questions derived from the aims and objectives of the study, the literature review, as well as emergent issues raised by the participants. The coding framework was discussed and reviewed with research colleagues at the Centre of Islamic Studies, as well as at research meetings with key stakeholders. During the coding process, inductive codes, or those emerging from the data were added to the coding framework if they described a new theme or expanded a predetermined code.
3. Indexing – the themes in the data were then used as labels for codes, which were then applied to the whole data set. This was done systematically to ensure all the

[20] Green and Thorogood (2000), 114–116.

[21] Ritchie and Lewis (2003), 56.

[22] Ibid.

data were accurately coded using NVivo version 10.[23] The process of generating themes and indexing continued until the point of data saturation. Data saturation was assessed at the point where 'no new information or themes'[24] were observed in the data. After this point only indexing continued until all of the data had been coded. See Appendix 2 for a complete list of codes used.

4. Charting (descriptive accounts) – after having coded the data according to the identified themes, the data was then charted to assist in the generation of descriptive accounts where verbatim text was reduced from its raw form. This involved a rearrangement of the data according to the thematic content by comparing data within and between interviews. Once judged to be comprehensive, each main theme was charted by completing a matrix where each interview has its own row and columns representing the subtopics. These charts contain summaries of data that can be referenced back to the original transcript. This enabled a presentation of the range and diversity of views. Key quotes were recorded, and certain themes were listed in the participants' own language. This was then followed by a refinement of categories to address overlap and to develop typologies that assisted in the collation of the related themes helping to divide and unite the participants' views. A schematic of the coding framework is illustrated in Appendix 3.
5. Mapping and interpretation (developing exploratory accounts) – The charts were then used to examine the data for patterns and connections. This stage was influenced by the original aims and objectives of the study as well as emergent issues from the data. Here patterns in the data were identified to then derive explanations of participants' experiences and views. An account was developed to explain reasons behind the differences and similarities captured between and within participant accounts to arrive at an understanding of Muslim perspectives on end-of-life care. For example, recurrent themes were identified and the reasons for these were explored. Explanations and reasoning given by participants were also studied in order to distinguish these from my own analysis as the investigator (reflexivity).

## 8.7 Data Analysis and the Process of Developing the Main Themes

Having analysed the literature and studied the transcripts using a framework analysis, I identified two main themes and four subthemes that helped me organize the insights emerging from the data. Although the data could have been presented in

---

[23] NVivo version 10 is a qualitative data analysis software used by researchers working with rich text-based data where the data can be systematically coded, searched and analysed. This is available from QRS International: http://www.qsrinternational.com/nvivo/support-overview/downloads/nvivo-10-for-windows

[24] Guest, Bunce, and Johnson (2006): 59.

multiple ways and I drafted several versions of the data tables, the themes outlined below ultimately functioned best as organizing concepts for the data I gathered from the participants I interviewed. The themes are as follows:

(A) End-of-life care decision-making in modern healthcare systems: values, norms and ontologies:

1. Understandings of death and dying;
2. Evidenced-based end-of-life care: Advanced Care Planning (ACP).

(B) Muslim values, beliefs and practice in end-of-life care decision-making: sources, languages and authorities:

1. Beliefs about suffering and understandings of what is a 'good death';
2. Religious versus clinical knowledge and language: conferring of trust in end-of-life care decision-making.

Whilst these themes emerged as being important from my analysis of participant accounts, they also provided a framework through which the data and discussion from this chapter could be related back to the broader discussion and aims of this volume in addressing the normative implications of the juxtaposition of Islam and biomedicine.[25]

## 8.8 Analysing the Role of Faith

As the focus of the study was on Muslim perspectives on end-of-life care, participants were chosen and asked about their experiences and understandings of the impact of Islam and the beliefs, values and practices of Muslims within end-of-life care decision-making. Discussions with some participants who were not Muslim (for example, doctors, nurses and multifaith chaplains) did inevitably include descriptions of their own faith commitments and how they entered into their deliberations and understandings of end-of-life care. Although such accounts were incredibly rich and helpful in providing an important backdrop to participants' narrative accounts, I did not employ such descriptions to develop a comparative analysis of different faith accounts. The latter would be very valuable; however, it was outside the scope of this study. Thus, within the presentation of the data, the faith of a participant is only listed in cases of Muslim participants as all other participant accounts were analysed primarily on their role (as nurses or multifaith chaplains) and not their religious background.

[25] Chenail (1995): 1–9. See also, Sandelowski (1998): 375.

## 8.9 Presenting the Data – How Quotes Were Chosen

For evidencing the findings and illustrating perspectives of participants,[26] quotes were carefully chosen for presentation in this chapter. However, in keeping with the 'aesthetics and ethics'[27] of qualitative research reporting, as some of the participant explanations were lengthy, quotes had to be selected that were relevant for each section and sometimes edited further for brevity. I was careful, however, to select and edit quotes that retained the overall message of each transcript from which they were extracted. I kept detailed memos during the coding process to assist the selection of appropriate quotes.

## 8.10 Findings

(A) ***End-of-life care decision-making in modern healthcare systems: values, norms and ontologies***

An analysis of 70+ interview transcripts has revealed the importance of discussions about death and dying when healthcare practitioners are deliberating end-of-life care with Muslim patients and families. Here some of the participants' views will be presented highlighting the challenges that arise when healthcare practitioners are communicating using biomedical *gnosis* and *praxis* and the recipients of care rely on metaphysical understandings rooted in Islamic theology and philosophy.

1. ***Understandings of death and dying***

A senior palliative care nurse described the importance of explaining to patients and families the process of dying and how she communicates this using her biochemical knowledge of gradual organ dysfunction and tissue degradation:

> It's like when you try and have a conversation with them about how people die. That's something that's a very common question. You talk about people gradually deteriorating, organs failing, organs becoming weaker, not the need to eat and drink, things like that. It's like they understand that, but that is in parallel to when your God takes you … I approach Muslim patients as I would approach all my other patients with the caveat considering that there is this parallel … They know there's a role for medicine, but it's like it runs in parallel. [As] soon as you start talking about dying, it's like, 'You don't decide that. You're not going to decide when I die.' We're not trying to decide when you die, but we can see the pattern. (*Interview 3, Senior Hospice Nurse, London*)

The nurse and other participants explained the challenges of explaining processes of death and dying to patients who did not rely only on understandings based on biomedical and/or physical processes of death. Healthcare professionals often described

[26] Sandelowski (1994): 479–482.

[27] Ibid.: 480–81.

feeling challenged when providing such information and in particular prognostic information:

> We're not trying to decide when you die, but we can see the pattern. One of the things that we are skilled in, is recognizing dying and when it's happening. We're not always that good at prognosticating. Sometimes we'll say, 'We think it might be three or four days.' Sometimes someone will last a week, but we recognize that they are in that dying phase, but it's that point there where they'll say, 'Well, fine, I hear you recognize that from a medical point of view, but actually, this is where my faith comes in … They want certain information, but they then … You can almost see them clicking with their faith. It's like they'll ask so many things but they won't ask. They would never ask a question like, 'How will I die? What will the end look like? Will I be in pain?' All of those things, they won't ask … I acknowledge their faith. I always say to them, 'This runs alongside your beliefs. I can help you with what I know from medicine. Obviously, you have your beliefs and if you need help with correlating that with your beliefs, then I can get someone to come and help. You can get your faith minister, whoever, to come along. (*Interview 3, Senior Hospice Nurse, London*)

She and other healthcare professionals explained how their role and information giving is limited to biomedical *gnosis* and *praxis*, and that if patients and families are reliant on faith-based understandings of death and dying, such conversations would require additional interlocutors, including chaplains and community-based faith leaders.

A Muslim patient explained his understanding of death and how throughout his life and during his terminal illness, meaning-making for him centred around his theological commitments and in particular a metaphysical understanding of the role of the soul in determining life and death:

> 'My faith, clearly mentioned in the Qur'an 'Every soul shall taste death' [Qur'an 3:185, *Āl 'Imrān*] … Anyone who is born is going to die. I'm very strong [in] believing that it isn't the end of the line … (*Interview 48, Patient, Muslim*)

He spoke about death being a part of his understanding of life and that death would come when God ordained it, and he was not dependent on physical parameters, such as organ dysfunction and tissue degradation, as death was a necessary transition into an afterlife.

Another participant also described the challenges he faced in receiving a diagnosis and despite his poor prognosis was spiritually committed and reliant on God:

> When I first went from the hospital they had not found it unfortunately. It is my Allāh … my Allāh. Anyway they said [then it was straight] to my liver. When they gave me the … they do not have any no spiritual power … They say 'Mr X will be dying today.' No one can say. Nobody can say. Only my God can say … (*Interview 68, Patient, Muslim*)

Other participants, particularly Muslim healthcare professionals, explained how they shared this metaphysical understanding and conceptualized death through a theological conception of the soul departing from the body.

> My understanding of death is based on the way that I've been taught – our religion teaches it, which is the permanent departure of the soul from the body. We know that the soul leaves when one sleeps, but that doesn't mean that they're dead. But, if they die, their soul goes. They reach a point in their life where the soul leaves the body and doesn't come back. It's

> probably never going to come back to their body. That's how I see death. That's what we [Muslims] define as dead. (*Interview 45, GP, Birmingham, Muslim*)

Participants explained that this understanding and definition of death raised questions for them within the biomedical sphere as it is not possible to determine when the soul has departed the body.[28] One of the participants explained how he personally reconciled the two spheres of *gnosis* and *praxis*:

> They may look 'alive' but they're not alive. As a doctor how can I measure that? What's the point? It's really hard, obviously. I think there are different [Muslim] scholars who have said different things about the way we can measure death and how you measure the proxy by which death has occurred. That is essentially permanent death or brainstem death. So, that's my understanding as to when you can define death. Philosophically, it's the departure of the soul ... But, medically it's when one's heart stops beating permanently, or when there's brainstem death. (*Interview 45, GP, Birmingham, Muslim*)

His deliberation reveals an important tension in how biomedicine and Islam are relied upon, within end-of-life care, to derive understandings of death and dying; and that informed participants (clinicians with deep knowledge of their own theology like this one) appear to resolve these tensions by concurrently relying on both sources.

Another participant explained the challenges of negotiating ceilings of treatment when patients were reluctant to accept prognostic information:

> If they don't want to go there, in that conversation, it's hard to offer the range of choices. If somebody is saying to you, 'I want every single bit of treatment right up until the minute I draw my last breath, because my God says, never give up and every minute of life is precious, so keep on battling.' You can't get past that to then talk about, but if the treatment doesn't work, even with all the treatment you are in your last two weeks. When I've tried to talk to people about prognosis, it's often, 'You can't play God: you don't know.' You know, I do get it wrong, of course I do. I know most of the time. At least I know the ballpark. Some people close their own options, or close off the discussion of their own options. (*Interview 6, Senior Hospital and Hospice Palliative Care Nurse and Care Coordinator, London*)

Such conversations reveal tensions that arise when healthcare practitioners who are reliant on their empirical expertise are conveying their expert knowledge to patients whose theological commitments mean they are unable to accept such advice. Many participants explained that such hesitance on the part of Muslim patients and families to accept biomedical understandings of processes of death and dying, as well as prognostic information, was not simply a particular example of grieving on hearing bad news, such as denial and anger.[29] Rather, what they explained was that such encounters revealed deep religious convictions and theodicies that patients and families relied on to express an understanding of death and dying that was not incognizant of their faith.

One of the patients described his reliance on God's mercy whilst also having an expectation from healthcare professionals' informing him about his disease and prognosis:

---

[28] On the difficulty of defining death, see Chap. 9, 'The Intersection between Science and Sunnī Theological and Legal Discourse in Defining Medical Death,' by Rafaqat Rashid in this book.

[29] Kübler-Ross and Kessler (2014).

> Love mercy … only Allāh can grant me the mercy. No one else. No man, no doctor can do that for me. But, why did my doctors not find out? It took me six months before I got told, 'You have cancer. You've got a large mass.' They said, 'We don't know whether it's cancer, or if it's some other kind of rubbish.' But, when they did the biopsy on me, they said it's 100% cancer, and the only option is operation.
>
> … It's very, very difficult. But then … Allāh gave me the disease, and it's only Allāh can take the disease off of me. I have very strong faith in Allāh since I found out I have cancer. My faith got stronger, *Inshā᾿ Allāh*. No one'll probably believe me, but I know how my heart feels. People can think what they like, but my heart … I know what my heart says. (*Interview 61, Patient, Muslim*)

He spoke about the difficulties of accessing care and making his beliefs known and understood by healthcare professionals and others. He did, however, describe his reliance on the healthcare system to provide him information about his condition as well as options for treatment and palliation. Again, his experience reveals an important juxtaposition of Islam and biomedicine, and the strength that a believer accrues from the former and the reliance he has on the latter.

The data shows that healthcare professionals, who are not informed about Islam, who are charged with caring for Muslim patients and families, however, require additional interlocutors to support their information-giving and care at an end-of-life situation. The role and contributions of these stakeholders will be explored in forthcoming sections, though it is important to mention here how the differences in the understanding of death and dying between biomedicine and Islam, as presented below, might lead to schisms in the traditional healthcare-professional/patient relationship. Although the addition of other stakeholders is welcome in such circumstances, it does raise questions about the ability and scope of relationship building between patients and healthcare professionals and the capacity for establishing trust. The latter will be explored further in subsequent sections.

Another patient explained this concurrent reliance on science and God as follows:

> Allāh says I gave everything to you. You try. You try. Whatever science. Science, who create? It's not people who create. It's created by Allāh. It's created by God. So that's why I'm following both. I'm turning to Allāh and I'm following His instruction. So that's why I'm taking the medication and science system and I'm praying to Allāh as well. (*Interview 68, Patient, Muslim*)

Again his beliefs and understanding reveal not a hierarchy, but a synchronicity between biomedicine and Islam, where in his case the harmony was due to his belief that God is the source of science, therefore, his reliance on science was ultimately connected to his reliance on God.

Overall, the data shows that the 'meaning-threatening potential of death-awareness'[30] that is encountered in end-of-life care demonstrates the reliance that patients and families have on religious meaning-making. The participants' views emphasize that healthcare practitioners who are familiar with such contributions to patients' and families' religious meaning-making, in the face of an existential threat,

[30] Abeyta et al. (2015): 973.

are more likely to able to accommodate such views and be able to, in parallel, present biomedical offers of understanding more sensitively.

2. ***Evidenced-based end-of-life care: Advanced Care Planning (ACP)***

Participants also described how patients' and families' religious values and beliefs often raised challenges when negotiating care plans. A systematic review has shown that Advanced Care Planning (ACP) can 'positively impact' the quality of end-of-life care.[31] A randomized controlled trial has also shown that 'advance care planning improves end-of-life care and patient and family satisfaction and reduces stress, anxiety, and depression in surviving relatives.'[32] Very few of these studies, however, focus on the views and preferences of minority ethnic and faith groups such as Muslims. Participants in this study described limitations of written document-based Advanced Care Planning when caring for Muslim patients and families:

> I still struggle with the Muslim patients often ... it's more of a struggle with this group of patients. And I suspect it's because they feel that these things are left in God's hands. I get that from patients a lot of time, what will happen will happen. And we want everything. So they want the patient, the relative or the patient themselves wants to be in hospital. Even though it may not from the perspective of what the hospital can do for the patient and comfort it may not be the right thing for the patient. But mostly the families want their loved one in hospital. (*Interview 31, GP and CCG End-of-Life Care Lead, London*)

Advanced Care Planning, that is carried out by hospice teams and general practitioners (GPs) in the community rely on co-operation from patients and families. One of the aims of the planning process is to record patients' and families' wishes to ensure that the care provided is aligned with their wishes. GPs explained that it was often difficult for them to negotiate advanced care plans with Muslim patients and families. Care plans are normative interventions aimed at reducing hospital admissions and establishing 'do not attempt resuscitation orders' (DNARs).[33] GPs described how it was challenging to ensure that such conversations were open to patients' and families' values and beliefs, whilst aligning with end-of-life care evidenced-based practice guidance. When patients and families were unwilling to accept such planning, healthcare professionals in the community and hospice setting often described such conversations as a 'tick-box' or 'detached' exercise, one where clinical and patient/family goals were unaligned. The reasons for such challenges include: patients' and families' commitments in God, relying on God's mercy and ability to cure. Although respectful of healthcare professionals' need to plan and provide care, many nurses and physicians describe how patients and families reject Advanced Care Planning as it contravenes their commitment to relying on God. Healthcare professionals explained how this reliance in God is manifest, from

---

[31] Brinkman-Stoppelenburg et al. (2014): 1000–1025.

[32] Detering et al. (2010): 1.

[33] Brinkman-Stoppelenburg et al. (2014): 1001.

the perspective of patients and families, and described that it may practically be discernible by a commitment in hospital admission and intervention:

> Well it's very hard but you have to be guided by the patient and their wishes and the family. So I can only explain the facts and this is what I do because one has to be careful that we don't put our own beliefs and backgrounds onto patients, so it unfortunately becomes in a way sort of a detached conversation … I'll give you an example of a classic case of dementia … the Muslim dementia patients are generally well cared for in the community. There's lots out there to help them but they don't take it up. The families want to do everything themselves, which is fine if you've got that support. But the end-of-life planning is always more tricky for these patients. Because even right to the end the recurrent pneumonia, aspirations, they want hospital admission every time. And a patient who's demented this can be quite unsettling for them, different environment, if they've got an infection they're more confused than usual and it becomes quite traumatic all around for the hospital staff, because they don't know the patient, the family because they feel their loved one is worse … And trying to persuade the family that actually perhaps the dementia is making obviously the move to the hospital not comfortable for the patient and if we were able to manage their loved one at home, giving them the support they need, they may fare better. Their symptom control may be better because they're going to be less confused in the surrounding that they are familiar with. But I do find that generally, and of course I'm generalizing, they want hospital admission every time where it may not be practical. And what happens unfortunately hospital admission these days is they get to casualty, they get given IV antibiotics, they get tossed out again. I see that patient comes home again, they're much worse because they're more confused, more disoriented and it becomes very challenging for everybody. (*Interview 31, GP and CCG End-of-Life Care Lead, London*)

GPs also explained how they have admitted patients despite their own clinical assessment of biochemical and radiological results as patients and families were keen for further intervention. Participants often described that such decisions were often linked to patients' and families' beliefs and explicit expressions around hope and reliance on God. Although respectful of their views, healthcare practitioners described that their conceding to such wishes has led to inappropriate hospital admissions and often discharge within 24 hours. Such admissions are a burden on scarce healthcare resources and can also be physically and emotionally stressful for patients and families alike. Their experiences highlight the implication of divergent views or epistemic differences, around Advanced Care Planning leading to harm.

The data shows that resistance to Advanced Care Planning, which is commonly aimed at reducing medical care and to encourage death at home or outside the hospital setting, may partly be due to patients' and families' faith commitments to do everything possible to preserve life and/or to adhere to a reliance on God. However, one participant explained how this commitment to intervention stemmed from her biomedical training. She described how despite being aware of the limitations and harms of hospital admission, in an acute context, she erred towards intervention despite her grandmother's preference to die at home accepting God's will:

> … we always think we can do a little bit more. Actually, I think of my own grandmother towards the end of her life … The last few months of her life, she was like, 'No, I want to stay at home.' I remember forcing her to hospital once or twice, because I just thought, 'We can do something about this. You know, you shouldn't be like … Your blood sugar shouldn't be going down. We can do something about this.' The last time, I knew that she was dying. I knew that she was dying. I think we all knew that she was dying. She was hypothermic.

> Her blood sugar was down. We sat down and we had a meeting. We said, 'Actually, we should really have one last go at sorting this out.' And we called the ambulance, even though we knew she didn't want to go. And the look she gave us was just ... was awful, actually. Was awful. It was just ... And I think having faith that you are meeting your Lord and that you want to go in a certain way and then being able to ... because I think medics will always try a little bit more. We always think there's a mechanical solution to death, that if we did something a little bit more, then it would be all right. (*Interview 8, Doctor, London, Muslim*)

Such participant views in the study highlight that although informed by faith, Muslims also rely on other sources of knowledge and understanding to arrive at end-of-life decisions, including epistemic influences of biomedicine.

Only recently have there been calls for re-establishing end-of-life care in the community, whereas societies have been increasingly dependent on the medicalization of death.[34] Transformation of end-of-life care will have to include the timeframe that is essential for the kinds of changes in cultural and infrastructural systems that are required, and there are likely to be lags in the uptake of such changes. For example, the wish to be admitted to hospital at the end of life is not distinct to Muslim patients and families and may be reflective of a prevailing social biomedical dependency around death and dying. Healthcare practitioners may, therefore, encounter a two-fold commitment to medicalization in the case of Muslim patients and families: firstly, that it is a faith-based commitment to the preservation of life and/or reliance on God; and secondly due to a social reliance on and expectations around modern healthcare and the promises of biomedical science.

Although Advanced Care Planning has been designed to dispel myths around expectations of healthcare, where practitioners convey disease prognosis and the unlikelihood of the success of various biomedical treatments and interventions. When conversing with Muslim patients and families, however, such discussions may not be as effective in enabling negotiations of care plans as practitioners may be unaware of the two factors (faith in preservation of life and biomedical dependence) being augmentative, where the latter enhances commitment to the former. Healthcare practitioners, thus, describe an inability to arrive at satisfactory decisions and remain unsure of the goals of Advanced Care Planning in such cases:

> It's difficult. I guess because we always want ... Our work is that we want things to be tidy. Sometimes it's not like that and we have to accept that. I guess we always want to ... A big part of our work and especially as part of care is Advanced Care Planning. Making sure that the patient's voice is heard. Sometimes, I have to take a step back and think to myself, 'Is this for me not for the patient?'... Me, explaining about why I don't want to resuscitate him is almost meaningless because he's like, 'I understand what you're saying and I understand you have a job to do. When God is ready to take me, then he will take me,' so your conversation is irrelevant ... (*Interview 3, Senior Hospice Nurse, London*)

The above quote and such contexts, therefore, highlight limitations of Advanced Care Planning and may also emphasize a need for adapting or redefining such processes for patients and families whose beliefs and values do not easily align with

[34] Illich (1974).

healthcare practitioners' care goals. Participants described how a lack of appropriate training and resources for dealing with patients and families from different religious backgrounds has led to a lack of clarity. The latter results in misunderstandings between GPs, hospice staff and patients and families. Participants also described the frustrations they endure as they rely on biomedical *gnosis* and *praxis* whilst trying to ensure that patients' and families' religious and other preferences are heard and met through shared decision-making.

Such cases also highlight the paradoxes that may coexist within healthcare decision-making, where transformations of biomedical *gnosis* and *praxis* reveal concurrence of well-established yet less evidence-based cultures and practices, running alongside more innovative ways of knowing and practising. Such cohabitations of biomedical *gnosis* and *praxis* mean what is normative in biomedicine currently is not only reflected by evidence-based practices, rather they are accompanied by variegated preferences and practices that are historically normative. In terms of the tensions arising from negotiations around Advanced Care Planning, this study shows that the integration of biomedical *gnosis* and *praxis* and Muslim theological understandings within end-of-life care are nuanced. Neither are they opposing or linearly concurrent within the deliberations and practices of Muslim patients, families and healthcare professionals. Although, on the one hand, there is a misalignment of emerging biomedical goals and Muslim patients' and families' theological preferences, such non-conformity may partly be due to biomedicine's own historical methods of *gnosis* and *praxis*. The apparent divergence here does not, therefore, render one source as being primary or secondary, when Muslim patients, families and healthcare staff are negotiating advanced care plans, rather the diachronicity of biomedicine means that they are intrinsically linked and co-dependent.

### (B) *Muslim values, beliefs and practice in end-of-life care decision-making: sources, languages, and authorities*

#### 1. *Beliefs about suffering and understandings of what is a 'good death'*

One of the key themes emerging from the data is the importance that Muslim patients and families place on ensuring that decision-making within the healthcare context is not incongruous with their faith. Many explained their theological commitments to beliefs in an afterlife and how illness and disease within their Islamic worldview are manifestations of suffering or a test, which offers a means of spiritual cleansing or of elevating the devotee:[35]

> What I mean is that Allāh's testing me. He's testing me to see how much … I got in me, to see if I've still got faith in Him or not. Do I keep to my *Ṣalāt*, or do I not? … Do I go astray? Which I haven't. I haven't … I am scared. I'm not gonna lie. I'm scared about losing my life. Have I done the right things in life? Will Allāh forgive me for my sins? Or, will Allāh not forgive me for my sins? That's the most important thing I'm worried about, mainly. I'm not scared to die … I've been through hell, myself, all my life. I've been through nothing

[35] On the theological discussion in the Muslim tradition of illness being seen as a 'test' from God, see for example, Chap. 3, 'The Piety of Health: The Making of Health in Islamic Religious Narratives,' by Ahmed Ragab in this book.

> but hell, but never mind, it's Allāh's choice. Maybe this is what Allāh wants for me, then so be it then … He's testing us all, in wealth, in health, in everything. (*Interview 61, Patient, Muslim*)

Another patient explained his understanding of his own suffering through the example of the Prophet Job.[36] He explained how God delivered Job from his suffering and that he believed that God would provide him the same deliverance, if he upheld Job's virtue of forbearance:

> He suffered about 18 years … After that my God gave him everything. So it is possible. Maybe I am suffering … the five or four years or two years. I don't know. Maybe my God will release me. (*Interview 68, Patient, Muslim*)

A multifaith chaplain explained how he understood his Muslim patients' faith commitments through conversations with them and deliberating their obligations over time:

> … my learning in that situation as it was shared with me that the pain, the suffering that he was experiencing was a cleansing of him and preparing him for that other life … That is how it was shared with me, that the Muslim perspective is that his suffering, I suppose in my terms, his suffering is not without meaning, his suffering means that his soul is cleansed as it journeys to that other place … But in some ways it focused on the suffering and trying to find meaning to that suffering, and of course as you will know sometimes we are unable to actually mitigate the pain. Sometimes the pain a patient is in, whether it's existential, whether it's total pain, whatever name they want to give it, sometimes there is no medication which will touch it. (*Interview 19, Hospice Chaplain, London*)

Healthcare professionals, however, often confessed an inability to understanding such commitments; and views around suffering raised tensions within end-of-life care decision-making:

> I'm just ruminating here, but that's why I think these people don't get … It's not just a transmission thing, it's a reception thing. We, on our part, I am very clear. I say, 'We will not resuscitate. That means this. They will die. They will not suffer. They will be pain-free, anxiety-free, but they will die … They also made a point of emphasizing when they were speaking over and over again that they felt that it was their father's choice and he would have made the choice, even if the treatments had meant him suffering, it would have been what he would wanted because suffering was a route to heaven … If a patient wanted to suffer in their life or in their route to death, that was entirely the patient's decision and I would always treat anybody I could. However, me or my colleagues, nursing or whatever, couldn't be party or collude with intentional suffering … That was another point that I go on, that no matter what their choice is, if their choice is suffering, I could not be party to that. We can't, nurses or doctors, we can't do that. No one in the caring profession would do that. (*Interview 45, Intensive Care Unit Consultant, Cambridge*)

Participants also described how Muslim patients' and families' understanding of suffering around death informed their uptake of palliative care interventions such as pain relief. Their theological understanding of the process of death and beliefs about the soul's departure meant they were less concerned about the physical symptoms

[36] The story of the trials and patience of Prophet Job (Ayyūb) appears, for example, in the Qur'an 21:83–84 (*al-Anbiyā'*) and 38:41–44 (*Ṣād*).

and biochemical and/or scientific markers that healthcare professionals were reliant on. They in some cases discouraged the use of pain relief as it would prevent their recognition of the process of death:

> They say, they're suffering, some family, when they even see the suffering, that suffering is in this *sakrat al-mawt* (agony of death),[37] because this is the last suffering. She's not going to suffer or he's not going to suffer afterwards. They believe that this is *sakrat al-mawt*, the suffering. There are the nurses, they don't want to experience this because they get traumatized, psychologically, they get affected when they see somebody in pain and making this noise … this treatment, when they put this morphine, patient don't say anything, they became really numbed. Not even moving at all … working in NHS for [the] last 18 years, before the injection wasn't really powerful, they used to see this noise of the person passing away … There are traumatized effects, what's happening to the nurses … But, again, for the Muslims, this is not acceptable. (*Interview 24, Hospital Chaplain, Muslim, London*)

Some participants explained how, such as in the quote above, transformations in end-of-life care has meant there have been changes in how suffering is understood and addressed in the biomedical context. Healthcare professionals describe a commitment to ensuring a 'good death,' which they often describe as one that is 'comfortable,' 'symptom free' or 'pain-free.' For Muslim patients and families, understandings of suffering and stages of dying and what is meant by a 'good death' is theologically rooted in hopes of attaining an auspicious transition to the afterlife, and not necessarily for physical pain relief:

> Islam is a very practical, logical religion. Therefore, if life is going to end, as long as you die well … that you die remembering God … without taking your own life, and it's a natural death … (*Interview 1, Hospital Chaplain, Muslim, London*)

Several participants explained that for Muslim patients and families a 'good death' is centred around being able to complete rituals of dying including the remembrance of God (*dhikr*) and invocations of testimonies of faith (*shahāda*). Opiates such as morphine are offered as part of the end-of-life care treatment plan to address pain and reduce anxiety; such interventions, however, can also induce altered consciousness. The latter causes anxiety for Muslim patients and families as they worry that the patient will be unable to recite prayers necessary for their harmonious transition. Healthcare professionals, thus, encounter challenges in being able to provide end-of-life care that they would consider as 'good death.' The juxtaposition of beliefs and values that are rooted in scientific understandings and those in religious beliefs thus result in a display of differential clinical goals, at least in the hospital setting.

One of the participants (Interview 24 above) explained that healthcare professionals' commitment to ensuring a patient is comfortable at the end of life within the current biomedical context may be as much to do with patient preferences as that of healthcare professionals themselves. When the latter encounter patients and families whose preferences do not match their own, this does raise tensions about notions of suffering and meaning-making at the end of life. Such differential beliefs

---

[37] *Sakrat al-mawt* (sing.) or *sakarāt al-mawt* (pl.), sometimes translated as 'in the throes of death' is a Qur'anic term referring to the unconscious moment when one is about to die. This is based on the Muslim understanding that death causes suffering and agony at the point when the soul is leaving the body, and there is no escaping this condition. See Qur'an 50:19 (*Qāf*).

and understandings require further study to ensure that healthcare professionals are adequately equipped to deal with such needs and are emotionally supported with regards to their own aftercare. For Muslim patients and families, being able to develop relationships with healthcare staff where their varying needs are understood is likely to lead to perceptions of receiving good care. Such differences also highlight that end-of-life care ought to be structured around relationship building and not decision-making. It is relationships that can accommodate for differences whilst decision-making may emphasize differences.

2. ***Religious versus clinical knowledge and language: conferring of trust in end-of-life care decision-making***

As stated earlier, when healthcare professionals encounter patients and families whose values and beliefs contravene normative biomedical *gnosis* and *praxis* they may rely on intermediary interlocutors to assist in end-of-life care decision-making. For example, a hospital chaplain explained the myriad roles that he undertakes when dealing with Muslim patients and families:

> … the doctors had said, 'We think that he should not be resuscitated if he has a cardiac arrest again. We are going to put in a DNAR [Do Not Attempt Resuscitation order] form.' They asked me is that okay, and they gave me all the conditions … Based on that, do you think it's the correct opinion? I think DNAR is only put in place when the doctors feel that the treatment is going to be futile. From a religious perspective, that's fine. I kind of reassure them that if the doctors are saying the treatment is going to be futile, then the DNAR, from a religious perspective, there's no issues. (*Interview 1, Hospital Chaplain, Muslim, London*)

As Muslim patients and families are informed by their religious commitments in all facets of life, they will usually rely on experts conversant in religious knowledge and language when they encounter the clinical context. Here the chaplain is explaining how he superimposes clinical decisions onto a religious framework to translate to patients and families the acceptability of the healthcare teams' evaluation. He also explained how formal training and familiarity with Islamic jurisprudential deliberations around seeking of treatment allows him to reassure families about the validity of accepting the scope and implications of clinical uncertainty:

> … I think from a religious perspective I've learnt from [Muslim] scholars and teachers that the basis of taking medicine or not taking medicine, and we look at that issue first. Is it *farḍ* [obligation], is it compulsory, is it *wājib* [compulsory] for a person to take medicine? The scholars say that if the medicine is definitely going to benefit you in a positive way, 100%, then you have to take it, it's *farḍ*. If there's doubt, 90%, 80% it might work, or 70%, then it's recommended, but it's not necessary. On that basis, any medicine, and majority of the times, it's not necessary to take. CPR is not going to work 100% all of the times. Therefore CPR [cardiopulmonary resuscitation] is not a 100% guaranteed medicine, or a method of keeping somebody alive is not guaranteed. Based on that, if the doctors feel that this person's condition is XYZ, and therefore if we are going to do CPR, it's going to cause more harm, because of the way we are going to do the CPR. CPR is not something which is just putting a small injection, or just giving a tablet, it is an aggressive [intervention]. You have to see the human dignity as well, weighed up with the likelihood of CPR working … I think from my perspective as an *ʿālim* [a Muslim scholar], I'm quite comfortable if the doctors have weighed it up, so I do rely on the doctors. (*Interview 1, Hospital Chaplain, Muslim, London*)

He emphasized that although many patients and families were committed to the value of 'seeking cure' for every disease, they had very little understanding of what this meant in practice. He explained that often Muslim patients and families enacted this value by simply demanding more intervention. By describing to them the risks of intervention and the unlikelihood of success, alongside their being no religious obligation to undertake interventions in such instances, he was able to reassure patients and families regarding the withholding of certain clinical interventions.

As patients and families rely on religious values, beliefs and rituals to construct meaning, they depend on those conversant in such tenets to assist in their deliberations. Decision-making for them is not simply negotiations around scientific data and biomedical trends offering information about prognosis, rather they require a deep consideration of their theological values to ensure their evaluation is cognizant with their faith. Some may argue that the above deliberation offered by the chaplain is simply a post-hoc rationalization of clinical decisions for appeasing patients' and families' religious commitment. However, the research shows that such reflections highlight the sensitive and complex nature of end-of-life care decision-making and offers insights into the types of resources around communication, language, knowledge, and trust building that may enable patients and families to deal with the existential realities encountered within end-of-life care. Such deliberations also emphasize that though healthcare professionals may be experts in biomedical *gnosis* and *praxis*, patients and families are experts of their histories, languages, values, beliefs and contexts. They, therefore, make decisions surrounding end of life in light of their particular understanding of death and dying. It also underlines that end-of-life care decision-making, in particular, involves careful negotiations and may include stakeholders that offer religious knowledge and moral support alongside that of the expertise of healthcare professionals.

Many participants remarked that access to chaplains who are sufficiently trained and knowledgeable about Islamic theological perspectives and are also adequately familiar with the clinical context is rare. Participants explained that when such expertise is unavailable, either due to lack of resources or time constraints in the hospital context, they are often unable to accommodate such beliefs and preferences. Others also described how relying on community-based faith leaders, who are afforded a social authority by patients and families, may err on the side of intervention, being unfamiliar with the clinical milieu. Such interactions often raise challenges for clinical staff where there is an inadequate interpretation between the language and knowledge of biomedicine and that of the patients' and families' religious commitments.

## 8.11 Conclusion

Analysis of the qualitative data presented here reveals that Islam, its texts and lived practice, finds growing importance within the British end-of-life care discourse as there is an increasing Muslim population and burgeoning interest in the role of faith and spirituality in healthcare decision-making. End-of-life care and its associated existential implications offer a singular lens through which the interaction between biomedicine and Islam can be investigated.

Here the discussions highlight key interfaces within end-of-life care where the interactions between Islam and biomedicine are acute. Firstly, such encounters revealed deep religious convictions and theodicies that patients and families relied on to express an understanding of death and dying that was cognizant with their faith. The 'meaning-threatening potential of death-awareness'[38] that is encountered in end-of-life care demonstrates the reliance that patients and families have on religious meaning-making. Biomedical *gnosis* and *praxis* only offer one language and framework for meaning-making, and the participants in this study highlight that people may rely on multiple rational, moral and theological sources of meaning-making. Normatively, for the practice of biomedicine, the study shows that those who are familiar with such contributions to patients' and families' religious meaning-making, in the face of existential threat, are more likely to able to accommodate such views and be able to, in parallel, present biomedical offers of understanding more sensitively.

Secondly, Advanced Care Planning as a normative biomedical tool for end-of-life care decision-making raises challenges and questions for Muslim patients and families and healthcare professionals. In terms of the tensions arising from negotiations around Advanced Care Planning, the study shows that the integration of biomedical *gnosis* and *praxis* and Muslim theological understandings within end-of-life care are nuanced. Neither are they simply opposing or linearly concurrent within the deliberations and practices of Muslim patients, families and healthcare professionals. Although, on the one hand, there is a misalignment of emerging biomedical goals and Muslim patients' and families' theological preferences, such non-conformity may partly be due to biomedicine's own historical methods of *gnosis* and *praxis*. The conflict here does not, therefore, render one source as being primary or secondary, when Muslim patients, families and healthcare staff are negotiating advanced care plans, rather the diachronicity of biomedicine means that they are intrinsically linked and co-dependent.

Thirdly, beliefs around suffering and notions of what is a 'good death' emphasize disparities between biomedical and Islamic theological ontologies. Patients and families committed to an afterlife may be less concerned with physical suffering and more committed to ensuring ritualistic practices for safeguarding a harmonious transition. In support of such views and values, healthcare staff, who may be challenged by witnessing physical suffering, may require appropriate training and support for their own aftercare.

Finally, the study shows that Muslim chaplains with a dual expertise in clinical contexts and theological knowledge are relied upon by patients, families and clinical teams alike to offer interpretation of clinical decisions. Such interpretation is not simply a post-hoc rationalization of clinical decisions for appeasing patients' and families' religious commitments. The research shows that such reflections highlight the sensitive and complex nature of end-of-life care decision-making and offers

[38] Abeyta et al. (2015): 973.

insights into the types of resources around communication, language, knowledge and trust building that may enable patients and families to deal with the existential realities encountered within end-of-life care. Such deliberations also emphasize that though healthcare professionals may be experts in biomedical *gnosis* and *praxis*, patients and families are more knowledgeable of their histories, languages, values, beliefs and contexts. They, therefore, make decisions about end-of-life in light of their particular understanding of death and dying. It also underlines that end-of-life care decision-making, in particular, involves careful negotiations and may include stakeholders that offer theological knowledge and support alongside healthcare professionals. Again, the deliberations highlight not a hierarchy but a synchronicity between Islam and biomedicine in end-of-life care decision-making. Normatively, for Islam and Muslims, such synchronicity emphasizes a growing need for experts who are able to adequately navigate the two spheres of knowledge, understanding and practice. This dual expertise will enable appropriate translation of values, beliefs and practices of faith alongside the evaluation of scientific data and deliberations of clinical goals. It is through the commune of corresponding skills and knowledge in the two fields that appropriate relationships will be harnessed to ensure better care.

## Appendices

### *Appendix 1: Draft Interview Guide for Semi-structured In-depth Interviews with Policy Makers, Healthcare Staff, Muslim Patients, Families, Islamic Scholars, Imams and Chaplains*

**Part A: Introduction and a brief description of what the research is about**

'Thank you very much for agreeing to participate in this study which aims to capture views of Muslims on end-of-life care or the views of those who have experience of taking care of Muslim patients and families at the end of life. Firstly, have you had a chance to read the information sheet? Do you have any questions or concerns about the information you were provided? Are you happy to participate in the study? I will be recording the interview, as stated in the information sheet. Are you happy with that? I will also be asking questions on a case-by-case basis and based on your responses.'

**Part B: End of life and end-of-life care services**

(a) **What is their experience of end-of-life care?**

   (i) 'To begin with could you please tell me a little about yourself, how you got into this role and what you do?'
   (ii) 'To begin with could you please tell me a little about yourself and your experience of end-of-life care?'

(b) **What are your experiences of end-of-life care?**

(i) 'Can you tell me a little bit about your experience of end-of-life care?'
(ii) 'Who was involved?'
(iii) 'What happened?'
(iv) 'Were there difficult decisions to be made? Can you tell me more about these?'

(c) **What resources do you have to navigate these questions and concerns?**

**Part C: Faith and end of life**

(a) **In your experience, does your faith or the faith of your patients affect your practice, experience and/views on end-of-life care?**

(i) If yes, then please can you tell me more about this?
(ii) Does it affect how you define death?

- Do you consider death to be:
  - The irreversible cessation of cardiac and respiratory function?
  - The irreversible loss of 'personhood'?
  - The irreversible loss of 'consciousness'?
  - The irreversible loss of brain stem function?
  - Brain stem and/or cardiac death (both are the same)?
  - When the soul departs the body

    Defined by brain stem death
    Defined by cardiac death
    Defined by either brain stem and/or cardiac death
    Defined by neither of these. If other, please explain

(iii) Does it affect the types of people who are involved in end-of-life care decisions?
(iv) Does it affect the type of care that is provided at the end of life?

**Part D: Faith, end of life and beliefs about the value of life**

(a) **In your experience, does your faith or the faith of your patients affect views about whether the value of human life is linked to quality of life?**

(i) If yes, then please can you tell me more about this?
(ii) Are views about human life and quality of life associated with understandings of death and dying? If so how? If not, why not?
(iii) Are views about human life and quality of life associated with views about an afterlife? If so how? If not, why not?
(iv) Are views about human life and quality of life associated views and beliefs about illness and suffering? If so how? If not, why not?

**Part E: Religious beliefs and making decisions about end-of-life care services**

(a) **In your understanding and experience, does your faith or the faith of your patients affect views about:**

(i) Withholding of life-sustaining treatment
(ii) Withdrawing of life-sustaining treatment
(iii) Euthanasia/Physician assisted suicide
(iv) Are these views associated with your ideas and concerns for the patients' quality of life? If so how? If not, why not?

(b) **In your experience, does your faith or the faith of your patients affect views about:**

(i) Meeting a patient's request to withhold treatment at the end of life
(ii) Meeting a patient's or family's request to withdraw treatment at the end of life
(iii) Meeting a patient's or family's request to continue treatment at the end of life
(iv) Considering a patient's request to end their life. Has this ever happened? Can you tell me more about it?

**Part F: Role of spiritual/religious leaders in end-of-life care**

(a) **Have you ever consulted an Imam, Chaplain or Islamic scholar when making decisions about end-of-life care?**

(i) If yes, then please can you tell me more about this?
(ii) Who were they and what was their role?
(iii) Why did you feel it was necessary to consult them? What happened?
(iv) How did you find their involvement in the overall experience of end-of-life-care decision-making?

**Part G: Potential impact of policy changes in the UK, such as an 'Assisted Dying Bill'**

(a) **Did you hear about the UK government's consideration of an 'Assisted Dying Bill' in 2015?**

(i) If yes, then please can you tell me more about this?
(ii) What did you understand about the Bill?
(iii) If the Bill or similar legislation is passed in the future, how would it impact your work/experience of the healthcare services?

- Would it impact how you would view the healthcare services in the UK?
- Would it impact how you would provide and/or access services?
- Would it impact your relationship with healthcare workers/patients?

**Part H: Questions and concluding remarks**

'Before we finish do you have any questions or concerns you would like to raise about what we have discussed? Are you still happy for me to use the data I have collected from this interview for my study? If you wish to withdraw at any point, then please do not hesitate to let me know. Finally, thank you so much for your time and generosity.'

## *Appendix 2: NVivo Version 10 Coding Frame*

Codes for NVivo Version 10

1. Islamic normative sources
   (a) Belief in God
   (b) Beliefs about death
      (i) Belief in the *ākhira* (hereafter)
      (ii) Islamic understanding of death
      (iii) 'Every soul shall taste death' (Qur'an 3:185, *Āl ʿImrān*)
      (iv) Stages of EOLC
   (c) *Ḥadīth* (tradition of the Prophet)
   (d) Islamic law
   (e) Qur'anic reference
   (f) Role of Islamic scholars
   (g) Other sources
2. Medical interventions
   (a) Organ donation
   (b) Defining death
      (i) Brain death diagnosis
   (c) 'Do Not Attempt Resuscitation' (DNAR)
   (d) Withdrawal of treatment
   (e) Withholding treatment
   (f) Treatment versus care
   (g) Administration of intensive care
   (h) Special issues
      (i) Assisted dying
      (ii) Euthanasia
      (iii) Advanced Care Plans

1. Role of healthcare staff
   (a) Informing about process of death
   (b) Different views re: death and dying
      (i) When God decrees
      (ii) Reliance on God
      (iii) Need for control
   (c) Prognostication
      (i) Challenges re: prognostication
2. Uptake from patients and families
3. Challenges
   (a) Wanting to hold on to theological commitments
   (b) Lack of trust

(i) Other interventions

3. Role of hospice
   (a) Care
      (i) Nursing care
      (ii) Medical care
   (b) Spiritual support
      (i) Chaplaincy in hospice
      (ii) Community volunteers
   (c) Bereavement support
   (d) Having diverse staff
   (e) Supporting family
   (f) Fulfilling patients' wishes
   (g) Working with community
   (h) Meeting religious needs
   (i) Meeting cultural needs
   (j) Meeting diverse needs
      (i) Diverse population in London
      (ii) Diverse population in Birmingham
   (k) Staff encountering Muslim patients and families
      (i) Needs
      (ii) Challenges
         1. Cases
         2. Resources they have
         3. Resources they don't have
         4. Resources/training they need

    (iii) Emerging challenges
        1. Value deliberations
        2. Staff needing more training and education re: Muslim theological commitments
            (a) Going beyond fulfilling ritual requirements
  (l) Perception about hospice services
    (i) Place to die
    (ii) For people of other faith
    (iii) For people of other ethnicity
  (m) Other

4. Hospital EOLC
   (a) How staff encounter Muslim patients and families
      (i) Cases
      (ii) Challenges
      (iii) Decision makers
         1. Resources they have
         2. Resources they don't have
         3. Resources/training they need
   (b) Role of palliative care
   (c) Role of allied healthcare staff
      (i) Clinical psychologist
      (ii) Other
   (d) Other
5. GP EOLC
   (a) Advanced Care Planning
   (b) Cases
   (c) Challenges
   (d) Decision makers
      1. Resources they have
      2. Resources they don't have
      3. Resources/training they need
   (e) Need for community chaplaincy
   (f) Other
6. EOLC cases

7. Personal faith
   (a) Patients
      (i) Values
      (ii) Qur'anic reference
      (iii) Other
   (b) Families
      (i) Values
      (ii) Qur'anic reference
      (iii) Other
   (c) Staff
      (i) Values
      (ii) Qur'anic reference
      (iii) Other
   (d) Other
8. Ethical deliberations
   (a) Harms of treatment
      (i) Side effects
   (b) Limitations of treatment
   (c) Best interests
      (i) Expectations or goals of intervention
   (d) Quality of life
      (i) Extending life
   (e) Patient autonomy
      (i) Female patients and challenges with protecting autonomy
      (ii) English proficiency
      (iii) Role of translators
      (iv) Patient refusing treatment
         1. Fatalism vs acceptance
   (f) Respecting patient and family values
      (i) Understandings about suffering
      (ii) Understandings about pain relief
      (iii) Understandings about hydration
      (iv) Understandings about nutrition

(g) Contentions issues
    (i) Futility
    (ii) Whose perspective(s)
(h) Role of court in deliberating ethical issues and clinical decisions
(i) Resource allocation
(j) Nature; and what is 'natural'
(k) Artificial
(l) Suffering
(m) Truth telling and collusion
(n) Care
(o) Phronesis
(p) Moral anxiety
(q) Moral frustration
(r) Moral conflict
(s) Other

9. Chaplaincy
    (a) History of chaplaincy
        (i) Changing landscape of chaplaincy
    (b) Multifaith Chaplaincy
        (i) Need for diversity
        (ii) Resource issues
        (iii) Trust
        (iv) Meaning-making
        (v) Existential questions
    (c) Muslim chaplaincy
        (i) Challenges in Muslim chaplaincy
            1. Duration of chaplaincy posts
            2. Number of chaplaincy posts
            3. Career progression
            4. Management in chaplaincy
            5. How involvement occurs
            6. Other
        (ii) Issues that require consultation/role of Muslim chaplaincy
            1. Existential questions
            2. Islamic legal permission for treatment
            3. Interpretation of religious values
                (a) Life as scared
                (b) Hope

(c) Acceptance
(d) Seeking cure
(e) Other

4. Pastoral role
    (a) Dealing with existential questions
5. Advice re: organ donation
6. Religious deliberation about withdrawal of treatment
7. Religious deliberation about withholding of treatment
8. Permissibility of medicines
9. Community chaplaincy role
    (a) Home visits
    (b) Prayers
    (c) Advice regarding EOLC
        (i) Death certification
        (ii) GP visit (prevent ambulance call outs)
        (iii) Burial
        (iv) Funeral prayer
        (v) Educating community
        (vi) Empowering community
    (d) Gap in community chaplaincy role
10. Other

(iii) Motivations for providing service

1. Reward for helping people

(iv) Negotiating between family and clinical team

1. Offering advice
2. Offering support
3. Offering religious guidance/interpretation
4. Liaising with community (Imam/scholar/family)
5. Imam versus chaplain advice
6. Challenges re: negotiation
    (a) Building trust
    (b) Competing voices
    (c) Difficult context
    (d) Delaying withdrawal of treatment
    (e) Medical versus Islamic view
7. On call emergency service
    (a) Support and advice when the patient is dying
    (b) Giving advice at bedside

(c) Marriage at bedside
(d) Prayers at bedside
(e) Support at bedside
(f) Visiting

8. Other

(v) Support and advice after death

1. Funeral arrangements

(vi) Bereavement support
(vii) Post mortem advice
(viii) Training and education of Muslim chaplains
(ix) Other

10. Values that are negotiated

(a) Best interests

(i) Theology

1. Hope
2. Seeking cure
3. Acceptance
4. Preserving life/life as sacred

(b) Quality of life

(i) Theology

1. Beliefs about suffering
2. Beliefs about afterlife
3. Reliance on God
4. What constitutes 'taking life'

(c) Life as a test
(d) Life as limited
(e) The five Islamic ethico-legal principles (*maqāṣid*)
(f) Balancing opposing Islamic values
(g) Custom or *ʿurf*
(h) Islamic versus 'secular'/ 'Western' values

(i) *Imān* or belief
(ii) Reliance on God's knowledge
(iii) Reliance on God's power
(iv) Belief in cure

(i) Dignity

(j) 'Good death'/dying well

   (i) Suffering
   (ii) Pain
   (iii) Level of *imān* or belief
   (iv) Purpose of life is worship

(k) Family values

   (i) Role of family

      1. Support of family
      2. Duty of family

(l) Community support
(m) Society and loneliness
(n) Virtues
(o) Duties
(p) Consequences
(q) Value deliberations

   (i) Suffering versus making comfortable
   (ii) Pain versus pain-free
   (iii) Caring, curing, letting die

(r) Other

11. Muslim EOLC challenges

   (a) Migration
   (b) Language
   (c) Education
   (d) Isolation and loneliness
   (e) Dealing with healthcare issues

      (i) Diagnosis

         1. Limitations of tools e.g., MMSE (no equivalent terms in Punjabi for 'imagine')

      (ii) Prognosis
      (iii) Uncertainty
      (iv) Healthcare logistics

         1. Referral
         2. Information
         3. Co-ordination of care
         4. Access to services

      (v) Relationship with GP
      (vi) Relationship with hospital staff
      (vii) Relationship with hospice

(viii) Understanding treatment
(ix) Understanding palliation
(x) Understanding clinical management

1. Withdrawal of interventions
2. Withholding interventions
3. Negotiating ceilings of treatment

(xi) Respecting teams
(xii) Unmet needs

(f) Dealing with religious issues

(i) Wanting to uphold religious values

1. Prayers
2. Other rituals
3. Ḥalāl food
4. Visitation by family and others
5. Values (hope, seeking cure, etc.)
6. Identity as a convert to faith
7. Hardship challenging faith
8. Faith as support in hardship

(ii) Understanding religious values
(iii) Unmet needs

(g) Dealing with unexpected needs

(i) Needing help at home
(ii) Loss of employment

1. Loss of identity

(iii) Migration status
(iv) Chaperone
(v) Legal requirements

1. Wills
2. Statutory requirements

(vi) Impact of illness

1. Physical
2. Mental
3. Familial
4. Social
5. Spiritual

(h) Patriarchy
(i) Intergenerational differences
(j) Services Muslim families may not take up

(k) Needs of Muslim patients and families

    (i) Religious needs

        1. Values
        2. Rituals
        3. People

    (ii) Cultural needs
    (iii) Other

(l) Genetic diseases
(m) Muslim diversity
(n) Rumours
(o) Challenging family dynamics
(p) Sensitive conditions

    (i) HIV/AIDS

(q) EOLC communication challenges

    (i) Language
    (ii) Values
    (iii) Roles
    (iv) Other

(r) Other

12. Decision makers

    (a) Role of patient
    (b) Role of family

        (i) Religious values
        (ii) Cultural values
        (iii) Duty to care for parents
        (iv) Duty to care for the ill

    (c) Role of Islamic scholars
    (d) Role of chaplains
    (e) Role of healthcare team
    (f) Role of community

        (i) Role of mosques
        (ii) Role of Imam
        (iii) Role of community
        (iv) Role of funeral services
        (v) Role of volunteers
        (vi) Islamic values re: community

            1. Social welfare (*farḍ kifāya*)

(g) Managing different needs
    (i) Needs of patient
    (ii) Needs of family
    (iii) Needs of healthcare staff
        1. Wanting to know they have done a 'good job'
        2. Following best practice guidance
        3. Aftercare for staff
        4. Support for staff
    (iv) Conflicting needs
    (v) Other
(h) Other

13. Trust building
    (a) Religious knowledge
    (b) Religious language
    (c) Religious authority
    (d) Clinical knowledge
    (e) Clinical language
    (f) Clinical authority
    (g) Dealing with uncertainty in clinical knowledge
        (i) Need for education
    (h) Dealing with uncertainty in religious knowledge
        (i) Need for more scholarship
    (i) Chaplaincy authority
    (j) Islamic scholarly authority
    (k) Authority of Muslim doctors
    (l) Other
14. Religion versus culture
    (a) Flying the body home
    (b) Role of women
    (c) Appropriation of religion
        (i) Role of religious authority in cultural practices
    (d) Other cultural practices
15. Children and young people in EOLC
    (a) Children
        (i) Role of mother
        (ii) Bereavement

(b) Young adults

(i) Religious views
(ii) Cultural views
(iii) Role of parents and family
(iv) Role of healthcare professionals
(v) Challenges

1. Sexuality and intimacy

(vi) Other

16. Post mortems and coroner services

(a) How staff encounter Muslim patients and families

(i) Cases
(ii) Challenges
(iii) Decision makers

1. Resources they have
2. Resources they don't have
3. Resources/training they need

(b) Other

17. Funeral services
18. Bereavement services
19. Gaps (in Muslim perspectives on EOLC)

(a) Need for research
(b) Need for training
(c) Need for education
(d) Case based learning
(e) Talking about death
(f) Other

20. Reflexivity on my role as researcher

(a) My identity

(i) Female
(ii) Visibly Muslim

(b) My tacit understanding
(c) Need to probe
(d) Being asked my views/perceptions
(e) Other

## *Appendix 3: A Schematic of the Coding Framework Used for the Data Presented*

| Codes and quotes | Themes or descriptive accounts | Exploratory accounts | Main themes or aspects |
|---|---|---|---|
| – Process of death:<br>'You talk about people gradually deteriorating, organs failing, organs becoming weaker...'<br>– Prognostication:<br>'We're not trying to decide when you die, but we can see the pattern ...'<br>'... recognize that they are in that dying phase ...'<br>– Theological commitments and prognostication:<br>'... when your God takes you ...'<br>'... You can almost see them clicking with their faith ...'<br>' ... You can't play God you don't know.' | 1. Biochemical knowledge of gradual organ dysfunction and tissue degradation<br>2. Prognostic information and challenges of conveying and accepting prognostic information:<br>– Nurses rely on biomedical knowledge and training<br>– Nurses rely on the experiential knowledge of the 'dying phase'<br>3. Time of death as God's knowledge<br>4. Ready to go when God decrees<br>– Patients and families by contrast rely on theological commitments | Understandings of Death and Dying | EOLC decision-making in modern healthcare systems: values, norms and ontologies |
| When nurses describe challenges of having ACP conversations.<br>GPs talk about challenges and not wanting to force ACP decisions.<br>Reasons for challenges:<br>– Theological commitments:<br>'in God's hands'<br>'what will happen will happen'<br>Not aligned with patients' values e.g., hope, reliance on God<br>– Negotiating ceilings of treatment:<br>'we want everything'<br>Subsequent harms:<br>– Inappropriate hospital admissions<br>– Rapid discharge<br>– Utilization of scare resources<br>Patient's don't consider ACP conversations as relevant to them. | 1. Advanced Care Plans<br>2. Theological commitments<br>3. Consequences of lack of understanding and ineffective negotiation/ communication<br>4. Importance of patient's voice in ACPs<br>5. ACPs perceived as being counter to theological commitments to hope and reliance on God | Evidenced-based EOLC: Advanced Care Planning | |

(continued)

| Codes and quotes | Themes or descriptive accounts | Exploratory accounts | Main themes or aspects |
|---|---|---|---|
| Beliefs about suffering:<br>– Beliefs in an afterlife<br>– Illness and disease as suffering<br>– Suffering as a means of cleansing<br>– Suffering as means of spiritual elevation<br>– Suffering as a preparation for afterlife:<br>'… the suffering that he was experiencing was a cleansing of him …'<br>Understanding about pain:<br>– Physical pain<br>– Spiritual pain/existential pain<br>Healthcare professionals' inability to understand such theological commitments to suffering:<br>'… It's not just a transmission thing, it's a reception thing'<br>Healthcare professionals' ethical commitment to not collude with suffering:<br>'… me or my colleagues … couldn't be party or collude with suffering'<br>Beliefs about suffering impacting uptake of interventions e.g., pain relief<br>Beliefs about a 'good death':<br>– Fulfilling rituals of death<br>– Remembering God (*dhikr*)<br>– Fulfilling debts<br>Concerns around sedation<br>Less concern (from patients and families) around agony of death<br>Staff morally challenged by witnessing patients' suffering; their notions of a 'good death' about patient being 'comfortable,' 'pain free' | 1. Suffering:<br>Theological beliefs about suffering<br>Healthcare professionals' ethical commitment to not collude with suffering<br>Uptake of pain relief<br>2. 'Good death':<br>Concerns around sedation<br>Concerns around being able to fulfil rituals<br>Healthcare professionals' distress at witnessing patient suffering | Beliefs about suffering and understandings of what is a 'good death' | Muslim values, beliefs and practice in EOLC decision-making: sources, languages and authorities |
| Chaplains being asked about healthcare interventions, e.g., DNAR<br>Chaplains and Islamic scholars being asked about withholding and/or withdrawal of treatment<br>Role of chaplains and Islamic scholars to interpret Islamic values, e.g., 'life as sacred'; 'seeking cures' | 1. Religious meaning-making<br>2. Interpretation of religious meaning-making in a clinical context<br>3. Role of interlocutors skilled in translating religious knowledge and language in a clinical setting<br>4. Lack of skilled interlocutors | Religious versus clinical knowledge and language: conferring of trust in EOLC decision-making | |

## References

Abeyta, Andrew A., Clay Routledge, Jacob Juhl, and Michael D. Robinson. 2015. 'Finding Meaning Through Emotional Understanding: Emotional Clarity Predicts Meaning in Life and Adjustment to Existential Threat.' *Motivation and Emotion* 39 (6): 973–983.

Ali, Sundas, ed. 2015. *British Muslim in Numbers: A Demographic, Socio-economic and Health Profile of Muslims in Britain Drawing on the 2011 Census*. London: Muslim Council of Britain.

Brinkman-Stoppelenburg, Arianne, Judith A. C. Rietjens, and Agnes van der Heide. 2014. 'The Effects of Advance Care Planning on End-of-life Care: A Systematic Review.' *Palliative Medicine* 28 (8): 1000–1025.

Chenail, Ronald J. 1995. 'Presenting Qualitative Data.' *The Qualitative Report* 2 (3): 1–9.

Detering, Karen M., Andrew D. Hancock, Michael C. Reade, and William Silvester. 2010. 'The Impact of Advance Care Planning on End of Life Care in Elderly Patients: Randomised Controlled Trial.' *British Medical Journal* 340 (7751): 1–9.

Engel, George L. 1977. 'The Need for a New Medical Model: A Challenge for Biomedicine.' *Science* 196 (4286): 129–136.

Frosch, D.L., and R.M. Kaplan. 1999. 'Shared Decision Making in Clinical Medicine: Past Research and Future Directions.' *American Journal of Preventive Medicine* 17 (4): 285–294.

Gale, Nicola K., Gemma Heath, Elaine Cameron, Sabina Rashid, and Sabi Redwood. 2013. 'Using the Framework Method for the Analysis of Qualitative Data in Multi-disciplinary Health Research.' *BMC Medical Research Methodology* 13 (117): 1–8.

Gaveras, Eleni Margareta, Maria Kristiansen, Allison Worth, Tasneem Irshad, and Aziz Sheikh. 2014. 'Social Support for South Asian Muslim Parents with Life-limiting Illness Living in Scotland: A Multiperspective Qualitative Study.' *BMJ Open* 4 (2): 1–11.

Good, Phillip, Russell Richard, William Syrmis, Sue Jenkins-Marsh, and Jane Stephens. 2014. 'Medically Assisted Nutrition for Adult Palliative Care Patients.' *Cochrane Database of Systematic Reviews* 4 (CD006274): 1–16.

Green, Judith, and Nicki Thorogood. 2009. *Qualitative Methods for Health Research*. 2nd ed. Los Angeles, CA: Sage.

Guest, Greg, Arwen Bunce, and Laura Johnson. 2006. 'How Many Interviews Are Enough?: An Experiment with Data Saturation and Variability.' *Field Methods* 18 (1): 59–82.

Heath, Iona. 2006. 'Commentary: Patients Are Not Commodities.' *British Medical Journal* 332 (7545): 846–847.

Illich, Ivan. 1974. *Medical Nemesis: The Expropriation of Health*. London: Calder and Boyars.

Kettani, Houssain. 2010. 'World Muslim Population.' In *Proceedings of the 8th Hawaii International Conference on Arts and Humanities, Honolulu, Hawaii*. Available at http://hichumanities.org/wp-content/uploads/proceedings-library/AH2010.pdf.

Kübler-Ross, Elisabeth, and David Kessler. 2014. *On Grief and Grieving: Finding the Meaning of Grief Through the Five Stages of Loss*. New York, NY: Scribner.

Mahdi, Sundus, Obadah Ghannam, Sydeaka Watson, and Aasim I. Padela. 2016. 'Predictors of Physician Recommendation for Ethically Controversial Medical Procedures: Findings from an Exploratory National Survey of American Muslim Physicians.' *Journal of Religion and Health* 55 (2): 403–421.

O'Neill, Onora. 2002. *Autonomy and Trust in Bioethics: The Gifford Lectures, University of Edinburgh, 2001*. Cambridge: Cambridge University Press.

Padela, Aasim I., Katie Gunter, Amal Killawi, and Michele Heisler. 2012. 'Religious Values and Healthcare Accommodations: Voices from the American Muslim Community.' *Journal of General Internal Medicine* 27 (6): 708–715.

Ritchie, Jane, and Jane Lewis, eds. 2003. *Qualitative Research Practice: A Guide for Social Science Students and Researchers*. London: Sage.

Sackett, David L. 2005. 'Evidence-based Medicine.' In *Encyclopedia of Biostatistics*, eds. Peter Armitage and Theodore Colton. 2nd ed. 8 vols. London: Wiley.

Sandelowski, Margarete. 1994. 'Focus on Qualitative Methods: The Use of Quotes in Qualitative Research.' *Research in Nursing ad Health* 17 (6): 479–482.

———. 1998. 'Writing a Good Read: Strategies for Re-presenting Qualitative Data.' *Research in Nursing and Health* 21 (4): 375–382.

Stange, Kurt C. 2010. 'Power to Advocate for Health.' *The Annals of Family Medicine* 8 (2): 100–107.

**Dr Mehrunisha Suleman** is a physician and bioethicist conducting postdoctoral research at the University of Cambridge on the ethics of end-of-life care. She is an expert for UNESCO's Ethics Teacher Training Programme and is a council member at the Nuffield Council on Bioethics. She has an *'Alimiyyah* degree in traditional Islamic studies.

# Chapter 9
# The Intersection between Science and Sunnī Theological and Legal Discourse in Defining Medical Death

**Rafaqat Rashid**

## 9.1 Introduction

This chapter engages with the ongoing conversations within the long Islamic intellectual tradition on the definition and meaning of death. Using medicalized dying as the context for discussion, I will consider epistemological and metaphysical matters and examine issues from ethico-legal and theological perspectives. There are several pragmatic implications of death for Muslims that go beyond simply harvesting organs for transplantation or withdrawing life support. There are also many gaps in the understanding of medical death in the Islamic legal corpus. The questions of what it is to be alive, to be human, and to be a person have not been adequately or systematically addressed in a way that allows us to see them not only as part of the majority Sunnī theological tradition, but also to place the Islamic understanding of these questions in a coherent dialogue with both scientific and philosophical inquiry. I will therefore explore the relationship between body, soul and mind in order to articulate the Islamic theological responses addressing notions of human personhood and how they fare at their intersections with biomedical science. The aim is to support an understanding of how the meaning and definition of death can be pragmatically and medically identified from an Islamic perspective.

That is why a study of the Islamic tradition and its philosophical nature is needed to clarify or verify any metaphysical and/or theological alignment with the physicalist view of a definitive indicator of death of the individual's being 'brain dead.' Here, I argue that the traditional understanding of death as the irreversible loss of cardiopulmonary function is not an accurate account of death. I shall argue that death is marked by the permanent cessation of higher-brain functioning, i.e., having permanently lost the capacity for sentience, volition, reasoning and all other

R. Rashid (✉)
Al-Balagh Academy, Bradford, UK
e-mail: drrafaqat@albalaghacademy.com



A. al-Akiti, A. I. Padela (eds.), *Islam and Biomedicine*, Philosophy and Medicine 137, https://doi.org/10.1007/978-3-030-53801-9_9

higher-brain functionalities. These lost functions correspond metaphysicially to the departure of the rational soul. Yet even after loss of this functioning, as I will demonstrate, the human organism has an intrinsic value – a moral value without the rational soul, when the *person* is dead but the *body* is alive.

## 9.2 Investigation of Human Death

The investigation of human death has focused on two important questions:

1. What is human death?
2. How can we determine that it has occurred?

The first question is ontological, requiring a definition or conceptualization of death. The second is epistemological, employing a general definition (or criterion) for determining that death has occurred with specific clinical tests that ensure the definition has been met.[1] The first question has led to a number of diverse conceptualizations of death. While these conceptions vary, definitions of death are tied to physiological markers and fall into one of three categories:[2]

1. those relating to the irreversible loss of vital fluid flow caused by cessation of heart and lung function, as determined by apnoea and absence of pulse. This is generally considered the traditional standard;
2. those based on either whole-brain or brainstem criteria marked by the irreversible loss of integrating capacity, consciousness, and capacity to breathe;[3] and finally,
3. those involving a higher-brain notion of death, defined by the irreversible loss of 'personhood,' identified as cessation of higher-brain *function* leading to the absence of responsiveness, sentience, voluntary movements, volition and all associated functionalities of the cerebral cortex.

Whole-brain death refers to the destruction of the entire brain, both the higher brain and the brainstem. The most powerful case for the whole-brain criterion appeals to two considerations:[4]

1. an *organismic* definition of death; and

---

[1] DeGrazia (2017).

[2] There may be some slight variants to these, but essentially these three broad accounts sum up all.

[3] Two sets of criteria for the diagnosis of brain death have been accepted. The first is the landmark Harvard code-of-practice definition for 'whole-brain' death with the requirement for ancillary testing in addition to contemporary criteria. The second is the original UK criteria of the irreversible loss of the capacity to breathe, combined with the irreversible loss of the capacity for consciousness satisfied through the loss of brainstem function. See Wijdicks (2001): 1215–21; Pallis and Harley (1996).

[4] DeGrazia (2017).

2. an emphasis on the brain's role as the *primary integrator* of overall bodily functioning.

The organismic definition of death is the irreversible loss of functioning of the organism as a whole.[5] Death is emphasized as a biological or physiological occurrence common to all organisms as a whole and goes beyond life and death of individual cells and organs. The functional component as an integrated unit breaks down, changing a living dynamic organism into one that no longer functions and so disintegrates and decays. It is the collapse of this integrated bodily functioning which leads to death. Some may argue that this conception of death is predominantly a positivist, physicalist view of death and precludes any metaphysical or theistic approach.[6] A study of the Islamic theological tradition and its philosophical nature is what is needed to clarify or verify any metaphysical and theological alignment with the physicalist view of death restricted to the brain.

It is important to emphasize that determining death is not as clear as some may assume. One can hope to be certain, but that is not always the case, nor is there any recourse which can assure that it is. For Muslims, the Qur'an and the Prophetic tradition or *ḥadīth* are not explicit about signs of death. As a result, some Muslim scholars argue that the whole-brain definition for death is not an acceptable standard for determining death. It is speculative, uncertain and doubtful. The person is alive, and we are certain about this, and death is uncertain, so this certainty of life cannot be overruled by the inherent uncertainty within the diagnosis of neurological death.[7] What these positions overlook is that Islam is predominantly a legal tradition and Islamic law (*fiqh*) is the determining factor that allows us to make the right moral decisions.[8] What is agreed upon is that the Qur'an and Prophetic tradition are not explicit in their definition or diagnosis of death, and it is therefore left to *ijtihād* (legal juristic effort) to deduce rulings from these texts and reach a legal opinion (*fatwā*) on the definition of death. Laws derived from *ijtihād* are considered *ẓannī* (predominant conjecture or an approximation), which is quite distinct from *qaṭʿī* (definitive or conclusive knowledge).[9] What is essential here is to acknowledge that although the epistemological precepts of Islamic law allow for some possibility of error in legal reasoning, which indeed is inevitable, the law must be accepted as the authoritative corpus in determining normative legal values.

That death must be determined with certainty (*yaqīn*), from a legal epistemological perspective, as some Muslim scholars assert, is not possible, as death cannot be determined at such a level of absoluteness. This has been shown not only in some of the claims of Muslim jurists, but would also be acknowledged by anyone with a

[5] Becker (1975): 334–59; Bernat, Culver, and Gert (1981): 389–94.

[6] Bedir and Aksoy (2011): 290–294.

[7] Al-Wāʿī (1987): 255.

[8] Jackson (2003).

[9] Al-Āmidī (1984), 4:396.

grasp of pragmatism and reality.[10] Classical Muslim jurists relied on sources other than religious scripture to indicate the physical signs which are recorded in the books of *fiqh*, and these sources relate to the experience and expertise of their time. Signs of death are listed such as limpness of the spine and limbs with an inability to actively move,[11] motionlessness, change of skin colour, glaring of eyes or their inability to constrict, depression of temples, slanting of nose, opening of the lips, lucidness of skin of the face, looseness of wrists from arms, ascending of the testicles with drooping of the (scrotal) skin.[12] Those signs are abstruse, diverse, subjective, rely on observer bias, and raise doubts as to the level of accuracy, especially when a person dies from conditions which may mask these signs.[13] What jurists try to achieve is a state of approximation, or its equivalence to certainty, where we can be assured that we are doing the right thing having sought Islamic legal authority. The great Damascene jurist of the Ḥanafī school, Ibn ʿĀbidīn (d. 1252/1836),[14] even warned that, 'many of those who have been considered dead due to their motionlessness are buried alive because it is difficult to determine death conclusively except with the best medical experts.'[15] When we turn to Islamic legal authority we can see that the tradition at times describes '*yaqīn,*' when used in the legal sense here in determining death, yet we know that we are unable to achieve absolute certainty. Rather our recourse is to *ijtihād*, which is considered *ẓannī*, or an approximation. This falls at the epistemic level of predominant conjecture (*ghalabat al-ẓann*), and not *yaqīn*. *Ghalabat al-ẓann* is described as a legal approximation of when 'there is a possibility of two matters: one is preferred above the other when assessing the proofs of the situation and what is apparent from the sources.'[16] These legal terms can at times be used interchangeably and can be confused. *Ghalabat al-ẓann* in applied legal theory is what suffices here with regards to determining human death.[17] Bearing these epistemic points in mind, we can now investigate how to determine a legal standard by which one can be treated as dead by Islamic law.

---

[10] Al-Saʿīdān (n.d.), 4.

[11] Al-Zaylaʿī (2000), 1:234; Ibn al-Humām (2003), 2:102; al-Shāfiʿī (2001), 1:322; al-Nawawī (1996), 5:110; Ibn Qudāma (2007), 2:162; al-Buhūtī (2015), 1:343.

[12] Ibn al-Humām (2003), 2:102; Ibn ʿĀbidīn (1994), 2:189; al-Kharashī (1975), 2:122; al-Shirbīnī (2000), 1:332; al-Buhūtī (1983), 2:84–5; Ibn Qudāma (2007), 2:162; al-Buhūtī (2015), 1:343; al-Nawawī (1996), 5:110.

[13] Abū Zayd (1997), 1:227; al-Nawawī (2003), 2:98 and 5:54; al-Ḥadīthī (1997), 24; Ibn Qudāma (2007), 2:337 and 5:110; Qalʿahjī (2007), 1:852; Ibn Rushd (1994), 1:164.

[14] He was a prominent Islamic scholar and jurist who lived in the city of Damascus during the Ottoman era. He was an authority of the Ḥanafī school of Islamic law. His most famous work was *Radd al-muḥtār* (*The Response to the Baffled*), which is still considered the authoritative text of Ḥanafī *fiqh*.

[15] Ibn ʿĀbidīn (1994), 1:275.

[16] Al-Saʿīdān (n.d.).

[17] Al-Jurjanī (2004), 144 and 128; al-Tahānawī (1996), 2:780; Ibn al-Farrā' (1993), 1:83; al-Bājī (2001), 11; al-Zarkashī (1992), 1:77; Ibn al-Najjār (1993), 1:74.

## 9.3 The Soul and Integrated Bodily Functioning

One notion that Muslim scholars agree upon is that death or end of life occurs at the time the soul[18] leaves the body, and this departure of the soul is seen as the main event that determines that the person has died.[19] We can consider this metaphysical departure of the soul from the body as equivalent to the collapse of integrated bodily functioning. On this account, the soul would be functionally equivalent to the brain as the primary integrator of bodily functioning and hence, death of the *person* would be ascribed to the death of the brain.

As stated in the Qur'an,

> And they ask you [O' Muhammad], about the soul (*rūḥ*). Say, 'The soul is part of my Lord's affair. You have only been given a little knowledge.[20]

The reality of the metaphysical nature of the departure of the soul from the body at the time of death is only known to God. To attempt to study the arrival and departure of the soul from the body is considered permissible; what is questioned is whether it is achievable.[21] There is some reference to the departure of the soul from the body in the Qur'an and Prophetic tradition, but it is not explicit or clear enough to give us a scientific, physiological or biological, account of the process.

> If you could only see the wicked in their death agonies, as the angels stretch out their hands [to them], saying: Let out your souls ...[22]

> The Prophet, when he entered upon Abū Salāma (who died) and his eyes were open and the Messenger closed them, then the Messenger said, 'when the soul is taken the eyes follow it.'[23]

There are also descriptions related to the kind of death or types of death:

> God takes the souls at the time of their death, and the souls of the living while they sleep. He keeps hold of those whose death He has decreed and sends the others back until their appointed time: there truly are signs in this for those who reflect.[24]

So, death is like eternal sleep in that the soul departs from the body just like it does during sleep, except death is eternal.[25] Muslim theologians, however, differentiate between death and sleep with regard to the soul, as one of allegory (*tashbīh*) in the

---

[18] It should be noted that the terms *nafs* (soul) and *rūḥ* (spirit) are used interchangeably in the Qur'an, generally referring to the soul. The former may also mean 'self,' 'blood' and 'living body,' while the latter may also mean 'physical breath' or even 'wind.' To avoid confusion, I translate both as 'soul.'

[19] Al-Nawawī (1996), 5:94, Ibn Qudāma (2007), 3:367, Niẓām (2000), 1:157.

[20] Qur'an 17:85 (*al-Isrā'*).

[21] Al-Qurṭubī (2006), 8:284–7; al-Ghazālī (2005), 1840.

[22] Qur'an 6:93 (*al-An'ām*).

[23] Related by Muslim (2006), 1:409 (*ḥadīth* no. 920); and Ibn Mājah (1952–1953), 1:467 (*ḥadīth* no. 1454).

[24] Qur'an 39:42 (*al-Zumar*).

[25] See Qur'an 39:42 (*al-Zumar*) and 6:60 (*al-An'ām*).

figurative sense and not equivalence (*tamāthīl*) in the real sense. The metaphysical connection (*ʿalāqa*) between the soul and body is described as one of completeness, whereas this connection is weakened during sleep. Sleep is not death in reality but rather a minor death (*al-wafāt al-ṣughrā*).[26]

Any approach in determining a standard for death must be in line with the spirit of juristic principles accepted as the corpus of authority derived from Qur'an and Prophetic tradition. This can be achieved by referring back to the approach of authorities amongst Muslim theologians and jurists and what they relied upon. Muslim scholars throughout history have attempted to explain in some detail the relationship between body and soul. It is with those descriptions that we can begin to get some account of the soul, how science can relate to it, and how this bodily manifestation can be picked up by clinical tests. Muslim jurists have listed indefinite physical signs in their *fiqh* books, relying on experience and expertise, after having accepted that there may be doubts. After all, what else could they do? They did not have the technology or the medical knowledge we have today and so addressed the issue the best way they knew. If we were to make sense of the soul's departure from the body and how this would manifest itself physically so we could use clinical tests to detect when it does so, this would be no more inaccurate than the approach of classical Muslim jurists, and in fact would arguably be more accurate, as more is known and the technology is more advanced.

From the theological perspective, al-Ghazālī (d. 505/1111)[27] explains:

> The meaning of the soul parting from the body is the separation (*taṣarraf*) of the control of its actions from the body. The organs are tools of the soul to be used by it such as drying with hands, listening with ears, seeing with eyes and learning the truth of things by themselves. Death is the failure of all, and all organs are tools used by the soul. The meaning of death is the separation of actions from the body and departing from the body as an instrument for the soul.[28]

So when the soul is unable to control these actions, that is death. This is further supported by what Ibn Qayyim al-Jawziyya (d. 751/1350)[29] asserts:

> The meaning of the parting of the soul from body is the separation (*taṣarraf*) of the stimulation of it [the soul] from the body due to the exiting of the body from its control … It can

[26] Al-Ashqar (1991), 373–4; Faraj (2010); al-Daqr (1997), 97.

[27] Abū Ḥāmid Muḥammad ibn Muḥammad al-Ghazālī considered to be the *mujaddid* (reviver) of his age, a Sunnī, Shāfiʿī jurist, Ashʿarī theologian, philosopher, and Ṣūfī master of Persian descent. His major work, the *Iḥyāʾ ʿulūm al-dīn* (*The Revival of the Religious Sciences*), was well-received universally by Islamic scholars such as al-Nawawī (d. 676/1277) who famously remarked, 'Were the books of Islam all to be lost, except the *Iḥyāʾ*, it would suffice to replace them all.' See Lumbard (2009), 291.

[28] Al-Ghazālī (2005), 1840.

[29] Shams al-Dīn Abū ʿAbd Allāh Muḥammad ibn Abī Bakr al-Zurʿī al-Dimashqī al-Ḥanbalī, commonly known as Ibn Qayyim al-Jawziyya. He was an important Sunnī medieval Islamic jurisconsult, theologian, and spiritual writer, belonging to the Ḥanbalī school of orthodox Sunnī jurisprudence, of which he is regarded as 'one of the most important thinkers.' See Livingston (1971), 96–103.

be determined that it is the soul that controls volition, voluntary actions and movements (*al-ḥarakāt al-irādiyya*) and perceives and feels sensation (*al-ḥiss*).[30]

Theologians like al-Ghazālī, Ibn Qayyim, and others,[31] who are also recognized authorities in Islamic law, describe a dualistic view of the soul, where the soul is described as either immaterial, or a subtle body (*al-jism al-laṭīf*), that can exist in a disembodied state, such that when the body has no causative relationship with the soul then this is death.[32] This dualist conception of the soul is the most accepted traditional view in Islam.[33] Ibn Qayyim provides detailed proofs from the Islamic scriptural sources in support of this definition in his well-known work *Kitāb al-Rūḥ* (*The Book of the Soul*).[34] This causative relationship is described in terms of *idrāk* (voluntary actions, volition, sentience, and will and all other associated capacities which determine moral actions). It does not necessarily extend to the broader conception of the permanent loss of the integrative bodily functioning, indicating that when the soul has no control of the *critical functions* of the body, the *mukallaf* no longer resides, and the *person* is to be considered dead. A *mukallaf* is a person who meets the minimal legal prerequisites to be considered obligated by Islamic law to discharge a legal duty. The use of the term here is in the broadest sense indicating the minimal requirements of capacity for a person to be held accountable morally as an *insān* (a human being or a moral human person) who has the capacity for the critical-functional human and rational components of the person.

## 9.4 Different Kinds of Life

Although heartbeat and breathing normally *indicate* life, they do not *constitute* life. Life involves the integrated functioning of the whole organism. The brain makes all these vital functions possible. But there are problems with conceiving of the brain as the primary integrator of bodily functioning, with the soul resembling the brain in this account. Many of our integrative functions like anti-entropic mutual

[30] Ibn Qayyim al-Jawziyya (1994), 288–289.

[31] Ibn Ḥajar al-ʿAsqalānī (2015), 2:67; Ibn Kathīr (1990), 14:202–4; al-Shawkānī (n.d.), 2:143. Other theologians include: Fakhr al-Dīn al-Rāzī (d. 604/1210), Sayf al-Dīn al-Āmidī (d. 631/1223), al-Bayḍāwī (d. 685/1286), and Saʿd al-Dīn al-Taftāzānī (d. 793/1390). See al-Ījī (1970), 229.

[32] This is also the Platonic conception of the soul. Plato (d. *ca.* 347 BC) in his *Phaedo* presents a dualist account of the soul, with a disembodied soul, or mind (*psyche*), with the person. See *Phaedo*, in Plato (1980), 63e-69e.

[33] For a fuller account of the soul in the Islamic tradition, see for example, Chap. 7, 'Where the Two Oceans Meet: The Theology of Islam and the Philosophy of Psychiatric Medicine in Exploring the Human Self,' by Asim Yusuf and Afifi al-Akiti in this book.

[34] He claims, 'The human soul is material but differs in quiddity (*al-māhiyya*) from the sensible body, being a body that is luminous, elevated, light, alive, and in motion. It penetrates the substance of the bodily organs, flowing therein in the way water flows in roses, oil in olives, and fire in charcoal,' in Ibn Qayyim al-Jawziyya (2014), 1:85.

interaction of cells and tissues, homeostasis, assimilation of nutrients, are not mediated by the brain and can therefore persist in individuals who meet the whole-brain criteria for death by standard clinical tests.[35] These integrative functions are not what constitute life and are not critical to rationality and human functioning. It is the cessation of the critical integrated brain functionality, not cessation of all isolated brain activity nor these integrative functions external to the brain, that relate to the actions of the soul. Hence, not every aspect of the brain is necessary to maintain the integrated critical system of the organism specific to the soul.

An irreversible cessation of the brain's capacity for consciousness as the *critical* brain's integrated higher-brain functioning would prove more befitting, rather than whole-brain functioning. 'Consciousness' here is to be used in the broad sense including subjective experience during wakefulness and dreaming states. When it comes to different aspects of consciousness like 'alertness,' considered as the *level* of consciousness, then it is fundamentally under the control of the ascending reticular activating system of the brainstem, which controls our sleep-wake cycle and is independent of the cerebral cortex. Other aspects of consciousness related to 'awareness' and 'wakefulness,' related to our higher-brain functioning, considered as the *content* of consciousness, are subject to the control and regulation of the cerebral cortex.[36]

The 'rational soul' has control over most conscious activities and 'resembles' the cerebral cortex's higher-brain functioning. According to Abū Bakr al-Rāzī (d. *ca.* 313/925)[37] the animal soul refers to unconscious activities, while the rational soul refers to conscious activities. The rational soul for al-Rāzī comprises *nafs* (the soul) described in the functional sense as the human (*insāniyya*) component or rational (*nāṭiqa*) soul, which has the role of the intellect relating to actions (*ʿāmila*) and cognitive intellect (*ʿālima*). The soul's intellective activity and cognitive involvement relates to the world of matter and intellect, and of body-and-mind (the physical world), but when the body is no longer, the soul reverts to the purely intellectual world of abstraction. Then there is the animal (*ḥayawāniyya*) component to the soul which controls motion (*muḥarrika*) and perception (*mudrika*), and finally the vegetative (*nabātiyya*) soul which relates to nutrition (*ghadhiyya*), growth (*nāmiyya*) and reproduction (*muwāllida*). The human and animal components of the soul relate to conscious activities such as sentience and volition, i.e., higher-brain functions, and the vegetative component relates to nutrition, growth and reproduction, i.e., the unconscious activities.[38] The different functional roles of the soul (rational, animal, vegetative) cohere with the views of many Muslim theologians in that they indicate

---

[35] Shewmon (2001): 457–478; See also, Potts (2001): 479–491.

[36] Laureys et al. (2009), 2:1133–1142.

[37] Abū Bakr Muḥammad ibn Zakariyyā al-Rāzī, known as Rhazes to Europeans, was born in Rayy, a Persian city near present-day Tehran. He was one of the most important and influential of all medieval Islamic physicians. He wrote on many different subjects related to medicine, ethics, and philosophy. His *Kitāb al-Ḥāwī fī al-ṭibb* (*The Comprehensive Book on Medicine*) was assembled by his students after his death and is preserved today. For more, see Adamson (2017), 63–82

[38] Al-Attas (1995), 143–176.

a separation of the centres of reason, volition and sentience from those components of the physical body that are effective of, responsive to, and subservient to such controls. The purpose of the soul is to know and obey God and be accountable to Him as an obligated agent (*mukallaf*). It follows that the rational soul is the primary component that is responsible and accountable for such obligations. The animal and vegetative souls would merely be those components that control and regulate movement and sensory organs, and so have a more bodily dependent role that allows the body to engage with its environment and hence to allow the soul to achieve its purpose.[39] The cerebral cortex has divisions, subdivisions and sub-regions that are known to control aspects of emotion, hearing, vision, personality and all voluntary actions. It also directs the conscious or volitional motor functions of the body and is the centre of sensory perception, memory, thoughts, judgement, and speech and language. Similarly, these attributes of voluntary bodily functioning and higher-brain functioning related to volition and sentience have also been ascribed to the soul. What we can be sure about is that involuntary movements and reflexes and general biological growth, reproduction and nutrition, have been shown not to be critically or primarily controlled by the brainstem, cerebral cortex or the 'rational' soul,[40] as they can be artificially maintained and supported.

The cerebral cortex, the location of higher-brain functioning, is the nearest instrument and implement of the rational soul. The differences between the soul and the cerebral cortex become clear for Muslims when we refer to some of the abstract and subjective functions like emotions, reflection, and aspects of higher cognition, and even more so when it comes to intention, will, perception of universals, subjectivity, and intuitive feelings related to the ego. These differences, the details of which are beyond the scope of this chapter, are what make us obligated and hence accountable agents and are related to the *critical* purposes and functions of the soul.

The problem with consciousness, as the 'essence' of the soul's loss, at death, of control of the critical human and rational components of the functioning body, is the impossibility of drawing a clear line between sentient *persons* and sentient *non-persons*, i.e., in progressive dementia cases or with human newborns that have no content of consciousness, or such diminished consciousness that they would be considered dead according to a higher-brain functioning criterion for determination of death. Is a foetus prior to the emergence of a soul dead or alive? If it is alive, it would have a relatively lower moral value until it is ensouled (i.e., becomes a person) at around 40 to 120 days.[41] Its life before ensoulment would just be a

---

[39] Ibid., 170–176.

[40] Except maybe some voluntary regulatory role in changing circumstances through an overriding mechanism.

[41] There is a difference of opinion amongst Muslim scholars about when ensoulment occurs in the foetus. This is based on interpretations and acceptance of different Prophetic traditions which indicate 40–42 days in accordance to some *ḥadīths* and 120 days according to others, where the total of three consecutive 40 days add up to 120 days. For a discussion of the controversy surrounding the various ensoulment periods in the Muslim tradition, see Chap. 6, 'When Does a Human Foetus Become Human?' by Hamza Yusuf in this book.

physiological or biological life, having less intrinsic value. Muslim jurists permit the abortion of an embryo or foetus not yet ensouled, with caveats. This differentiates between the state before ensoulment, where it has a lower moral value, relative to post-ensoulment, when the foetus is considered a human *person* (*insān*). It then has a life of moral value equal to any other person's, and to take this life would thus be considered a greater crime.[42]

According to Ibn Qayyim, the foetus has two types of life: (1) *qabla-nafkh* (pre-ensoulment), similar to plant life, with growth and involuntary nourishment, related solely to the physiological body; and (2) *baʿda-nafkh* (post-ensoulment), when the soul has been blown into the body and there are sentience, volition and voluntary movements (i.e., higher-brain functions).[43] Studies of embryological and foetal development show that by week 11–15 from conception[44] (gestational age GA, 13–17 weeks), the first sulcus of the cerebrum appears and it is not until week 17 (GA 19 weeks), that the important layers of the developing cerebral cortex are developed. The first foetal movements felt by the mother, sometimes called *quickening*, often occur between 14 and 20 weeks (GA 16 to 22 weeks) of pregnancy. The heart develops in the 1st week (GA 3rd week); and at the end of the 2nd week (GA 4th week), the heartbeats of the embryo begin. It is by the 21st week (GA week 23) that the foetus demonstrates stimulus-induced heart-rate accelerations. As the pons, which is later to mature, mediates arousal, body movements, and vestibular and vibroacoustic perception from around the 18th to 25th weeks, the foetus responds with arousal and body movements to vibroacoustic and loud sounds delivered to the maternal abdomen. Cognitive brain activities and REM sleep cycles occur, interestingly, just after what some consider ensoulment (again, after around 16–17 weeks, or 120 days from conception).[45] The functional status of foetal organ development prior to ensoulment (in the scenario of less than 120 days) suggests that heartbeat, pulsation, and circulation of blood, as well as basic respiratory movements, can occur even pre-ensoulment. These are bodily functions that occur without the existence of the soul in the body. There are dissenting juristic views amongst Muslim scholars on the time of foetal ensoulment, mainly between 40 and 120 days. Even if we consider ensoulment at the earlier time of 40 days, we cannot escape the fact that what exists before ensoulment is considered a growing organism with some integrated functional capabilities consistent with life, some element of functional independence and intrinsic moral value.

---

[42] Ibn ʿĀbidīn (1994), 2:380 and 2:390; Ibn al-Humām (2003), 2:495.

[43] Ibn Qayyim al-Jawziyya (1994), 288–9.

[44] Note that embryological staging in the Qur'an begins at conception which is at fertilization. However gestational age (GA) is counted from the first day of the menstrual period, which is 14 days before conception/fertilization, and this is generally considered the earliest time for fertilization. Therefore, according to dating from the Islamic theological perspective, 40 days would be counted as 54 days gestation.

[45] A useful resource is Hill (2021).

A patient who has advanced dementia or is in a permanent vegetative state (PVS),[46] may show no evidence of consciousness on physical examination. Such patients are seemingly awake but lack any behavioural evidence of 'voluntary' or 'willed' behaviour. This is due to extensive and irreversible brain damage. Patients in a vegetative state may have awoken from a coma (related to different *levels* of consciousness), but still not have regained awareness (*content* of consciousness).[47] In the vegetative state, patients can open their eyelids occasionally and demonstrate sleep-wake cycles, but lack cognitive function and volition on physical examination and clinical testing. In my view, a patient in PVS or severe progressive dementia[48] who is spontaneously breathing and has circulating blood and exhibits a full range of brainstem reflexes would be alive, as this is like the state of a pre-ensouled foetus, that is a physiological, biological life, and hence at a relatively lower moral value of life. He would be a living body; but the *person* (the soul), if present, would have no control of the critical human and rational components of the body, and there would be no sentience and volition. Similar is the case of an anencephalic infant, one who is born without cerebral hemispheres and never had the capacity for sentience or volition (i.e., with no higher-brain functions). He would also be alive as a living physiological, biological body; yet his soul (if indeed he has one) – its instrument to control the critical human and rational components of the body – would have no capacity.

Some of our biological bodily functions may still be alive and able to function independently of our soul, and so the physiological body may still have integrated bodily functioning. The body, in this case, would have an intrinsic moral value without the soul, but less than that of a life with the soul.

## 9.5 Normative Legal Values and Death

There are Islamic legal cases mentioned in the books of *fiqh* that more specifically identify cessation of volition, sentience, and voluntary action (i.e., higher-brain functions) as determining factors in considering somebody as legally dead, and also in meeting out retaliatory punishment upon a murderer. Both these kinds of ruling require a substantial degree of certainty, and these cases suffice to provide

[46] This is due to extensive and irreversible brain damage, as opposed to a coma, which is a state of unconsciousness. Note the use of 'permanent' vegetative state rather than 'persistent.' The latter is potentially reversible, while the former is not.

[47] Laureys et al. (2010): 1–4.

[48] Most PVS patients are unresponsive to external stimuli, but their condition may be associated with different levels of consciousness. Some level of consciousness means a person can still respond in varying degrees to stimulation, though involuntarily as in the minimally conscious state (MCS). People in MCS display severe altered consciousness but can demonstrate some evidence of conscious awareness and higher-brain functioning. See Giacino et al. (2002): 349–353.

normative legal rules in enacting death behaviours.[49] The punishment of *qiṣāṣ* (retribution by death penalty) is meted out on the assaulter, accused of murder, on the basis that the victim has lost all sentience, volition, sight, speech, and voluntary movements (*ḥarakāt al-ikhtiyārī*) permanently. Interestingly, even in the situation where the attacker does not fully slit the throat of the victim, and the soul has not yet departed, *qiṣāṣ* will only be meted out on the accused if as a result the victim has permanent cessation of sentience and volition. Any apparent involuntary movements (*ḥarakāt al-iḍṭirārī*) or sentience detected is considered analogous to the movements seen after sacrificial slaughtering of an animal (*ḥarakāt al-madhbūḥ*) and is therefore not recognized as a sign of life.[50]

The Shāfiʿī jurist Badr al-Dīn al-Zarkashī (d. 794/1392) asserts that the state of sustained life (*al-ḥayāt al-mustaqarra*) is when the soul is connected to the body with voluntary movements and sentience. Involuntary movements alone are not to be considered as signs of life. This follows from the *ḥadīth* of the second caliph, ʿUmar ibn al-Khaṭṭāb (d. 23/644), who declared that after slitting the throat of a sacrificial animal, any movement is involuntary and is to be recognized as devoid of sight, speech, voluntary movement, sentience and volition (i.e., the higher-brain functions).[51] So all four Sunnī legal schools concede this to be a virtual or *de jure* death (*al-mawt al-ḥukmī*).[52] Preparing the funeral prayer (*janāza*), bathing (*ghusl*), shrouding (*kafan*), and burial (*dafn*), including taking into account the waiting period (*ʿidda*) of his wife and her remarriage, will all follow. He will not be able to inherit from others and all the rulings of death will apply.[53]

I believe the Islamic legal sources indicate that the irreversible loss of *higher-brain functioning* described as a loss of voluntary movement, sentience and volition, marks the commencement of death and the time when death behaviours becomes appropriate, regardless of any involuntary movement.[54] A state without higher-brain functioning would be analogous to the state of *ḥarakāt al-madhbūḥ*, where sentience, volition and higher cognitive functioning are absent, and this is when death behaviours can commence.

---

[49] The term 'death behaviours' has been borrowed from Veatch, who says that some behaviours traditionally associated with death can be unbundled, but also that other behaviours (including organ procurement) must continue to be associated with death. See Veatch (2005): 353–378.

Death behaviours in the Islamic tradition would include ritual acts/practices performed after death is announced, such as initiation of the three-day ritual mourning, ritual washing, shrouding, the funeral prayers, burial, distribution of inheritance, and all other associated actions after death.

[50] Niẓām (2000), 1:381; al-Dardīr (1986), 4:340; al-Nawawī (1996), 18:372; Ibn Qudāma (2007), 9:384.

[51] Al-Zarkashī (1982–5), 29:150.

[52] Examples of *mawt ḥukmī* include cases when someone has been missing for some time and a judge determines that s/he has died, i.e., presumptive death with high probability, which permits rulings of death to proceed. See al-Kharashī (1975), 2:145; al-Mardāwī (1955-8), 9:141; Ibn Nujaym (1997), 8:335; Yāsīn (1991), 413.

[53] Al-Shirbīnī (2000), 5:252–3; al-Nawawī (2003), 4:7; al-Ramlī (1993), 2:436–7.

[54] DeGrazia (2017).

I believe death behaviours can be started at two moral levels, or in two moral states. The first moral state is permanent loss of capacity for higher-brain functioning, which allows for all rulings of death. The second state is that when all breathing and circulation has permanently ceased after withdrawing all artificial support. The person is then to be considered already dead, and the body can now be shrouded, prayed over and buried.

## 9.6 Determining When Death Has Occurred

In summary, we may accept one of two ontological concepts of life related to the soul's departure:

1. The organismic (or physiological body) approach. This notes that a person comes into existence at conception and dies when organismic integrated functioning of the physiological body has broken down. This is based on what is necessary for the organism to continue to function as a whole and occurs when the body's vital functions cease. It is interpreted as either (i) the traditional definition of death related to irreversible loss of vital fluid flow, where death would be the loss of heart and lung function, since continued integrated functioning of the organism as a whole is not impossible with the loss of these organs; or (ii) the functional cessation of the whole brain, including the brainstem. Heart and lung function in itself is not what is essential for integrated life; rather, the loss of those capacities provides evidence that organismic integrated functioning has broken down. Once the whole brain ceases to function, the other organs necessarily fail. The brain is taken as the vital organ on which integrated functioning depends, rather than the heart and lungs. Here, the soul departs when the integrated functioning of the organism as a whole breaks down and the physiological body dies. This presents problems, as the soul has no instrumental control of the body once the higher-brain functioning has ceased and the body is not responsive to the soul and can continue living independently of the soul only if artificially maintained.
2. The higher-brain-function approach, which notes that a person comes into existence at the emergence of sentience and volition, since these are signs of higher-brain functioning, and dies before the organism (biological body) does. The soul has no instrumental control when the higher-brain function permanently ceases, and this is when death behaviours can commence.

Physiological death is not an event at some precise moment in time, but is a process. The common point of contention is knowing when to declare death. Should this be when the biological tissue has degenerated to the degree that putrefaction has occurred, or should it be at a point of no return when we are convinced that the death process is *irreversible*, or after the death cascade initiates and as soon as clinical signs are manifest enough for accurate positive clinical testing?

Historically, questions like this rarely arose because there was no technology that could either accurately detect the physiological process of death or to slow it. The interval between the initial cascade of the physiological death process to the end stage of death was so narrow that it was wrongly taken to be a precise moment in time. Today we have technology that can prolong the process or even reverse it.

Waiting for putrefaction is no longer needed. With putrefaction, the person died some considerable time before. Moreover, this does not actually address when death occurred; rather it is beyond the point when one is certain that death has already happened. We now have the technology to be able to determine death prior to this.

When the *capacity* of life has permanently ceased, and not merely physiological or electrical brain activity, then it can be said that the soul has lost control of the *critical* human and rational components of the body *permanently*, and death behaviours and legal rulings related to death can begin.

We have modern technology that can bring back a heart that ceases to beat. We have lifesaving mechanical support that can perfuse the brain if the heart stops beating. We have ventilation that supports the lungs when they fail. This was not the case before. If the heart or breathing stopped, the person had no pulse and perfusion, and as soon as this was recognized using somatic signs, the person was declared dead and preparations for burial were initiated; yet physiological activity was still present, ceased only gradually, and potentially could be reversed. We recognize that as the traditional definition of determining death. It is what the classical books of *fiqh* refer to when they describe somatic signs. These signs determined a point at which death could be declared legally, morally, or permanently *irreversible*, yet one at which we know now death/dying to be physiologically *reversible*.[55] Those who see the concept of death in biological terms believe that organisms whose physiological function could be restored should not be called dead, even though the function is permanently lost. This is not an accurate view of death, as death occurs when function loss is legally or morally irreversible, even though, physiologically, the process might be reversed. If we recognize that the person has lost the *capacity* for life, then this understanding has a broader appeal, for it identifies the time when the soul has permanently lost control of the critical human and rational components of the person.

So when does the soul actually depart during this death process, and how do we define the moment of permanent loss of capacity of higher-brain functioning in this death cascade, so as to declare death? As we explained earlier, the exact time of departure of the soul is not known with certainty, nor are we ever likely to know. What we can claim is that the soul departs sometime between the onset and the end of the physiological death process. Once the death cascade for this *permanent* loss of the capacity for higher-brain functioning initiates, the higher-brain functioning has permanently ceased, and death can be pronounced. This can be detected as soon as somatic signs are manifest enough for positive clinical testing. There is no accurate positive clinical test or anatomical criterion for a higher-brain formulation of death, since determining self-consciousness and the subjective first-person

[55] Veatch and Ross (2016), 37–49.

experience requires clinical evaluation that is limited to patients' responsiveness to the environment.[56] This would prove difficult, as such patients' responsiveness to the environment has either ceased or severely diminished to a degree that such tests would be either inaccurate or of no value. The precautionary step with today's technology would be to maintain the closest and most accurate form of clinical testing that could be an indicator that higher-brain functioning had permanently ceased because consciousness has permanently ceased. In that case, the person (the soul), if present, would have no control of the critical human and rational components of the body and there would be no sentience or volition. The current brainstem death criterion which can be accurately tested and is indicative of permanent loss of consciousness, would be the most accurate and closest method to achieving this. Despite the apparent differences between brainstem death and whole-brain death in defining death, the clinical testing of both is identical, even though the role of confirmatory investigations is different. This form of testing would also apply to higher-brain functioning criteria until new technology is able to give a more precise positive clinical testing or an anatomical criterion defined for a higher-brain formulation of death. Muslims will need to articulate precisely what components of human higher-brain functioning are ascribed to the soul in order to determine which testing for higher-brain formulation of death is the most appropriate, and how this question relates to the different ontologies of consciousness, especially given the ethical complexities that will arise with advancing technology.

## 9.7 Conclusion

Physiological death is in fact a *process*, whereas it has previously been viewed by many as occurring at a precise moment in time. The latter view is the more traditional one and is deeply embedded in society through the arts, literature, and law. To escape entirely from such a conception of death can prove difficult and affect moral sensibilities. With the medical technology we have today, this process can be delayed and prolonged through artificial means, and even reversed.

We can conclude that death is the *permanent loss of capacity of higher-brain functioning*. This occurs when there is no volition or sentience attributed to higher-brain functioning and the 'rational soul' has permanently lost its capacity of control of the critical human and rational components of the body, so that the soul, as defined by Muslim theologians, has become 'independent' or 'separated' from the body. Once the death cascade has been initiated, there is permanent loss of capacity for higher-brain functioning, and as soon as somatic signs are detected, relying on the most accurate and precise tests easily available, the person can be declared dead. At present, there is no accurate anatomical criterion for a higher-brain formulation of death. Thus the brainstem criterion for death is the closest and most accurate,

[56] Laureys (2005): 899–909.

because it is a marker that consciousness has permanently ceased. All Islamic rulings related to marriage, the waiting period and inheritance would be executed at this point. Organs can be procured and life support withdrawn when the breathing and circulation of the biological body has permanently ceased after withdrawing all artificial support. Then burial rituals can ensue.

There is a need for further research and thought to determine more precisely how the soul ties into the *content* of consciousness of higher-brain functioning. There is equally a need to ascertain which diagnostic tests would give an accurate account of the absence of the 'soul-related functioning' of the cerebral cortex.

Finally, it is worth remembering that the boundary between life and death is not perfectly sharp. Whatever definition of death is adopted, there will always remain the possibility of misdiagnosis. What is ultimately important is the Muslim public's acceptance of when those death behaviours can begin.

## References

Abū Zayd, Bakr ibn ʿAbd Allāh. 1997. *Fiqh al-nawāzil: Qaḍāyā fiqhiyya muʿāṣira*. 2 vols. Beirut: Mu'assasat al-Risāla.

Adamson, Peter. 2017. 'Abū Bakr al-Rāzī (d. 925), *The Spiritual Medicine*.' In *The Oxford Handbook of Islamic Philosophy*, eds. Khaled El-Rouayheb and Sabine Schmidtke. Oxford: Oxford University Press.

al-Āmidī. 1984. *al-Iḥkām fī uṣūl al-aḥkām*, ed. al-Sayyid al-Jumaylī. 4 vols. Beirut: Dār al-Kitāb al-ʿArabī.

al-Ashqar, ʿUmar Sulaymān. 1991. '*Baḥth muqaddam*.' In *al-Ḥayāt al-insāniyya: Bidāyatuhā wa-nihāyatuhā fī al-mafhūm al-Islāmī: Thabat kāmil li-aʿmāl Nadwat al-Ḥayāt al-Insāniyya: Bidāyatihā wa-Nihāyatihā fī al-Mafhūm al-Islāmī, al-munʿaqida bi-tārīkh al-Thulāthāʾ 24 Rabīʿ al-Ākhir 1405 H, al-muwāfiq 15 Yanāyir 1985 M*, eds. ʿAbd al-Raḥmān al-ʿAwaḍī and Khālid Madhkūr. Kuwait: al-Munaẓẓama al-Islāmiyya lil-ʿUlūm al-Ṭibbiyya.

al-Attas, Syed Naquib. 1995. *Prolegomena to the Metaphysics of Islām: An Exposition of the Fundamental Elements of the Worldview of Islām*. Kuala Lumpur: ISTAC.

al-Bājī. 2001. *al-Minhāj fī tartīb al-ḥijāj*, ed. ʿAbd al-Majīd Turkī. Beirut: Dār al-Gharb al-Islāmiyya.

Becker, Lawrence C. 1975. 'Human Being: The Boundaries of the Concept.' *Philosophy and Public Affairs* 4 (4): 334–59.

Bedir, Ahmet, and Şahin Aksoy. 2011. 'Brain Death Revisited: It Is Not "Complete Death" According to Islamic Sources.' *Journal of Medical Ethics* 37 (5): 290–294.

Bernat, James L., Charles M. Culver, and Bernard Gert. 1981. 'On the Definition and Criterion of Death.' *Annals of Internal Medicine* 94 (3): 389–94.

al-Buhūtī. 1983. *Kashshāf al-qināʿ ʿan al-Iqnāʿ*. 6 vols. Beirut: ʿĀlam al-Kutub.

———. 2015. *Sharḥ Muntahā al-irādāt al-musammā Daqāʾiq ūlī al-nuhā li-sharḥ al-Muntahā*, ed. ʿAbd Allāh ibn ʿAbd al-Muḥsin al-Turkī. Beirut: Muʾassasat al-Risāla.

al-Daqr, Nadā Muḥammad Naʿīm. 1997. *Mawt al-dimāgh bayn al-ṭibb wa-al-Islām*. Beirut: Dār al-Fikr al-Muʿāṣir.

al-Dardīr. 1986. *al-Sharḥ al-ṣaghīr ʿalā Aqrab al-masālik ilá madhhab al-Imām Mālik*, ed. Muṣṭafā Kamāl Waṣfī. 4 vols. Cairo: Dār al-Maʿārif.

DeGrazia, David. 2017. 'The Definition of Death.' In *The Stanford Encyclopedia of Philosophy*, ed. Edward N. Zalta. Spring 2017 ed. Available at https://plato.stanford.edu/entries/death-definition/

Faraj, Muḥammad Ibrāhīm al-Nādī. 2010. *Mawt al-dimāgh wa-mawqif al-fiqh al-Islāmī minh: Dirāsah muqārana*. Alexandria: Dār al-Fikr al-Jāmiʿī.
al-Ghazālī. 2005. *Iḥyāʾ al-ʿulūm al-dīn*. Beirut: Dār Ibn Ḥazm.
Giacino, Joseph T., S. Ashwal, N. Childs, R. Cranford, B. Jennett, D. I. Katz, J. P. Kelly, J. H. Rosenberg, J. Whyte, R. D. Zafonte, and N. D. Zasler. 2002. 'The Minimally Conscious State: Definition and Diagnostic Criteria.' *Neurology* 58 (3): 349–353.
al-Ḥadīthī, ʿAbd Allāh. 1997. *al-Wafāt wa al-ʿalāmātuhā bayn al-fuqaḥāʾ wa-l-aṭibbāʾ*. Beirut: Dār al-Muslim.
Hill, Mark A. 16 March 2021. '*Embryology: Timeline Human Development*.' Available at https://embryology.med.unsw.edu.au/embryology/index.php/Timeline_human_development
Ibn ʿĀbidīn. 1994. *Radd al-muḥtār ʿalā al-Durr al-mukhtār sharḥ Tanwīr al-abṣār*, eds. ʿĀdil Aḥmad ʿAbd al-Mawjūd and ʿAlī Muḥammad Muʿawwad. 6 vols. Beirut: Dār al-Fikr.
Ibn al-Farrāʾ, Abū Yaʿlāʾ. 1993. *al-ʿUdda fī uṣūl al-fiqh*, ed. Aḥmad ibn ʿAlī Sayr al-Mubārakī. 5 vols. Riyadh: Sayr al-Mubārakī.
Ibn Ḥajar al-ʿAsqalānī. 2015. *Fatḥ al-bārī bi-sharḥ Ṣaḥīḥ al-Bukhārī*, eds. ʿAbd al-ʿAzīz ibn ʿAbd Allāh ibn Bāz, ʿAlī ibn ʿAbd al-ʿAzīz al-Shibl, and Muḥammad Fuʾād ʿAbd al-Bāqī. 13 vols. Cairo: al-Maktaba al-Salafiyya.
Ibn al-Humām. 2003. *Fatḥ al-Qadīr Sharḥ Fatḥ al-qadīr ʿala al-Ḥidāya*, ed. ʿAbd al-Razzāq Ghālib al-Mahdī. 10 vols. Beirut: Dār al-Kutub al-ʿIlmiyya.
Ibn Kathīr. 1990. *al-Bidāya wa-al-Nihāya*. 15 vols. Beirut: Maktabat al-Maʿārif.
Ibn Mājah. 1952–1953. *Sunan Ibn Māja*, ed. Muḥammad Fuʾād ʿAbd al-Bāqī. 2 vols. Cairo: Dār Iḥyāʾ al-Kutub al-ʿArabiyya.
Ibn al-Najjār. 1993. *Sharḥ al-Kawkab al-munīr al-musammā bi-Mukhtaṣar al-Taḥrīr*, eds. Muḥammad al-Zuḥaylī and Nazīh Ḥammād. 4 vols. Riyadh: Wizārat al-Awqāf al-Saʿūdiyya.
Ibn Nujaym. 1997. *al-Baḥr al-rāʾiq Sharḥ Kanz al-daqāʾiq fī furūʿ al-Ḥanafiyya*, ed. Zakariyyā ʿUmayrāt. 9 vols. Beirut: Dār al-Kutub al-ʿIlmiyya.
Ibn Qayyim al-Jawziyya. 1994. *al-Tibyān fī aqsām al-Qurʾān*, ed. Fawwāz Aḥmad Zamarlī. Beirut: Dār al-Kitāb al-ʿArabī.
———. 2014. *Kitāb al-Rūḥ*, eds. Muḥammad Ajmal al-Iṣlāḥī, Kamāl ibn Muḥammad Qālimī and Bakr ibn ʿAbd Allāh Bū Zayd. 2 vols. Mecca: Dār ʿĀlam al-Fawāʾid.
Ibn Qudāma. 2007. *al-Mughnī*, eds. ʿAbd Allāh ibn ʿAbd al-Muḥsin al-Turkī and ʿAbd al-Fattāḥ Muḥammad al-Hulw. 15 vols. Riyadh: Dār ʿĀlam al-Kutub.
Ibn Rushd. 1994. *Bidāyat al-mujtahid wa-nihāyat al-muqtaṣid*, ed. Muḥammad Ṣubḥī Ḥasan Ḥallāq. 4 vols. Cairo: Maktabat Ibn Taymiyya.
al-Ījī, ʿAḍud al-Dīn. 1970. *al-Mawāqif fī ʿilm al-kalām*. Beirut: ʿĀlam al-Kutub.
Jackson, Sherman A. 2003. 'Shariʿah, Democracy, and the Modern Nation-State: Some Reflections on Islam, Popular Rule, and Pluralism.' *Fordham International Law Journal* 27 (1): 88–107.
al-Jurjanī. 2004. *Muʿjam al-taʿrīfāt*, ed. Muḥammad Ṣiddīq al-Minshāwī. Cairo: Dār al-Faḍīla.
al-Kharashī. 1975. *al-Kharashī ʿalā Mukhtaṣar Sīdī Khalīl*. 8 vols. Beirut: Dār al-Ṣādir.
Laureys, Steven. 2005. 'Science and Society: Death, Unconsciousness and the Brain.' *Nature Reviews Neuroscience* 6 (11): 899–909.
Laureys, Steven, M. Boly, G. Moonen, and P. Maquet. 2009. 'Coma.' In *Encyclopedia of Neuroscience*, ed. Larry R. Squire. 10 vols. Amsterdam: Elsevier.
Laureys, Steven, Gastone G. Celesia, Francois Cohadon, Jan Lavrijsen, José León-Carrión, Walter G. Sannita, Leon Sazbon, Erich Schmutzhard, Klaus R. von Wild, Adam Zeman, Giuliano Dolce, and the European Task Force on Disorders of Consciousness. 2010. 'Unresponsive Wakefulness Syndrome: A New Name for the Vegetative State or Apallic Syndrome.' *BMC Medicine* 8 (68): 1–4.
Livingston, John W. 1971. 'Ibn Qayyim al-Jawziyyah: A Fourteenth Century Defense Against Astrological Divination and Alchemical Transmutation.' *Journal of the American Oriental Society* 91 (1): 96–103.
Lumbard, Joseph E. B, ed. 2009. *Islam, Fundamentalism, and the Betrayal of Tradition: Essays by Western Muslim Scholars*. Bloomington, IN: World Wisdom.

al-Mardāwī. 1955–8. *al-Inṣāf fī ma'rifat al-rājiḥ min al-khilāf 'alā madhhab al-Imām Aḥmad Ibn Ḥanbal*, ed. Muḥammad Ḥāmid al-Faqī. 12 vols. Cairo: Maṭba'at al-Sunna al-Muḥammadiyya.

Muslim ibn al-Ḥajjāj. 2006. *Ṣaḥīḥ Muslim*, ed. Abū Qutayba Naẓar Muḥammad al-Fāryābi. 2 vols. Riyadh: Dār Ṭayba.

al-Nawawī. 1996. *al-Majmū' sharḥ al-Muhadhdhab*, ed. Maḥmūd al-Maṭrajī. 22 vols. Beirut: Dār al-Fikr.

———. 2003. *Rawḍat al-ṭālibīn*, eds. 'Ādil Aḥmad 'Abd al-Mawjūd and 'Alī Muḥammad Mu'awwaḍ. 8 vols. Beirut: Dār al-'Ālam al-Kutub.

Niẓām, al-Shaykh, ed. 2000. *al-Fatāwā al-Hindiyya al-ma'rūfa bi-al-Fatāwá al-'Ālamkīriyya fī madhhab al-Imām al-A'ẓam Abī Ḥanīfah al-Nu'mān*, ed. 'Abd al-Laṭīf Ḥasan 'Abd al-Raḥmān. 6 vols. Beirut: Dār al-Kutub al-'Ilmiyya.

Pallis, Christopher, and D. H. Harley. 1996. *ABC of Brainstem Death*. 2nd ed. London: BMJ Publishing.

Plato. 1980. *Plato: The Collected Dialogues*, eds. Edith Hamilton and Huntington Cairns. Princeton, NJ: Princeton University Press.

Potts, Michael. 2001. 'A Requiem for Whole Brain Death: A Response to D. Alan Shewmon's "The Brain and Somatic Integration."' *Journal of Medicine and Philosophy* 26 (5): 479–491.

Qal'ahjī, Muḥammad Rawwās. 2007. *Mawsū'āt fiqh al-Ḥasan al-Baṣrī* 2 vols. Beirut: Dār al-Nafā'is.

al-Qurṭubī. 2006. *al-Jāmi' li-aḥkām al-Qur'ān*, ed. 'Abd Allāh ibn 'Abd al-Muḥsin al-Turkī. 24 vols. Beirut: Mu'assasat al-Risāla.

al-Ramlī, Shams al-Dīn. 1993. *Niḥāyat al-Muhtāj ilā Sharḥ al-Minhāj fī al-fiqh 'ala madhhab al-Imām al-Shafi'ī*. 7 vols. Beirut: Dār al-Kutub al-'Ilmiyya.

al-Sa'īdān, Walīd ibn Rāshid. n.d. 'Risālat al-Iktifā' bi-al-'amal bi-ghalabat al-ẓann fī masā'il al-fiqh.' Self-published. Available at http://www.saaid.net/book/open.php?cat=4&book=1406.

al-Shāfi'ī. 2001. *al-Umm*, ed. Rif'at Fawzī 'Abd al-Muṭṭalib. 11 vols. Alexandria: Dār al-Wafā'.

al-Shawkānī. n.d. *al-Badr al-ṭāli' bi-mahāsin man ba'd al-qarn al-sābi'*, ed. Muḥammad ibn Muḥammad ibn Yaḥyá Zabārah al-Yamanī. 2 vols. Cairo: Dār al-Kitāb al-Islāmī.

Shewmon, D. Alan. 2001. 'The Brain and Somatic Integration: Insights into the Standard Biological Rationale for Equating "Brain Death" with Death.' *Journal of Medicine and Philosophy* 26 (5): 457–478.

al-Shirbīnī, al-Khaṭīb. 2000. *Mughnī al-muḥtāj ilā ma'rifat ma'ānī alfāẓ al-Minhāj*, eds. 'Alī Muḥammad Mu'awwaḍ and 'Ādil Aḥmad 'Abd al-Mawjūd. 6 vols. Beirut: Dār al-Kutub al-'Ilmiyya.

al-Tahānawī. 1996. *Mawsū'at kashshāf iṣṭilāḥāt al-funūn wa-al-'ulūm*, eds. Rafīq al-'Ajam and 'Alī Daḥrūj. 2 vols. Beirut: Maktabat Lubnān.

Veatch, Robert M. 2005. 'The Death of Whole-Brain Death: The Plague of the Disaggregators, Somaticists, and Mentalists.' *Journal of Medicine and Philosophy* 30 (4): 353–378.

Veatch, Robert M., and Lainie F. Ross. 2016. *Defining Death: The Case for Choice*. Washington, DC: Georgetown University Press.

al-Wā'ī, Tawfīq. 1987. 'Ḥaqīqat al-mawt wa al-ḥayāt fī al-Qur'ān wa al-aḥkām al-shar'īa.' *Majallat al-Majma' al-Fiqh al-Islāmī* 3: 255.

Wijdicks, Eelco F. M. 2001. 'The Diagnosis of Brain Death.' *The New England Journal of Medicine* 344 (16): 1215–21.

Yāsīn, Muḥammad Na'īm. 1991. 'Nihāyat al-ḥayāt al-insāniyya fī ḍaw' ijtihādāt al-'ulamā' al-muslimīn.' In *al-Ḥayāt al-insāniyya: Bidāyatuhā wa-nihāyatuhā fī al-mafhūm al-Islāmī: Thabat kāmil li-a'māl Nadwat al-Ḥayāt al-Insāniyya: Bidāyatihā wa-Nihāyatihā fī al-Mafhūm al-Islāmī, al-mun'aqida bi-tārīkh al-Thulāthā' 24 Rabī' al-Ākhir 1405 H, al-muwāfiq 15 Yanāyir 1985 M*, eds. 'Abd al-Raḥmān al-'Awaḍī and Khālid Madhkūr. Kuwait: al-Munaẓẓama al-Islāmiyya lil-'Ulūm al-Ṭibbiyya.

al-Zarkashī. 1982–5. *al-Manthūr fī al-qawā'id*, ed. Taysīr Fā'iq Aḥmad Maḥmūd. 3 vols. Kuwait: Wizārat al-Awqāf wa-al-Shu'ūn al-Islāmiyya.

———. 1992. *al-Baḥr al-muḥīṭ fī uṣūl al-fiqh*, eds. ʿAbd al-Qādir ʿAbd Allāh al-ʿĀnī and ʿUmar Sulaymān Ashqar. 6 vols. Kuwait: Wizārat al-Awqāf wa-al-Shuʾūn al-Islāmiyya.
al-Zaylaʿī. 2000. *Tabyīn al-ḥaqāʾiq sharḥ Kanz al-daqāʾiq*, ed. Aḥmad ʿIzzū ʿInāya. 7 vols. Beirut: Dār al-Kutub al-ʿIlmiyya.

**Dr Rafaqat Rashid** is a physician, a traditionally-trained Muslim scholar, and an academic in the field of Islamic medical ethics and medical law. He is the co-founder of Al-Balagh Academy and is a Senior Lecturer at the JKN Institute, Bradford, UK.

# Part III
# Interfacing Biomedical Knowledge and Islamic Theology

# Chapter 10
# Islam and Science: Reorienting the Discourse

**Omar Qureshi, Afifi al-Akiti, and Aasim I. Padela**

## 10.1 Introduction

### *10.1.1 Science and Religion*

The idea of a conflict between religion and science has generated a vast amount of literature.[1] Diverse solutions and models for the apparent conflict are set out, usually with a discussion of how the problem should be resolved. One such solution is the principle of Non-overlapping Magisteria (NOMA) proposed by Stephen Jay Gould (d. 2002). Briefly, a magisterium 'is a domain where one form of teaching holds the appropriate tools for meaningful discourse and resolution.'[2] Science in this model is concerned with the empirical realm, which embraces both fact and theory. Religion, on the other hand, covers questions of ultimate meaning and moral value. While this model secures a place for both religion and science, it entails that neither one informs the other. Moreover, a particular conception of religion is assumed where

[1] For example, see Brooke (2014), Brooke and Numbers (2011), and Morvillo (2010).

[2] Gould (1999), 6.

O. Qureshi (✉)
Zaytuna College, Berkeley, CA, USA
e-mail: oqureshi@zaytuna.edu

A. al-Akiti
Oxford Centre for Islamic Studies, Oxford, UK
e-mail: afifi.al-akiti@worc.ox.ac.uk

A. I. Padela
Department of Emergency Medicine & Institute for Health and Equity, Medical College of Wisconsin, Milwaukee, WI, USA
e-mail: apadela@mcw.edu


A. al-Akiti, A. I. Padela (eds.), *Islam and Biomedicine*, Philosophy and Medicine 137, https://doi.org/10.1007/978-3-030-53801-9_10

the epistemological framework does not account for empirical knowledge. Further solutions have taken a more categorical position, in which only one of the two can lead to the truth.

When examined through the doctrines of an Islamic theological school, or *kalām*, these solutions are found wanting, and another model is called for. In this chapter, we propose a new model that takes into account the historical aspects of science as well as the diverse methodological and metaphysical commitments that both science and Islam bring into the investigation. We believe that conflicts between 'Islam' and 'science' do not occur at the level of empirical observation, but that they emerge from the differing epistemological and ontological commitments found in the various scientific approaches and those of the several Islamic theological schools. Reorienting dialogues about Islam and science towards a deeper and more fruitful engagement requires investigating them from the vantage-point of a particular school of Islamic theology, and attending to the historical and philosophical natures of scientific inquiry.

## 10.2 Which Islam?

In the 2003 issue of the journal *Islam and Science*, Dimitri Gutas questioned the validity of the title of the journal. Gutas' main objection was that the title assumed the existence of an immutable Islam throughout the Muslim world for the past fourteen centuries. In his view there is no such monolithic and timeless Islam, rather Islamic doctrines are negotiated and Muslim praxis evolves, and consequently the assumption of an immutable 'Islam' frustrates attempts to understand the relationships between various Islamic doctrines and science.[3] In response to Gutas, Muzaffar Iqbal answers the question 'Is there anything that can be called normative Islam?' in the affirmative. When discussing issues relating to Islam and science, Iqbal suggests that normative Islam

> 'is neither a historic construct, nor a social contract; it is a metaphysical, metahistorical construct which Islam shares with other monotheistic religions. Briefly stated, this essential Islam is none other than the first part of the *shahāda* which every Muslim proclaims numerous times during the course of his or her day: *Lā ilāha illa Llāh*; *there is no deity other than Allāh*.'[4]

Additionally, Iqbal notes, there are a set of beliefs about God and the human that form the essence of Islam.[5] Unfortunately, Iqbal does not address the various questions such an understanding of normative Islam generates for the dialogue between Islam and science, and his definition, while accurate enough, does not get us very far in understanding whether or not 'Islam' and 'science' conflict, or if they do

[3] Gutas (2003): 215–220.

[4] Iqbal (2003): 223.

[5] Iqbal (2003): 221–234.

conflict, where they do. In our view, to consider these questions one must specify the core set of claims that comprise an 'Islamic' worldview and then assess whether these are in conflict with science. These core sets of claims, in our view, are found within the schools of Islamic theology.

We would argue that discussions on Islam and science should be conducted at the methodological and metaphysical levels: for this is where most perceived conflicts exist and can be attended to. While schools of Islamic theology have much in common, they posses slightly different metaphysical, epistemological, and ontological frameworks. When these are kept in mind, conceptual rigour and substantive depth can be added to investigations into the compatibility of 'Islam' with science. Discourses at this deeper level are presently few and far between. To be clear, it is not that Iqbal's definition of normative Islam is incorrect. Rather, discussing the reception of the products of modern science within Islam requires a dialogue between the philosophies of science and the schools of Islamic theology. Such dialogues would allow for engaging in discussions about scientific and Islamic perspectives on the nature and makeup of reality, causation, knowledge and certainty, the definition of a species, the mind and its representations of the world, what kinds of things exist in the world, and matter and the nature of essences. The last section of this chapter will illustrate how one might attend to such questions from within a particular school of Islamic theology, namely the Ashʿarīs.

## 10.3 Which Science?

Science is a human activity that is conducted as part of, or situated within, philosophical traditions existing at particular historical moments. Therefore, when considering the possibility of conflict between the claims of Islamic theology and those of 'science,' one must be attentive to the fact that scientific claims might be modulated by underlying worldviews and philosophies.

For example, philosophers of science have described two broad frameworks that we might use to understand science and its implications. Empiricist and realist epistemologies of scientists bring to the fore a central metaphysical concern about the truth claims of science. The empiricist camp, which holds that knowledge is to be found only in the domain of sensory experience and the observable, is directly at odds with the realist camp, whose adherents use sense-data to make claims about the unobservable aspects of reality. 'The fundamental distinction,' writes Michael R. Matthews, 'is that the empiricists wish to confine the claims of science to what we can experience … [for them] the theoretical terms do not refer, and are not meant to refer, to existing entities.'[6] The aim of science according to empiricists is 'to produce theories that predict phenomena and connect … items to experience.'[7] This is

[6] Matthews (1994), 164.

[7] Ibid., 163.

in contrast to realists, who look for the underlying causes of the experience and hold these to be real entities. The law of gravitational attraction derived by Sir Isaac Newton (d. 1727), explains the planetary motions as described by Johannes Kepler (d. 1630), and is a good example of realist theorization that builds upon empirical claims. The realists go beyond just empirical observation and seek to explain phenomena at a deeper, yet more general level. For example, according to Newton, force is not just a mathematical construct for explaining motions of a body, rather, force is real (although not directly observable) and makes an object accelerate or change direction.

A fruitful dialogue about Islam and science requires specifying which conception of science one is using, because, as we saw above, there are different approaches to the study of the natural world and different meanings accorded to the knowledge produced by such investigation. Whichever perspective on science one adopts, one must realize that historical, cultural, philosophical, and theological variables play a role in what scientific questions we investigate and what answers we are willing to entertain. Science that presumes there are no immaterial souls, or no possibility of God's action in the world, will look different from science which permits such things. As a result, 'Western' science and science that is conducted by Muslims might have different methodological and metaphysical commitments, features, presuppositions, and conclusions.

## 10.4 From Natural Philosophy to Modern Science

As part of reflecting on the question 'which science?', Muslims engaging in dialogues about Islam and science need to consider the shifts in thinking that informed a 'modern' science as we know it. From the Ancient Greeks into the nineteenth century, the investigation of nature was known as 'natural philosophy,' and this form of inquiry was integrated with theology and broader philosophical reasoning. From the seventeenth to the nineteenth century, a transition from natural philosophy to modern science took place. According to Edward Grant (d. 2020), the term 'natural philosophy' began to refer to the study of nature in the thirteenth century as part of the translation of Greek texts, especially of Aristotelian works, into Latin, either via Arabic translations or directly.[8] Prior to that, the works of Plato (d. *ca.* 347 BC), in particular the *Timaeus*, informed much of the discussion on the study of nature, and the work of the Latin Encyclopedists, from Pliny the Elder (d. 79) and his first-century contemporaries to Isadore of Seville (d. 636) and into the Middle Ages, contributed greatly to the study of the natural world. As a result, the metaphysics that underlay the study of nature was largely Platonic or Platonizing – a metaphysics that included divine beings, Intellects and Souls, in a realm above the human. 'Natural philosophy' as a term was still unknown in Latin Europe. The case of

[8] Grant (2007), 105–106.

mathematical sciences is different, however. According to Robert E. Hall, the elaboration of statics and hydrostatics started in the sixteenth century, and those mathematical disciplines were joined with dynamics and kinematics from the philosophical tradition to form an early modern unified science of mechanics in the seventeenth century, all of which derived in part from the medieval Islamic tradition.[9]

Starting in the twelfth century, as the works of Aristotle (d. 322 BC) on natural philosophy entered Europe through translations made from Arabic and Greek to Latin, Aristotelian theories shaped the study of nature, and natural philosophy was refashioned in the Aristotelian mould. Aristotle's natural philosophy came to serve as the 'handmaid of theology' in the universities. With the wide development of experimentation in natural philosophy in the seventeenth century, numerous departures from the Aristotelian worldview were necessitated, since theory did not correspond well with observations of the natural world. Hence a 'modern' science emerged, and the term 'natural philosophy,' as referring to scientific inquiry about the natural world, was eventually discarded. Andrew Cunningham and Perry Williams place the invention of modern science (and the use of that term and the philosophy underlaying it) during the late eighteenth and nineteenth centuries; it is in 1833 when we first encounter the term 'scientist,' in the work of William Whewell (d. 1866).[10] As a result, modern science emerged as a new system for understanding the deep structure and functioning of the natural world.

Another shift seen in the change from pre-modern to modern science is in the essentialism or typological thinking which becomes displaced by the theory of evolution developed by Charles Darwin (d. 1882) and replaced with what Ernst Mayr (d. 2005) terms 'population thinking.' 'Essentialism' is a term applied to a variety of concepts, but generally refers to the idea that individuals are identical in their essence and any variations observed are accidental (in the philosophical sense). That idea, going back as far as Plato, can be seen in defining a triangle as having certain essential features that separate it from other shapes such as a square or a circle. The differences that may exist in an individual triangle, such as colours, lengths of the sides, and other attributes, are merely accidental qualities that play no role in understanding the essence of a triangle. For an essentialist, Whites, Blacks, and Asians are different variations of the human species. Applying this to biology, typological thinkers see species as constant, and all of the variations that exist amongst the members are purely incidental and not such as to take an organism outside of its species. With population thinking, individuals are assumed to be unique and the variations among them are real, and important to the level that one cannot make any generalizations about a group. Consequently, the species problem in biology is entirely a philosophical matter, one that is similar to the medieval debate over whether universals really exist or not.[11] Thus, when treating of natural species, Darwinism presents us with a form of philosophical nominalism when

[9] Hall (2001), 297–336.

[10] Cunningham and Williams (1993): 407–432.

[11] Mayr (2007), 171–193.

studying the natural world that has replaced the essentialist approach to nature in pre-modern science.

From the above, we can see the dimensions of science which history and philosophy bring to light. These dimensions are rarely included in general curricula or even in the training of scientists. What we come to appreciate when delving into the history and philosophy of science is that the activity called 'science' was conducted with different methodological and metaphysical commitments through various time periods. So any discussion about religion and science must account for those commitments.

## 10.5 A Case Study of Islam and Science

In this section we will explore some of the methodological and metaphysical commitments of scientific activity and engage with them as they appear within the Islamic tradition. This engagement inside a particular school of Muslim theology, or *kalām*, illustrates how a philosophical framework contends with the deliverables of science, and shows also the multiplicity of ways in which one can draw upon the Islamic, as well as the scientific, tradition. This is an alternative model to current ones in the discourse on Islam and science. It will serve to move the discussions to a more meaningful engagement, one that ultimately demonstrates the futility of the conflict thesis.

Abdelhamid I. Sabra (d. 2013) has studied the engagement of ʿAḍud al-Dīn al-Ījī (d. 756/1355), a leading Ashʿarī theologian, with science by presenting his arguments in his major theological work, *al-Mawāqif fī ʿilm al-kalām* (*Waypoints in Theology*), on the Ashʿarīs, his Islamic theological school. Al-Ījī's writings present an example of engaging with the deliverables of science from within his school of Islamic theology. In the section on substances, al-Ījī engages the position of the Aristotelianizing philosophers (*falsafa*; read: 'scientists') that:

> Form is constitutive of body (it being possible that accidents, like forms, may succeed one another indefinitely in the same substrate): 'It may be argued [against us] that a heated body turns cold again by nature, and therefore, that something persists which is a principle of the quality (cold). To this we say: why should it follow that this something be a constituent of body? And why do you deny the attribution of this (reversion to cold) to The Free Agent?'[12]

Arguing on the basis of the Ashʿarī doctrine of atomism, al-Ījī opposes the *falsafa's* conception of nature, which denies the existence of an indivisible substance, and holds that matter is composed of substance and form. As Sabra notes, it is al-Ījī's question at the end of this passage that:

> strikes at the heart of Aristotelian physics by dissolving Aristotelian substance into a conglomerate of bare atoms in which properties succeed one another in a pattern determined by a free transcendent will. And it is this constant affirmation of an uncompromisingly contingent view of the world and of everything happening in it that characterized, in my view, the Ashʿarite attitude to the 'science of nature.' The attitude is given explicit and general

[12] Sabra (1994): 33, quoting al-Ījī (1938), 198.

expression in the principle succinctly formulated by al-Ījī himself earlier in his book – that 'there is no necessity from or over God (*lā wujūba ʿan Allāhī wa lā ʿalayhi*).'[13]

It is important to note here that the empirically observed phenomena of the natural world are not being contested by al-Ījī. Rather, it is the metaphysical question of the nature of matter and the theological implications of God's being a free agent that al-Ījī is addressing.

That same methodology is also observed when al-Ījī engages with the Ptolemaic picture of the cosmos, in which the total number of spherical bodies was 24, a number which has been established apparently by observation. Their number is not contested by al-Ījī. Rather, what he contests is the relative positions of Venus and the Sun, which was based on the 'premises that the body of the heavens is incapable of being pierced [i.e., penetrated], "otherwise, it would be possible to attribute the (planet's) movement to the planet itself as a swimmer in water."'[14] Here al-Ījī questions this reasoning. He asks, 'Why not allow the planets to be placed in rings (*niṭāqāt*, belts), rather than complete spheres or spherical shells, which would move either by themselves, or by an impulsion (*iʿtimād*) exerted on them by the planets?'[15] Sabra concludes that what we see here is that Ashʿarī atomism continued to hold sway during the 'age of science' in Islamic civilization and was a locus of dialogue between Muslim theologians and Greek-inspired philosophers-cum-scientists. This indeed remains part of the library of the Islamic intellectual tradition, which may one day be recovered and built upon in order to explain better the realities around us.

Here, we should draw attention to the Ashʿarī epistemological framework, which enabled al-Ījī to move between the deliverables of science and those of religion, and thereby relate truth-claims emerging from empirical science to truth-claims from religion. A proposition, or *ḥukm*, is the affirmation or denial of one thing predicated of another, such as the proposition, 'the sky is grey.' According to the Ashʿarī school, the claim that emerges in any proposition belongs to either one of three types: legal (*sharʿī*), rational (*ʿaqlī*), or empirical (*ʿādī* or *ʿurfī*).[16] A legal truth is one whose source is Divine revelation (*sharʿī*), such as the proposition, 'fasting in Ramadan is an obligation.' Such a proposition is known only from Divine revelation through the Prophets. A rational truth, such as '2 + 2 = 4,' can be known without Divine revelation and is not based on empirical observations. Lastly, an empirical truth is one that can be made only from the domain of sensory experience and the observable through one or more of the senses, which includes experimentation, for example, 'Quinine treats malaria.'

It is this Ashʿarī epistemological understanding of the relationships between empirical and rational truth-claims that allowed al-Ījī to engage with the deliverables of science. According to this school of Islamic theology, all types of empirical truth-claims must be rationally possible (*mumkināt*).[17] Anything that is rationally

[13] Sabra (1994): 33, quoting al-Ījī (1938), 28.

[14] Sabra (1994): 35, quoting al-Ījī (1938), 200.

[15] Al-Ījī (1938), 200; cf. Sabra (1994): 35.

[16] Al-Sanūsī (2019), 111–146.

[17] Al-Sanūsī (2019), 130–137; cf. al-Ījī (1938), 58.

impossible, i.e., a proposition that contradicts a necessary truth, such as '2+2=5,' cannot exist. Thus all that exists in the world is rationally possible. Divine power (*qudra*), in the Ashʿarī view, relates only to that which is rationally possible.[18] This entails that all empirically known things exist by virtue of God's power. Therefore, the world and its phenomena are the acts of God, and natural events cannot be in conflict with Divine revelation. Any conflict is only apparent and perceived, and results from interpretation of observed phenomena through theology or metaphysics. Hence the relationship between empirical, rational, and legal truth-claims allows for recognizing where a potential conflict is located, so that one's engagement with science can be made at the appropriate level.

Returning to Sabra's evidence of the fourteenth-century example of a dialogue between Ashʿarī *kalām* and science, he observes that:

> Science was not a direct competitor of *kalām* in the way that *falsafa* was, and generally the specialized scientific disciplines were not as such perceived as posing a threat to religion. And yet *they had to be reinterpreted in the light of the prevailing* kalām *metaphysics and given new foundations and new definitions of their scope and value.*[19]

It is in the methodological and metaphysical commitments that conflicts between Islam and science may appear to exist, and it is towards those commitments that the discourse needs to be reoriented.

This analysis of the dialogue between Islam and science should be taken as a model that presents a nuanced and positive 'Islamic' engagement with the deliverables of science. It transcends the current approaches in that discourse. It clearly illustrates the futility of the conflict thesis.

## 10.6 Conclusion

Scholarly investigations of Islam and science have been conducted with insufficiently examined conceptions of both. While they have yielded certain fruits, they should be seen as only the first stage of the investigation. Many important questions relating to causality, epistemology, speciation, scientific reasoning, logic, and conceptions of nature have either not been treated, or else treated in an unsatisfactory brief manner. In order to move the investigation towards more substantial issues, fuller conceptions of 'Islam' and 'science,' which emphasize methodological and metaphysical commitments, are required. In this chapter, we have argued that treating these issues from the standpoint of a particular school of theology and a particular philosophy of science will allow theologians and scientists to move in that direction. In adopting this model, we should be able to detect the actual areas of apparent conflict and thus reorient the discourse and move the investigation forward.

---

[18] Al-Sanūsī (2019), 242–43.

[19] Sabra (1994): 41 (emphasis ours).

## References


Brooke, John Hedley. 2014. *Science and Religion: Some Historical Perspectives*. Cambridge: Cambridge University Press.

Brooke, John Hedley, and Ronald L. Numbers, eds. 2011. *Science and Religion around the World*. Oxford: Oxford University Press.

Cunningham, Andrew, and Perry Williams. 1993. 'De-Centring the "Big Picture": "The Origins of Modern Science" and the Modern Origins of Science.' *The British Journal for the History of Science* 26 (4): 407–432.

Gould, Stephen Jay. 1999. *Rocks of Ages: Science and Religion in the Fullness of Life*. New York, NY: Ballantine Books.

Grant, Edward. 2007. *A History of Natural Philosophy: From the Ancient World to the Nineteenth Century*. Cambridge: Cambridge University Press.

Gutas, Dimitri. 2003. 'Islam and Science: A False Statement of the Problem.' *Islam and Science* 1 (2): 215–220.

Hall, Robert E. 2001. 'Mechanics.' In *Science and Technology in Islam*, Part 1: *The Exact and Natural Sciences*, eds. A. Y. al-Hassan, Maqbul Ahmed, and A. Z. Iskandar. Paris: UNESCO.

al-Ījī, ʿAḍud al-Dīn. 1938. *Mawāqif fī ʿilm al-kalām*, eds. Ibrāhīm al-Dasūqī ʿAṭiyya and Aḥmad Muḥammad al-Ḥanbūlī. Silsilat Maṭbūʿāt fī ʿIlm al-Kalām, no. 1. Cairo: Maṭbaʿat al-ʿUlūm.

Iqbal, Muzaffar. 2003. 'Islam and Science: Responding to a False Approach.' *Islam and Science* 1 (2): 221–234.

Matthews, Michael R. 1994. *Science Teaching: The Role of History and Philosophy of Science*. New York, NY: Routledge.

Mayr, Ernst. 2007. *What Makes Biology Unique?: Considerations on the Autonomy of a Scientific Discipline*. Cambridge: Cambridge University Press.

Morvillo, Nancy. 2010. *Science and Religion: Understanding the Issues*. Malden, MA: Wiley-Blackwell.

Sabra, Abdelhamid I. 1994. 'Science and Philosophy in Medieval Islamic Theology: The Evidence of the Fourteenth Century.' *Zeitschrift für Geschichte der Arabishe-Islamishen Wissenshaften* 9: 1–42.

al-Sanūsī. 2019. *Sharḥ al-muqaddimāt*, ed. Anas Muḥammad ʿAdnān al-Sharafāwī. Damascus: Dār al-Taqwá.



**Dr Omar Qureshi** is currently Provost and Assistant Professor of Islamic Law and Theology at Zaytuna College, USA. After obtaining his Bachelor of Arts in Microbiology, he went on to complete his Master of Education in Curriculum and Instruction – Science Education both from the University of Missouri – Columbia. Prior to Zaytuna College, for seven years Omar served as the principal and dean of academics for a parochial school located in Chicago's West suburbs. While in Chicago, Omar completed his PhD in Cultural and Educational Policy Studies: Philosophy of Education at Loyola University Chicago in 2016. His dissertation, entitled 'Badr al-Dīn Ibn Jamāʿa and the Highest Good of Islamic Education,' treats the topic of educational institutional identity in the United States.

**Dato' Dr Afifi al-Akiti** is the Kuwait Fellow in Islamic Studies at the Oxford Centre for Islamic Studies, and teaches in the Faculty of Theology, University of Oxford. He is a Fellow of Worcester College, Oxford. Dato' Afifi is trained as a theologian in both the Islamic and Western traditions. His areas of expertise are Islamic theology, law, and science. He has worked on several BBC documentaries, including the award-winning *Science and Islam* (2009). Since 2010, Dato' Dr Afifi has been listed in *The Muslim 500: The World's 500 Most Influential Muslims*.

**Dr Aasim I. Padela** is a clinician, health researcher, and bioethicist at the Medical College of Wisconsin. He utilizes methodologies from health services research, religious studies, and comparative ethics to examine the encounter of Islam with contemporary biomedicine through the lives of Muslim patients and clinicians, and in the writings of Islamic scholars. His scholarship develops intellectual frameworks through which Islamic theology (both moral and scholastic) can engage with contemporary natural and social scientific data.

# Chapter 11
# Science in the Framework of Islamic Legal Epistemology: An Exploratory Account

**Kamaluddin Ahmed**

## 11.1 Introduction

### *11.1.1 Science and Religion*

Science is a process to arrive at rigorous knowledge that provides answers about how nature works. It does so through the generation of hypotheses, testing these by accumulation of data, and drawing conclusions that are continually revisited. Scientists are sceptical about whether other approaches can discover any truth about natural phenomena. Religion, on the other hand, is not primarily concerned with material questions about how nature works. Instead, it provides a range of answers on immaterial existential and philosophical questions such as 'Is there a God?', 'Why do we exist?', and 'What is virtue?' Understood thus, science and religion would operate in different domains and little conflict would be presumed to exist between them. Steven Jay Gould (d. 2002) famously referred to this idea as the Non-Overlapping Magisteria (NOMA) between science and religion.[1]

Rejecting the idea that religion and science have separate domains, advocates of 'new atheism' maintain that science can play a role in answering the metaphysical questions addressed by religion, mainly by problematizing the questions themselves and falsifying the answers provided to them by religion.[2] They do so by attempting

[1] See Gould (1997) and (2002). Chapter 10 of this book, 'Islam and Science: Reorienting the Discourse,' by Omar Qureshi, Afifi al-Akiti, and Aasim I. Padela also touches upon the Gould's idea of NOMA, and also offers different strategies for thinking about the Islam and science discourses.

[2] See Dawkins (1998).

K. Ahmed (✉)
University of Oxford, Oxford, UK
e-mail: kamaluddin.ahmed@orinst.ox.ac.uk



A. al-Akiti, A. I. Padela (eds.), *Islam and Biomedicine*, Philosophy and Medicine 137, https://doi.org/10.1007/978-3-030-53801-9_11

to extend the process of the scientific method beyond the natural and material realms and insisting that knowledge acquired through revelation, scripture, and prophecy must, like any and all other forms of knowledge, be demonstrably falsifiable through empirical and rational methods in order to be considered valid. Otherwise, religious knowledge ought to be dismissed as mere conjecture or hypothesis and epistemological traditions of religion should be reduced to mythology and superstition. Simply put, their mantra is that 'that which is not falsifiable is itself false.'

Critics have labelled such an approach 'scientism' and argue that a philosophically grounded understanding of science does not support such claims.[3] According to them, science is conscious of its limits in understanding and 'knowing' non-material aspects of life. An empiricist scientism on the other hand declares emphatically that there are no immaterial facets to life and any such phenomena may be successfully reduced to material explanations without the need to search for a supreme being or a higher sense of purpose in life. Rigidly applied, scientism would dispense not only with religion but also philosophy, the aesthetic and creative arts, and all categories of knowledge not exclusively based on empiricism and rationalism.

On the other end of the spectrum, defenders of religion, who may perhaps be well-intentioned but are nonetheless misguided, adopt a rejectionist stance towards scientific explanations and advocate scepticism regarding even the most basic of self-evident truths. Proponents of this approach revel in finding instances in the history of science where long-held facts and theories were later found to be false. The corrections by Nicolaus Copernicus (d. 1543), and then by Galileo Galilei (d. 1642) to the Ptolemaic model is taken by those proponents as evidence that science disproves itself. It is sheer irony that it escapes the adherents of such anti-science dogma that Galileo is revered by modern scientists as the icon who symbolizes the transition from natural philosophy to modern science. Unfortunately, such radical views attract a disproportionate amount of attention and fanfare. In reality, most religious people readily acknowledge and accept the central role played by science in our knowledge about the natural and material realms. The extremely rare instances in which revelatory knowledge contravenes scientific knowledge are attributed not to any flaw in science, but rather to the omnipotent power of a Supreme Being and His Will to suspend the laws of science that He Created.

## 11.2 Islamic Epistemology Between Revelation and Reason

Well before Islam's encounter with modern science, Muslim scholars engaged the philosophical traditions (*falsafa*) of their time. The 'Graeco-Arabic translation movement' began under Abbasid rule as early as the eighth century, or second Islamic century. By the end of the ninth century, major works by Plato (d. *ca.* 347 BC), Aristotle (d. 322 BC), and Plotinus (d. 270), and others were being read and

---

[3] See Hayek (1942) and Popper (1979).

discussed in Arabic.[4] The disciplines through which Islamic scholarship first interacted with *falsafa* were speculative theology (*kalām*) and theosophical spirituality (*taṣawwuf*). Ṣūfīs, when confronted by the Neoplatonic and neo-Aristotelian philosophical movement, turned their direction as well to the nature of the material world. Some strands of Sufism conceptualized the entire material universe as having a shared affinity with the Creator, a doctrine known as *waḥdat al-wujūd*, or unity of being.[5]

The philosophies of Plato, Aristotle, and Plotinus that were transmitted to the Muslim world were further developed over two centuries by al-Kindī (d. 256/873), al-Rāzī (d. *ca.* 313/925), al-Fārābī (d. 339/950), and Ibn Sīnā (Lat. Avicenna; d. 428/1037) among others. In the later reception of these ideas, Islamic scholars who, for any number of reasons, held philosophical positions to be truths, attempted to reconcile philosophical ideas with religious precepts. For example, al-Fārābī and Ibn Sīna upheld the philosophers' position that the world was pre-eternal and uncreated, a tenet that directly contradicted religious belief that God is the Creator of all things, including the world itself. In his seminal work, the *Incoherence of the Philosophers* (*Tahāfut al-falāsifa*), al-Ghazālī (d. 505/1111) condemned this position as contrary to Muslim belief.[6] Ibn Rushd (Lat. Averroes; d. 595/1198) attempted to reconcile the stances of theologians like al-Ghazālī and philosophers like Ibn Sīna by positing that while God mostly Creates objects within the framework of time, He may Create them outside the framework of time and hence the world was timeless but not uncaused.[7] Ibn Rushd's attempts to mediate between philosophy and religion are not unlike contemporary efforts to reconcile science and religion. However, since many of the natural philosophy positions held by the philosophers and adopted by their Muslim defenders in the medieval period have now been disproven by modern science, *falsafa* is no longer the best candidate for us to locate our discussion on the place of science in Islamic epistemology.

Others have tried to frame the discussion of science in Islam as a contest between rationalism and traditionalism. The rationalist-traditionalist dichotomy has been forwarded by countless writers both from outside and within Islamic scholarship. Historically, these categories were often little more than a polemical tool employed to mar one's opponent. Nonetheless, many contemporary authors uncritically accept these categories to be binary. For example, Ibn Rushd is often lauded as a 'rationalist' who privileged reason (*ʿaql*) and al-Ghazālī is dubbed a traditionalist who was responsible for the demise of reason not only in philosophy, but in Islamic civilization as a whole.[8] Proponents of such historical revisionism often quote primary sources selectively or out of context. In defence of their thesis, they approvingly cite

---

[4] See Gutas (1998).

[5] This doctrine was developed in detail by the famous Andalusian mystic and scholar, Ibn al- ʿArabī (d. 638/1240).

[6] Al-Ghazālī (2000).

[7] Ibn Rushd (1959).

[8] For an erudite rebuttal of this view, see Griffel (2009), al-Akiti (2009) and Tamer (2015).

Ibn Rushd's concise work, *The Decisive Treatise on Determining the Connection between the Religion and Philosophy* (*Faṣl al-maqāl fī mā bayna al-sharīʿa wa ʾl-ḥikma min al-ittiṣāl*),[9] where Ibn Rushd outlines his position that reason and revelation may not contradict one another. Ibn Rushd is preceded, however, on this very issue by none other than al-Ghazālī who earlier wrote in his treatise entitled, *The Hermeneutical Principles of Scriptural Interpretation* (*Qānūn al-taʾwīl*), that transmitted revelatory texts (*naql*) and human rationality (*ʿaql*) when properly understood could never be in contradiction with one another.[10] All this is not to suggest that Ibn Rushd was merely copying al-Ghazālī. Rather, each had their own subtle understandings and definitions of rationality, and neither can be falsely accused of being anti-rationalist or rationalist at the expense of revelation.[11] As Sherman Jackson correctly observes, 'Traditionalism is no more devoid of the use of reason than Rationalism is of a reliance on tradition. As such, these two approaches are better understood as different traditions of reason.'[12] Clearly then, laying exclusive claims to rationalism or accusing others of anti-rationalism, has little to contribute to an analysis of science and religion in Islam.

Academics who have not fallen prey to such polemics often turn to *kalām*, or Islamic theology, indeed labelled by many as 'rationalist' theology, as the first place to start a discussion on Islam and science. I agree that the vast historical literature of *kalām* provides striking examples on how Muslim scholars employed epistemologies that did not originate in revelation or prophecy to understand matters traditionally held to be the exclusive domain of the latter. As a radical first step, early Islamic speculative theologians (*mutakallimūn*) removed matter and the material world from the exclusive domain of natural science and put forth a theory of matter as sacred.[13] Although some contemporary Muslims may dismiss these efforts as far-flung or even abstract, they nonetheless indicate Islam's longstanding historical engagement with the physical matter and substance of the material world, a domain that would in modern times be held to belong exclusively to science. Recent works that aim to draw upon the scholarly tradition of *kalām* to articulate the relationship between religion and science in Islam have looked at issues such as causality, cosmology, time and space, evolution and design, and even quantum physics.[14] These findings have in turn been placed in conversation with Western literature on religion and science that is written from a faith-based perspective. The works of well-regarded authors such as Ian Barbour (d. 2013), John Polkinghorne (d. 2021), Nancy Cartwright, Paul Davies, William Lane Craig, Robert Russell, and others are read by Muslim scholars who then attempt to incorporate, modify, and align their ideas

---

[9] Ibn Rushd (1959).

[10] Al-Ghazālī (2013). We will return to al-Ghazālī's views in Sect. 11.3 below.

[11] Two studies that skilfully compare and contrast al-Ghazālī and Ibn Rushd are Bello (1989) and Okumuş (2011).

[12] Jackson (2002), 17.

[13] Altaie (2010), 87–99.

[14] See Guessom (2011) and Altaie (2016).

with Islamic beliefs and scriptures.[15] This has been a beneficial and productive second step, after engaging the classical and medieval *kalām* literature, in exploring the intersection between science in Islam.

While *kalām* may have successfully integrated elements of Greek philosophy and logic into Islamic epistemology, the challenge of incorporating modern science may require us to venture beyond *kalām*. I propose to outline a tentative model for on how to better understand the relationship between science and Islam through the lens of Islamic law and legal epistemology (*fiqh* and *uṣūl al-fiqh*). The intellectual history of both *kalām* and *fiqh* establishes that they were so closely intertwined that any discussion of what constitutes Islamic epistemology that looks at one and not the other, as much Western scholarship on Islam has thus far done, would not only be inadequate but also misleading.[16] While the discussions in *kalām* can help us construct a paradigm by which to potentially incorporate science in the understanding of *metaphysical* matters, Islamic jurisprudence and legal epistemology (*fiqh*) would be better placed to offer a paradigm on how Islamic epistemology may incorporate scientific understanding of *physical* matters. The literature on Islam and science has yet to explore what the discipline of *fiqh* may offer in navigating science, beyond edicts and legal rulings.

## 11.3 Islamic Legal Epistemology

Most non-Muslims are likely to have encountered the term Sharīʿa for Islamic law and are less familiar with the terms *fiqh* and *uṣūl al-fiqh*. Understanding the linguistic definitions of these words can help in appreciating their terminological usage in Islamic scholarship. Lexically, *sharīʿa* means a way or path, *fiqh* describes a deep understanding arrived after much study and consideration, and *uṣūl* denotes the foundational principles of such understanding. The interplay between these terms may be summed up in the following way: The foundational principles (*uṣūl*) collectively comprise an epistemology for arriving at a deep understanding (*fiqh*) of the scriptural texts (*nuṣūṣ*) of Islam [the Qur'an and Prophetic reports (*ḥadīth*)], which in turn detail a way of life (*sharīʿa*) that seeks the pleasure (*riḍā*) of God.

Perhaps the most significant paradigm developed by Muslim jurists for generating such an understanding was a classification of sources and interpretations on the basis of certainty and probability. Two excellent discussions of this in the Western literature are by Bernard Weiss and Aron Zysow.[17] I will briefly outline the paradigm with an eye towards how I propose to use it for the incorporation of science into Islamic epistemology.

[15] See Yaran (2003).

[16] Two notable and welcome exceptions to this are: Vishanoff (2011) and Eissa (2017). Neither, however, discusses religion and science.

[17] See Weiss (1998) and Zysow (2013).

Sources of Islamic epistemology can be divided into three categories: (1) the primary sources of the revealed texts of scripture (Qur'an) and Prophetic teachings and practices (Sunna); (2) secondary sources such as analogical inference (*qiyās*) from the primary sources; and (3) tertiary sources such as an individual jurists' expert legal opinion (*ijtihād*), social welfare and utility (*maṣlaḥa*), equity and juristic preference (*istiḥsān*) and others. The authenticity of the Qur'an and certain Prophetic teachings are held with absolute certainty by Muslims, known as *qaṭʿ*. The rest of the sources fall on a sliding scale of probabilities known as *ẓann*. Interpretations of the meanings of the primary sources are similarly divided into these two categories, while the interpretation and application of the secondary and tertiary sources are all characterized as probabilistic. This should not be misunderstood or misrepresented, as some have, to suggest that all Islamic epistemology is speculative or arbitrary for that would be an incorrect notion.

Certainty and probability are to be understood relative to each other. Interestingly, the manner in which early jurists treated these categories resembles how they are treated in science. The grade of certainty is awarded only in the case of absolute certainty, which refers to God's knowledge that He revealed to humanity through scripture and rigorously authenticated (*ṣaḥīḥ*) and widely transmitted (*mutawātir*) Prophetic reports (*ḥadīth).* Relative to that, everything else is characterized as 'uncertain.' However, within this broad category there are many forms and sources of knowledge that are characterized as necessary knowledge because they are so highly plausible and accurate. After that are forms and sources of knowledge that are very plausible and these are acted upon if there is nothing within them that contradicts revelatory sources. Thereafter are forms and sources of knowledge that are judged as fairly plausible, merely possible, sceptical, doubtful, and impossible (i.e., certainly false). All of this is what I refer to as the hierarchy of *ẓann*. At the same time, within the realm of the 'uncertain,' and even in interpretations of the 'certain,' there is a multiplicity of views. Hence the various and at times competing interpretations/understandings (*fiqh*) of sources of knowledge as well as competing principles and methodologies (*uṣūl*) of epistemology is what I refer to as the multiplicity of the *ẓann*.

Two tertiary sources employed within the interpretive epistemology of Muslim jurists that have special relevance for identifying a role for science are *ʿaql* and *ʿurf*. *ʿAql* may be understood as applied human reasoning, specifically a rational understanding of *empirical* reality. When early classical scholars encountered neo-Aristotleian logic (*manṭiq*), several of them, including al-Ghazālī integrated these new and ostensibly foreign, mundane, and 'secular' forms of knowledge into their understanding of *ʿaql*. Al-Ghazālī's approach in the *Qānūn* is that revelatory knowledge transmitted through scripture and prophecy (collectively referred to as *naql*) and all human knowledge arrived at through other means (collectively referred to as *ʿaql*) are never contradictory to one another when placed in the context of fundamental Islamic theological beliefs such as the omnipotence and omniscience of the One Supreme Being.[18] A later scholar, Ibn Taymiyya (d. 728/1328), while vigor-

[18] See al-Ghazālī (2013).

ously disagreeing with al-Ghazālī's incorporation of Greek logic in conceiving of *ʿaql*, nonetheless equally strongly argued the same point in his major work, *The Refutation of the Contradiction of Reason and Revelation* (*Darʾ taʿāruḍ al-ʿaql wa-al-naql*).

*ʿUrf* refers to prevailing customs and practices between and amongst individuals and groups that constitute *social* reality. As the Muslim community spread geographically it encountered a vast variety of customs and norms in different societies and territories. Jurists as early as Muḥammad ibn al-Ḥasan al-Shaybānī (d. 189/805) and as late as the pre-modern jurist Ibn ʿĀbidīn (d. 1252/1836) incorporated these norms and practices in their considerations of Islamic law. For example, language (*lugha*) was accepted as a norm that indicated human expressions and perceptions of reality.

It is important here to note that legal rulings that were made on the basis of *ʿurf* were always susceptible to change if the custom changed. Thus, if we conceive of prevalent scientific understandings as *ʿurf*, then there is a precedent for legal rulings to change when such scientific understandings change. *Ceteris paribus*, or if all things remain the same in prevalent epistemologies, be they linguistic, scientific, or other, then there is no basis to question the determinations of earlier jurists. However, juristic positions that were informed by, or even dependent upon, particular epistemological understandings that have since changed or been refined will have to be re-examined. In the next section, I will outline how these concepts and categories, taken together, may provide an outline for the role of science in Islamic legal epistemology.

## 11.4 Interactions Between Science and Islamic Scriptural, Theological, and Legal Epistemologies

I propose that scientific theories and hypotheses can be plotted on the same scale of probabilities (*ẓann*) and certainties (*qaṭʿ*) that Muslim jurists use to classify sources of knowledge such as rational empiricism (*ʿaql*) and customary practices (*ʿurf*). Hence scientific claims are engaged in the same way as other sources of knowledge. Let me outline a typology for such engagement by providing several concrete examples as well as the accompanying legal implications below.

**Type One** An instance where science suggests a specific understanding (*fiqh* in the linguistic sense) about a matter based on its own methodological principles (*uṣūl*) *and* the primary, i.e., revelatory, sources of Islam make no claims about the matter. Further, there is nothing in the knowledge claims of science about the matter that contradicts any Islamic doctrine that is based on certain knowledge from Islamic scriptural sources.

**Example** Science articulates a theory about how neural networks guide muscle activity and coordination based on empirical data. An analogous example, not grounded in empirics but rather in customary practice (*ʿurf*), would be a chiropractor's longstanding experience with massage therapy and its efficacy in relieving muscle spasms.

**Juristic Rulings:**

1. Within the realm of scientific empirical knowledge, the understanding put forth by neuroscience is not as certain as basic facts such as the law of gravity. Thus this claim is graded as probabilistic, or *ẓannī,* within Islamic legal epistemology as is any knowledge that is even slightly less than absolutely certain.
2. However, as there is (i) no higher source of knowledge within the hierarchy of the *ẓann* that speaks about this matter, (ii) nor any competing interpretation from the biomedical sciences or other sources within the multiplicity of the *ẓann*, and (iii) there is no contradiction with any Islamic doctrine based in the realm of *qaṭʿ* knowledge, this knowledge will be treated as necessary knowledge that may be acted upon.

**Theological and Spiritual Context:**

1. The mechanism by which neural networks operate will be treated as an aspect of God's will which has been discovered through scientific knowledge.

**Type Two** An instance where science suggests an understanding based on its own methodological principles about a matter which is also discussed by Islamic sources. As in Type One, there is nothing in the knowledge claims of science that contradicts any of the certain knowledge of Islam. However, in this case the scientific knowledge interfaces with other, 'uncertain' (*ẓannī*) sources, and may even offer claims that conflict with these other sources.

**Example** Human genetics identifies behavioural genes that cause anger and envy through empirical study. Islamic sources consider anger and envy to be states of the heart or soul. An analogous example from customary practice (*ʿurf*) would be some Islamic jurists judging shrimp to be within the category of fish with respect to dietary laws, whereas a biological taxonomy would classify shrimp as crustaceans.

**Juristic Rulings:**

1. (As Type One above) Within the realm of scientific and empirical knowledge, the understanding put forth by the geneticist is not as certain as basic facts such as the law of gravity. Hence this knowledge is labelled and treated as probabilistic (*ẓannī*).
2. Since the scientific claim contradicts a claim based on the Islamic tradition, and both are within the realm of uncertainty, there is a need to develop a hermeneutical strategy to either harmonize and reconcile (*taṭbīq*) the two, perhaps by subsuming both under a broader meaning. Alternatively, one form of knowledge will

have to be preferred over the other (*tarjīḥ*) based on a legitimate and defensible principle.

**Theological and Spiritual Context:**

1. Such scientific discoveries may also be considered as knowledge revealed by God to His Creation as part of His Guidance (*hidāya*).

**Type Three** An instance where science presents an understanding based on its own methodological principles. In this instance the claims of science conflict with Islamic doctrines that are based on certain scriptural knowledge. The conflicting account given by science and by Islamic source-texts as to the origin of the human species, or to prevailing views about whether the Red Sea parted for the Prophet Moses and his followers, are but two of several examples.

**Juristic Rulings:**

1. If science itself accepts that its claim to knowledge is uncertain, then that which is deemed certain by Islamic knowledge will take preference.
2. However, if science claims that the knowledge is certain within its own paradigm, then one of the following will apply:
   (a) Were we to treat the scientific claim as based on rational empiricism and thus science as *ʿaql*, then according to al-Ghazālī, Ibn Rushd, and Ibn Taymiyya such a situation of conflict is not possible. The former two would advocate *taʾwīl*, or further interpretation beyond the apparent understanding of the evidence, both Islamic and scientific, until the contradiction disappears.
   (b) Were we to treat the scientific claim as emerging from social reality and thus science as *ʿurf*, then such a case would be referred to as *khilāf al-āda* where something is observed in social reality that is contrary to the norm. The perceived contradiction would be explained as a Divine miracle. Since science does not view miracles to be within the power or ability of any being or phenomena that it acknowledges, from a scientific standpoint such an occurrence would be labelled as 'impossible.'

Each of the aforementioned types require further elaboration and explanation. For the purposes of this exploratory account I would suggest that Type Two represents the most significant challenge and opportunity for a rigorous and productive engagement between science and religion. Therefore, I will now fill in certain lacunae in the second type by means of short case illustrations before I sketch out more fully how the aforementioned categorizations and typologies may generate a better understanding of humanity.

## 11.5 Knowledge and Tradition

Both Islamic scholars (*ʿulamāʾ*) and scientists are purveyors of knowledge and also members of networks and traditions. It is important to recognize science as a tradition, an ongoing intellectual conversation over observations and truth claims, because it engenders a non-dogmatic approach to dialogue with religion. In any case science as a tradition may replace other traditions that jurists have relied upon in the past when arriving at rulings. I will illustrate this through two examples.

### *11.5.1 The Curious Case of Shrimp*

As mentioned above (Sect. 11.4), many early jurists classified shrimp as fish and hence viewed shrimp as permissible to eat. The basis for classifying shrimp as fish was not a primary scriptural text nor even a secondary interpretative tool within Islamic law. Rather, it was the tradition of *lugha*, or language. Several linguists labelled shrimp as fish (*samak*) and jurists followed suit. At that time, this was perfectly acceptable and part of an established pattern of medieval jurists referring to experts in the field, in this case linguistics, to come to an understanding of physical phenomena. This was standard for matters relating to social and empirical reality (here again we see the concepts of *ʿaql* and *ʿurf*). Indeed, jurists have always referred to the best non-revelatory forms of knowledge of the time to inform their *fiqh*. In contemporary biomedical matters it is perfectly conventional then for jurists to avail themselves of scientific expertise when seeking to understand the matter at hand. In a sense then, science may replace language as the new *ʿurf*. This should not be taken up as a slogan, as it may easily lend itself to abuse and misinterpretation. Rather, the role of science in generating an understanding of the matter at hand and its legal implications should receive sustained scholarly interest and engagement.

### *11.5.2 Molecular Reality*

Another area where jurists relied upon non-revelatory knowledge was in determining whether impermissible substances had been transformed sufficiently to be judged permissible. This concept is known as *tabdīl māhiyya*, or the transmutation of the essential nature of something, and was borrowed from Greek philosophy. Jurists relied on the methods philosophers used to judge such transmutation. However, the scientific parallel today, which is much closer to empirical reality and hence of much greater probability than the methods employed by the Greek philosophers to discern transmutation in the past, would be of a rearrangement of atoms resulting in a change in the molecular structure of an object. At present, scientific technologies are able to discern such rearrangements with certainty or near-certainty. Accordingly, instead of using philosophical precepts, jurists may rely upon such modern scientific knowledge to judge when something impermissible, e.g., porcine, has sufficiently transmuted into a new material that becomes permissible to use.

## 11.6 Defining Humanity: The Overlap Between Religion and Science

The division of religion and science into the non-overlapping areas of the physical understanding of life and the metaphysical understanding of life fails in one critical area: an understanding of that unique phenomenon that is at once material, physical, and natural while also metaphysical, emotional, and spiritual; humanity itself. While all religions offer knowledge on the metaphysical and spiritual aspects of a human being, Islam displays perhaps the greatest interest in aspects of the material existence of human beings. Thus Islam is brought into a direct conversation with science, creating the opportunity for science and religion not only to achieve harmony, but to complement one another in arriving at a holistic understanding of humanity.[19] Questions arise, however. Would Islam as a religion allow science a role in understanding humanity, and if so, to what extent? Could science reciprocate and in any way be informed by Islam, or would it be a one-sided exchange?

The metaphysical and existential question of what constitutes the essence and origin of human life was traditionally approached by Muslim scholars with certain verses of the Qur'an along with Prophetic reports that discuss the development on an embryo and foetus, and notably, the infusion of the soul or spirit (*rūḥ*) by God into the foetus at 120 days of gestation. Meanwhile, genetics suggests that the fertilized zygote is uniquely *human* shortly after conception and well prior to the completion of 120 days. Recent and ongoing genetic research seeks to map human behaviour and emotions to the genetic coding that takes place at this early moment.

An Islamic understanding of humanity that emerges from the primary sources is that a human being is composed of material and immaterial aspects, as well as aspects that are interrelated. The purely material aspect is the physical body, or *jasad*, and the purely immaterial aspect is the spirit, or *rūḥ*. I would argue that the former may be understood entirely on the basis of scientific knowledge, while the latter may only be understood on the basis of religious knowledge. There are however, three more components to a human in the Islamic model, each of which has material and immaterial aspects and hence would benefit from being understood and 'known' through an epistemology shared between religion and science. The three are the *qalb* (heart), *ʿaql* (mind/brain), and *nafs* (desire, appetite, ego). The

[19] For an example of this engagement, highlighting the overlap between religion and science, see Chap. 7, 'Where the Two Oceans Meet: The Theology of Islam and the Philosophy of Psychiatric Medicine in Exploring the Human Self,' by Asim Yusuf and Afifi al-Akiti in this book.

material aspects of the first two are identical to those that a cardiologist and neurologist would identify. The material aspect of the third is, interestingly contested in both arenas. Muslim scholars have disagreed as to whether the *nafs* has a tangible (*ḥissī*) existence or is merely a metaphor for the passions and urges of a human. Those that postulate a physical aspect differ as to its nature and location within the body. While scientists are in agreement on asserting that there is no separate physical organ or location for human desires and urges, there is some variance as to where such desires originate physiologically.

Islamic epistemology recognizes an immaterial aspect to each of the three components. The *qalb* is the locus of human emotions and feelings, including the most powerful emotions of faith and belief in God and love for Him. The *ʿaql* is the locus of thoughts and analysis. Interestingly, both the *qalb* and *ʿaql* have been attributed in the Qur'an with the faculty of knowledge.[20] Finally, the *nafs*, as mentioned, is the locus of desires, urges, and passions. Science itself is not in agreement on the exact details of these matters. Psychologists and psychiatrists continue to disagree on whether certain behavioural disorders may be treated through therapy (i.e., by addressing the 'mind') or through psycho-active medicines (which target the 'brain'). Regardless, for the purpose of illustrating the preceding discussion we shall examine the origin and inception of life and the definition of when does a human being first become a human being.

Both the science of human embryology and the Qur'an mention stages of embryonic and foetal development. Genetics would suggest that at the very moment of conception the ensuing being is 'genetically' human as the zygote contains all the necessary 'programming' for a unique human being. A more nuanced position would suggest waiting two weeks after conception because the embryo may split into two genetically identical individuals. Here again, questions may be raised on using genetics alone as an indicator of humanity as although identical twins are genetically the same (at least initially, barring later epigenetic changes), they are certainly not identical as individuals.

Ethical and legal considerations compel scientists to further scrutinize the physical and material stages of human development to determine when abortion may be considered an acceptable method of birth control, and when it may be considered murder. Interestingly, the single demarcation point which is agreed upon has no biological basis, namely childbirth. Those who believe that third trimester abortion should be both legally and ethically acceptable would not allow the murder of a prematurely born baby at the same stage of human development. The differentiating factor here would be only whether the foetus/baby is inside the womb or outside.[21] Language may be employed to try to suggest a difference between the two as a seven-month old inside the womb is termed a foetus, while a seven-month old

[20] One of the most detailed expositions on these aspects can be found in al-Ghazālī (2010).

[21] Some bioethical arguments may turn on the idea of dependence, that a foetus is dependent on the womb fully and thus the womb-holder (pregnant woman) has certain rights. Some may say that the foetus turned baby is an independent being and thus accrues its own rights. However, one must acknowledge that the baby is also fully dependent on others for sustaining its life.

'born' two months prematurely is deemed a baby. Hence, inside the womb what is termed as late termination of pregnancy is, outside the womb, universally acknowledged as murder.

Another attempt at delineating a borderline stage in human development is to pinpoint certain physiological functions such as heartbeat or brain activity, or to identify when the foetus would feel pain. Basic brain function is held to start at 8 weeks, while response to external stimuli commences at 16 weeks. The heart is held to start beating at three weeks, yet it is noticeable only at six weeks. Would those who define death as the cessation of heart or brain function would then define life as the commencement of the same? Such consistency would be logical and scientific. However, the scientific community is not so consistent.

Knowledge gleaned from Islamic scriptural sources provides another benchmark. The infusion of the *rūḥ*, or spirit, into the foetus, often referred to as ensoulment is held to place at 120 days according to a Prophetic report largely accepted by scholars. Many Muslim scholars have chosen to pinpoint 120 days as the beginning of human life. Medieval jurists inflicted different criminal punishments on those who injured a pregnant woman and thereby caused a miscarriage based on whether they felt the foetus was younger or older than 120 days. Given all the frameworks we examined earlier in the chapter, what would be the result of a joint inquiry between Islam and science on the question of the origin of human life?

First, prior to enlisting scientific knowledge, the traditional position of the beginning of human life at 120 days needs to be examined closely. The Prophetic text which mentions the time of ensoulment is known in legal epistemology as a *khabar wāḥid*, or solitary report, which although it does represent a highly probable source of knowledge, it is not the highest on the scale of the *ẓann*. The prohibition on taking a human life is however indicated by absolute certain sources of knowledge, scriptural texts in the Qur'an, that are unequivocal (*muḥkam*) in meaning. Thus, according to Islamic legal epistemology itself, using a less than certain solitary report to qualify or specify a text of absolute certainty is highly problematic.

Second, even if one were to accept with certainty that ensoulment occurs at 120 days, that in and of itself does not singlehandedly establish the moment of the origin of human life. Instead, all it establishes is the moment of the fusion of the material aspect of a human being with their immaterial soul. The question would remain as to how to categorize the foetus before ensoulment. In other words, is a foetus that is 119 days old human? If not, what is it? Interestingly, there are no clear and direct sources of Islamic knowledge on this matter. If we were to follow the paradigm outlined in this chapter, one would turn to science for any inputs it might offer. As already mentioned, there are many characteristics, genetic and physiological, in the 119-day old foetus that would suggest that it is human according to genetics. Although, science itself does not profess certainty on this matter, there is high plausibility that a 119-day old foetus is genetically human. And as noted above there is some measure of uncertainty, in other words a lack of absolute certainty based on Islamic sources regarding the time of ensoulment when an entity would be deemed human. Combining these two pieces of evidence would strongly suggest that the scriptural texts upholding the sanctity of human life, which are unequivocal (*muḥkam*) and of the grade of absolutely certain (*qaṭʿ*), may not be qualified and specified but rather should be interpreted as broadly as possible.[22]

Finally, even if contemporary biomedicine does not provide a definitive answer to the origins of life, perhaps for ideological reasons and not scientific ones, the philosophical concept of *māhiyyat al-shayʾ* or the essential nature of a thing, when mated with genetics, would suggest that human essence is established at the very moment of conception, for this is when the entity, i.e., the zygote, is intrinsically unique. Both biologically and philosophically, it is also at this moment when the entity begins to have the unique potential and possibility (*quwwa* and *iḥtimāl*) of becoming a living human being.

Certainly there remains an interesting theological question as to whether a 119-day old foetus that for one reason or another is terminated or miscarried already had a *rūḥ* waiting to enter it. Such an understanding is not entirely implausible as scriptural texts in the Qur'an suggest that God Created all the souls in the far distant past, well before the universe was created. More importantly, although souls are originally created, they will live forever. Therefore, when one commits murder, one is only killing the body, not the *rūḥ*. If termination of the physical aspect of a human being is termed murder, then certainly the same would be true of a foetus prior to 120 days.

## 11.7 Conclusion

Science may be conceptualized in the same manner as earlier Muslim scholars conceived *ʿaql* and *ʿurf*. Within the limits prescribed by a scriptural understanding of religion, science may then be used as *ʿaql* and *ʿurf* were used, or perhaps as the 'new' *ʿaql* and *ʿurf*, to better inform our understanding of both *empirical* and *social* realities without resulting in a confrontation with scriptural revelation or prophecy.[23] *Kalām* may be combined with the juristic categories of *ʿaql* and *ʿurf* to provide a comprehensive epistemological framework by which Islamic scholars could develop new hermeneutical strategies to engage, accommodate, and at times circumscribe emerging avenues of knowledge emanating from the modern sciences including biomedicine. Such strategies will be of particular utility when scientific claims challenge, or are perceived to challenge, Islamic doctrines based on scripture, as well as the epistemological frameworks, of Islam. Theologically, scientific knowledge may contribute to and enrich our understanding of the wisdom (*ḥikma*) of the Divine and the wonders of His Creation. Spiritually, science may highlight

---

[22] For a more elaborated example of such theological reasoning at work, see Chap. 6, 'When Does a Human Foetus Become Human?' by Hamza Yusuf in this book. Through a careful engagement of both the scriptural materials and scientific evidence, he argues that the ensoulment of the foetus should be interpreted as taking place on the fortieth day or at the sixth week of gestation.

[23] For another non-conflict model of science and religion, see Chap. 10, 'Islam and Science: Reorienting the Discourse,' by Omar Qureshi, Afifi al-Akiti and Aasim I. Padela in this book.

and sharpen the contrast between the mundane and the sacred by providing a more informed understanding of the forms and natures of materiality. The more science provides a detailed understanding of the physical aspects of humanity, through genetics, neuroscience, pathology, and other disciplines, the sharper the contrast will be with the spiritual aspect of humanity represented by the *rūḥ*.

## References


al-Akiti, Afifi. 2009. 'The Good, the Bad, and the Ugly of *Falsafa*: Al-Ghazālī's *Maḍnūn, Tahāfut,* and *Maqāṣid,* with Particular Attention to Their *Falsafī* Treatments of God's Knowledge of Temporal Events.' In *Avicenna and His Legacy: A Golden Age of Science and Philosophy*, ed. Y. Tzvi Langermann. Cultural Encounters in Late Antiquity and the Middle Ages, no. 8. Turnhout: Brepols.

Altaie, M. Basil. 2010. 'Matter: An Islamic Perspective.' In *Matter and Meaning: Is Matter Sacred or Profane?*, ed. Michael Fuller. Newcastle-upon-Tyne: Cambridge Scholars Publishing.

———. 2016. *God, Nature, and the Cause: Essays on Islam and Science.* Abu Dhabi: Kalam Research and Media.

Bello, Iysa. 1989. *The Medieval Islamic Controversy Between Philosophy and Orthodoxy: Ijmāʿ and Taʾwīl in the Conflict between al-Ghazālī and Ibn Rushd.* Islamic Philosophy and Theology, no. 3. Leiden: Brill.

Dawkins, Richard. 1998. 'When Religion Steps on Science's Turf: The Alleged Separation Between the Two Is Not So Tidy.' *Free Inquiry* 18 (2): 18–19.

Eissa, Mohamed Ahmed Abdelrahman. 2017. *The Jurist and The Theologian: Speculative Theology in Shāfiʿī Legal Theory*. Islamic History and Thought, no. 5. Piscataway, NJ: Gorgias Press.

al-Ghazālī. 2000. *The Incoherence of the Philosophers [Tahāfut al-falāsifa]: A Parallel English-Arabic Text*, ed. and trans. Michael E. Marmura. Provo, UT: Brigham Young University Press.

———. 2010. *The Marvels of the Heart: Book 21 of the Iḥyāʾ 'ulūm al-dīn, the Revival of the Religious Sciences*, trans. Walter James Skellie. Louisville, KY: Fons Vitae.

———. 2013. *Qānūn al-taʾwīl. In Majmūʿat rasāʾil al-Imām al-Ghazālī*, ed. Aḥmad Shams al-Dīn. Beirut: Dār al-Kutub al-ʿIlmiyya.

Gould, Stephen Jay. 1997. 'Nonoverlapping Magisteria.' *Natural History* 106 (2): 16–22 and 60–62.

———. 2002. *Rocks of Ages: Science and Religion in the Fullness of Life*. New York, NY: Ballantine Books.

Griffel, Frank. 2009. *Al-Ghazālī's Philosophical Theology*. New York, NY: Oxford University Press.

Guessom, Nidhal. 2011. *Islam's Quantum Question: Reconciling Muslim Tradition and Modern Science*. London: I.B. Tauris.

Gutas, Dimitri. 1998. *Greek Thought, Arabic Culture: The Graeco-Arabic Translation Movement in Baghdad and Early Abbasid Society (2nd-4th/8th-10th centuries)*. London: Routledge.

Hayek, Friedrich August von. 1942. 'Scientism and the Study of Society. Part I.' *Economica* 9 (35): 267–291.

Ibn Rushd. 1959. *Kitāb faṣl al-maqāl*, ed. George F. Hourani. Leiden: Brill.

Jackson, Sherman. 2002. *On the Boundaries of Theological Tolerance in Islam: Abū Ḥāmid al-Ghazālī's Fayṣal al-Tafriqa*. Karachi: Oxford University Press.

Okumuş, Mesut. 2011. 'The Influence of al-Ghazzālī on the Hermeneutics of Ibn Rushd.' *Der Islam* 86 (2): 286–311.

Popper, Karl R. 1979. *Objective Knowledge: An Evolutionary Approach*. New York, NY: Oxford University Press.

Tamer, Georges, ed. 2015. *Islam and Rationalisty: The Impact of al-Ghazālī: Papers Collected on his 900th Anniversary, Vol. 1*. Leiden: Brill.

Vishanoff, David. 2011. *The Formation of Islamic Hermeneutics: How Sunni Legal Theorists Imagined a Revealed Law*. New Haven, CT: American Oriental Society.
Weiss, Bernard G. 1998. *The Spirit of Islamic Law*. Athens, GA: University of Georgia Press.
Yaran, Cafer S. 2003. *Islamic Thought on the Existence of God: Contributions and Contrasts with Contemporary Western Philosophy of Religion*. Washington, DC: The Council for Research in Values and Philosophy.
Zysow, Aron. 2013. *The Economy of Certainty: An Introduction to the Typology of Islamic Legal Theory*. Atlanta, GA: Lockwood Press.

**Kamaluddin Ahmed** is a DPhil scholar in Oriental Studies at the University of Oxford, an Islamic Bioethics researcher, and a classically trained Islamic scholar. His thesis focuses on the relationship between scriptural traditions and legal reasoning in the intellectual history of Islamic law in the ninth century, or third Islamic century.

# Chapter 12
# Interface between Islamic Law and Science: Ethico-Legal Construction of Science in Light of Islamic Bioethical Discourses on Genetic and Reproductive Technologies

**Ayman Shabana**

## 12.1 Introduction

Various applications of modern genetic and reproductive technologies have inspired solutions to hitherto impossible medical problems. While reproductive technology has overcome intractable infertility conditions, genetic technology ushered a new chapter in the history of medicine by enhancing the ability to anticipate disorders and even to chart therapeutic plans on the basis of individual needs and circumstances. Despite their impressive achievements, however, these technologies raise serious ethical concerns both at the individual and collective levels. Muslim responses to these concerns reveal a sober realization that these technologies pose significant challenges to various aspects of the inherited Islamic normative tradition. Chief among these challenges is the increasing power and authority of modern science, which requires proper evaluation of the latter in the process of juristic assessment. In general, Islamic bioethical discourses are presented as vouched on solid scientific understanding of the issues under investigation but this leaves the exact role of science rather obscure. While accurate scientific explanations of bioethical issues are considered indispensable, ultimate authority remains tied to Islamic normative values as well as the ethical ends of the Sharīʿa. This in turn raises a number of important questions such as: To what extent does science, particularly in its positivist sense that does not recognize religious or metaphysical assumptions,[1] play a role in Islamic bioethical deliberations? How is science understood and conceptualized in modern bioethical discourses? How can its role be characterized and

[1] For this definition of science, see Stearns (2011), 269.

A. Shabana (✉)
Georgetown University in Qatar, Doha, Qatar
e-mail: as2432@georgetown.edu


A. al-Akiti, A. I. Padela (eds.), *Islam and Biomedicine*, Philosophy and Medicine 137, https://doi.org/10.1007/978-3-030-53801-9_12

how can the relationship between the jurists and scientists or technical experts be defined? To what extent does science aid or challenge the normative authority of the Sharīʿa? And, finally, are these questions new? To what extent can precedents in the Islamic juridical corpus provide instructive insights for contemporary discourses?

This chapter investigates these questions by examining Islamic responses to some illustrative applications of genetic and reproductive technologies in the form of individual as well as collective *fatwās*. It argues that the general tendency in Islamic normative discourses leans more towards accommodating rather than challenging or denying the authority of modern science. This, however, does not mean that all applications of modern biomedicine are condoned or accepted. Scientific applications or procedures often undergo a process of legitimization through which they are scrutinized and subjected to certain conditions and stipulations to distinguish permissible and impermissible use. On the other hand, as discussed below, some applications and procedures are contested and even rejected outright. In general, while the technical knowledge gained through applied science is considered necessary for accurate understanding and characterization of the issue in question, applied scientific knowledge is viewed as playing a supportive rather than essential role in the process of normative assessment. Within Islamic bioethical deliberations scientific knowledge is perceived as contingent and subject to change in light of new research. Normative assessment, on the other hand, is perceived as grounded in divine revelation, which shapes and informs a comprehensive moral view of the world. This, in turn, reveals a continuation to, rather than, departure from, the attitude of pre-modern jurists towards the role of technical expertise in the legal process. The chapter suggests that normative juristic articulations in the modern period seek to provide an unofficial ethical gatekeeping function, which works in parallel with other types of formal gatekeeping measures undertaken by state-affiliated regulatory bodies.

## 12.2 Conceptualization of Science in Modern Islamic Discourses

The Arabic term *ʿilm* was used in the Islamic tradition to denote the general concept of knowledge. One of its famous definitions indicates that it stands for firm belief that corresponds to reality (*al-iʿtiqād al-jāzim al-muṭābiq lil-wāqiʿ*). Another definition indicates that it stands for perceiving something as it is or according to its reality (*idrāk al-shayʾ ʿalā mā huwa bi-hi*).[2] Some of the main classifications used include its division into either necessary or acquired knowledge. Necessary knowledge obtains immediately without the need for extensive reflection or contemplation, as is the case with one's knowledge of what is possible and impossible. Acquired knowledge, on the other hand, depends on learning and instruction. Knowledge was

[2] Al-Jurjānī (2009), 157.

also divided into theoretical (*naẓarī*) and practical (*ʿamalī*) types. The former stands for mere abstract knowledge, while the latter depends on actual practice as is the case with rituals. Another classification denotes the division between rational (*ʿaqlī*) knowledge, which is based on intellectual means and methods, and textual or scriptural (*samʿī*) knowledge, which is based on divine revelation.[3]

The emergence of new classifications of knowledge in the modern period and the consolidation of the authority as well as the prestige of the applied sciences as the domain of reliable empirical knowledge raised questions about the Islamic conceptualization of science. Surveys of the discourses on Islam and science identify multiple approaches throughout the Muslim world in the wake of the introduction of Western science during the nineteenth century, mainly under Western colonial rule. For example, Muzaffar Iqbal traces the emergence of two main approaches towards modern science in the post 1950s era. The first represents a continuation of the earlier apologetic discourse that was adopted by Muslim modernist thinkers and reformers during the nineteenth and early twentieth century, within which the compatibility between Islam and Western science was emphasized. The second approach takes a critical look at the philosophical underpinnings of modern science and highlights the specific epistemological and metaphysical dimensions of the Islamic conceptualization of science. This second approach was developed mainly by some Muslim intellectuals who gained considerable familiarity with modern science both as graduates of modern educational systems, but also through actual professional experience in the West.[4]

One of the most important aspects of the Islamic conceptualization of science has to do with the relationship between religious and non-religious/secular knowledge. This issue was the main topic of discussion during a special congress that was organized by the Islamic Organization for Medical Sciences (IOMS) in Kuwait in January 2001 in collaboration with the National Council for Culture, Arts, and Literature of Kuwait, the Islamic Educational, Scientific, and Cultural Organization (ISESCO), and the International Islamic Fiqh Academy of the Organisation of Islamic Cooperation (OIC).[5] Most of the participants were of the view that Islam does not espouse a sharp division between religious and scientific knowledge. By contrast, both types of knowledge are meant to support and complement each other. Several arguments have been used to substantiate this view, which appeal to both scriptural as well as historical evidence. For example, it is indicated that Islamic

[3] Rāghib al-Iṣfahānī (2010), 347–5. Theologians were divided on the general concept of *ʿilm* into three main opinions. The first opinion, argued by Fakhr al-Dīn al-Rāzī (d. 606/1210), indicates that *ʿilm* belongs to the category of the necessities, which means that it happens by itself without acquisition or contemplation as is the case with one's knowledge of one's own existence. The second opinion, argued by al-Juwaynī (d. 478/1085) and al-Ghazālī (d. 505/1111), indicates that *ʿilm* is not limited to the category of the necessities but it emphasizes the difficulty of delineating a specific definition for it. The third opinion indicates the possibility of delineating the meaning of *ʿilm*. This third opinion generated several definitions of *ʿilm* such as the ones mentioned above. See al-Ījī (1997), 1:48–52; al-Zarkashī (2010), 1:52–5.

[4] See Iqbal (2007), 160–78.

[5] See al-ʿAwaḍī and al-Jindī (2002).

foundational sources encourage acquisition of knowledge in the generic sense without any distinction between religious or natural sciences. Not only the first verse in the Qur'an includes an invitation to reading and learning but the entire text is replete with exhortations to explore divine manifestations in the universe. The root of the term *ʿilm* and its derivatives occur in the Qur'an more than 850 times and the term itself occurs about 94 times.[6] On the other hand, the Islamic civilization prides itself on the outstanding achievements of numerous scholar-scientists, which are often celebrated as part of humanity's common scientific heritage.[7]

Apart from these general statements that are usually adduced to demonstrate Islam's appreciation of science and scientific achievements, some scholars highlighted certain aspects of the Islamic conceptualization of knowledge. For example, in his keynote lecture, the Syrian physician Dr Muḥammad Haytham al-Khayyāṭ noted that the early generations of Muslims did not distinguish between religious and natural sciences but rather between useful or beneficial (*nāfiʿ*) sciences on the one hand and useless and harmful sciences on the other. For example, the Prophet used to implore God in his prayer to guide him to useful knowledge and to guard him from useless knowledge.[8] Moreover, the Qur'anic story of Hārūt and Mārūt, includes condemnation of harmful knowledge.[9] Therefore, argues al-Khayyāṭ, any beneficial knowledge should be seen as legitimate and can be considered 'Islamic.'[10] In terms of their utility and objectives, the former Mufti of Tunisia (1984–1998), Muḥammad al-Mukhtār al-Sallāmī (d. 1440/2019), distinguished four types of knowledge. The first includes what is considered obligatory knowledge, which each individual has to acquire in order to ensure success in this world and salvation in the hereafter. The most prominent example of this type is knowledge of religious obligations such as the five pillars of Islam. The second type includes the different branches of knowledge that are also obligatory but at the collective rather than individual level. This type of knowledge is important for the well-being of society and must be acquired at least by some. It covers almost all types of knowledge, which are essential for the various professions and fields such as medicine, engineering, and agriculture. The third type includes knowledge that enhances the quality of people's life, as is the case with music, athletics, and gardening. This type of knowl-

[6] ʿAbd al-Bāqī (2001), 576–91.

[7] See al-Shakʿa (2002).

[8] Al-Khayyāṭ (2002), 81. As noted above, the Qur'an contains numerous references to indicate the virtue of knowledge, including, for example, the elevated ranks of those who pursue knowledge [Qur'an 58:11 (*al-Mujādala*)], and instructing the Prophet to ask for an increase in knowledge [Qur'an 20:114 (*Ṭā Hā*)]. Similar references are frequently mentioned in the Sunna of the Prophet as well. Classical commentaries on these references tend to place more emphasis on religious knowledge. See, for example, Ibn Ḥajar al-ʿAsqalānī (n.d.), 1:140–1. Here, al-Khayyāṭ, however, emphasizes the extent to which knowledge (whether religious or secular) is deemed beneficial or harmful. He also refers to a Prophetic report in which pursuit of knowledge is described as an obligation on every Muslim. Although this report is contested among the scholars of *ḥadīth*, some have indicated that its meaning is supported by multiple other reports, see al-Qārī (2001), 1: 434–5.

[9] Qur'an 2:102 (*al-Baqara*).

[10] Al-Khayyāṭ (2002), 81.

edge is considered permissible and, depending on the need of the community, may even be recommended. The fourth includes all types of useless or harmful knowledge, as is the case with magic and talismans. In principle, this type of knowledge is prohibited but its status may change depending on the need of the community and the requirement to achieve self-sufficiency or to deter enemies.[11]

This broad conceptualization of science and its comparison to the general concept of knowledge is reminiscent of classical juristic and theological discourses in the Islamic tradition. For example, the famous theologian-jurist Abū Ḥāmid al-Ghazālī (d. 505/1111) divides sciences into two main types. The first includes the religious sciences (*sharʿiyya*), which draw on revelatory sources. The second includes the non-religious sciences (*ghayr sharʿiyya*), which do not depend on revelatory sources. They may depend instead on human reasoning (e.g., mathematics), experimentation (e.g., medicine), or oral transmission (e.g., language). Non-religious sciences can be categorized on the basis of their objectives and overall utility into recommended (*maḥmūd*) as is the case with medicine or agriculture, denounced (*madhmūm*) as is the case with magic and talismans, or neutral (*mubāḥ*) as is the case with decent poetry. Non-religious sciences can also fall under the category of the collective duty (*farḍ kifāya*), depending on social need as is the case again with mathematics and medicine, which are deemed indispensable for commercial transactions and preservation of physical health respectively.[12] Religious sciences, on the other hand, are divided into four types. The first includes the roots or foundations (*uṣūl*), which comprise four elements: the Qur'an, the Prophetic Sunna, juristic consensus, and reports of the Companions of the Prophet. The second includes the branches (*furūʿ*), which are derived from the above roots, as is the case with substantive law (*fiqh*). The third includes propaedeutic preliminary sciences (*muqaddimāt*), which are deemed important for the proper understanding of foundational texts, as is the case with linguistic sciences. The fourth includes the complementary sciences (*mutammimāt*) which build on all of the above as is the case with Qur'anic exegesis.[13]

One of the main points that the participating scholars in the congress of the Islamic Organization for Medical Sciences addressed was the modern positivist concept of science and the confusion it created in terms of its comparison with the more generic and comprehensive concept of knowledge from the Islamic perspective. For example, several scholars emphasized the specific Western context within which the modern concept of science emerged. According to this view modern science had to part ways with religion due to the struggle it had to undertake against Christianity.[14] The dichotomy between religion and science, therefore, reflects the historical struggle between modern science and the church in European history. While science in this sense is used mainly to denote empirical knowledge in the

[11] Al-Sallāmī (2002), 106–111.

[12] Al-Ghazālī (2010), 1:34.

[13] Ibid., 1:35.

[14] See, for example, Ḥatḥūt (2002), 127–31; and al-Taskhīrī (2002), 158–9.

domain of natural sciences, it cannot be applied to religious sciences. The modern concept of science in the positivist sense depends exclusively on empirical methods but the sources of knowledge in Islam include, in addition to empirical methods on the basis of human reasoning and sense perception, also verified reports of revelatory sources.[15] According to the Qatari-based Egyptian scholar Yūsuf al-Qaraḍāwī:

> Science that has been extolled in the Qur'an and reiterated in its verses includes any knowledge that reveals the reality of things and clears the veil of ignorance and doubt from the intellect, whether its subject matter is man, existence, or the unknown and whether its method is sense perception and experimentation, reasoning and demonstration, or revelation and prophethood.[16]

Accordingly, the concept of knowledge in Islam, as has also been reflected in Islamic history, is more comprehensive and the relationship between the different branches of knowledge is marked by complementarity rather than opposition and conflict. For example, the sciences of Sharīʿa are meant to guide, regulate and organize the various dimensions of human life, including all types of sciences, within the framework of the Islamic view of the world. Such a view of the world rests on human stewardship (*khilāfa*), through which man is to pursue knowledge for the service of humanity. From this perspective the stakes of divorcing science from religious morality are quite high, as a purely materialist approach to science may turn it into a self-destructive enterprise.[17]

Several scholars at the 2001 special congress emphasized the need for developing a new Islamic epistemology, which can incorporate all branches of knowledge including natural and applied sciences. For example, Aḥmad Fuʾād Bāshā, Professor of Physics at Cairo University, noted that such epistemology should transcend the duality of religion and science. Moreover, it should highlight the role of religious belief in promoting, rather than obstructing, the process of learning and discovery. Religious faith and God-consciousness can be important resources to promote a deeper understanding of the various phenomena in the universe.[18] One of the main points used, either by positivist scientists or conservative religious scholars, to highlight the dichotomy between religion and science, is the changing nature of science

[15] Al-Sallāmī (2002), 104.

[16] Al-Qaraḍāwī (2002), 279.

[17] Wāṣil (2002a), 251–3. The modest state of scientific progress in the Muslim world and the general lack of appreciation for science, as reflected in different social and economic indicators, was also discussed. Since the Islamic religion is perceived as encouraging the pursuit of knowledge in general, an explanation for this must rest on other factors. According to the Tunisian historian ʿAbd al-Jalīl al-Tamīmī, the answer lies in ineffective and overall corrupt politics. For example, he points out the dismal budgets allocated for educational programmes in the Arab world as well as the absence of the proper environment conducive to free and independent academic research. He laments the mushrooming of universities and educational institutions throughout the Arab world, but without significant achievements at the international level. See al-Tamīmī (2002), 233–43. It is important to note that al-Tamīmī's views were criticized by several other participants, who accused his views as being too pessimistic. Some have even asked him to retract this overly negative assessment of Arab educational institutions, see al-ʿAwaḍī and al-Jindī (2002), 269.

[18] Bāshā (2002), 177.

and the unchanging nature of religion. In response to this point, the Iranian scholar Muḥammad ʿAlī al-Taskhīrī, points out that all laws in the universe, including natural, cosmic, social, and also behavioural, are fixed because they have been instituted by God. They reveal God's way (*sunnat Allāh*) in his creation, which does not change. What changes, however, is man's knowledge of these laws, which is constantly evolving. Therefore, man's knowledge remains relative as it continues to approximate absolute divine knowledge.[19] Similarly, the well-known Syrian scholar Muḥammad Saʿīd Ramaḍān al-Būṭī (d. 1434/2013) notes that the Qur'an invites people to utilize their intellects to achieve deeper understanding of the world in light of the changing circumstances.[20] The concluding statement of the Islamic Organization for Medical Sciences special congress emphasized several points, which include: the comprehensiveness of the Islamic conception of science, which covers all types of cosmic and natural sciences in addition to religious sciences; inclusion of the cosmic and natural sciences within the category of collective duties, which have to be mastered at least by some; the importance of utilizing cosmic and natural sciences for the derivation of proper Sharīʿa-based rules, which in turn will require closer collaboration between religious scholars and technical experts.[21]

## 12.3 Islamic Law and the Mechanics of Legal Construction

Classical Muslim jurists devoted a great deal of attention to the issue of legal construction under several themes in legal theory such as analogy (*qiyās*) and independent legal reasoning (*ijtihād*).[22] Under *qiyās*, Muslim jurists discussed the extent to which a new case can be compared to an existing or previously studied one. This analogy is undertaken on the basis of a common operative cause (*ʿilla*). According to a famous juristic dictum, the legal ruling (*ḥukm*) revolves around its operative cause; that is to say, the ruling applies as long as its *ʿilla* exists and vice versa. This is the reason why the *ʿilla* is also called the anchor (*manāṭ*) of a ruling. A major part of the analogy-related discussions focuses on methods to evaluate operative causes of particular rulings. As the celebrated Shāfiʿī jurist al-Ghazālī notes, this process includes three types: actualization (*taḥqīq*), verification or careful examination (*tanqīḥ*), and extrapolation (*takhrīj*). Firstly, the actualization of an *ʿilla* involves the process of implementing legal rulings in specific cases. For instance, one of the conditions for the validity of prayer is facing the direction of the Kaʿba in Mecca,

[19] Al-Taskhīrī (2002), 160.

[20] Al-Būṭī (2002), 327.

[21] See al-ʿAwaḍī and al-Jindī (2002), 718–9. For an epistemological discussion on the place of scientific knowledge and its relationship with the Muslim legal tradition, see Chap. 11, 'Science in the Framework of Islamic Legal Epistemology: An Exploratory Essay,' by Kamaluddin Ahmed and Aasim I. Padela in this book.

[22] Other terms were also used such as *istinbāṭ*, *taḥarrī* and *istidlāl*; see *al-Mawsūʿa al-fiqhiyya* (1982-), 1:316.

which is based on a textual reference in the Qur'ān.[23] Thus, determining the exact direction whenever a Muslim has to pray is an example of the actualization of an *ʿilla*. Other examples include actual determination of unspecified values such as average or sufficient amounts, which depends on common standards in particular social contexts. Secondly, the careful examination of an *ʿilla* involves the process of targeting the most relevant aspect of a textual reference or legal precedent, which can then be extended to similar or relevant cases. For example, instructions given by the Prophet to some of his contemporaries would also be applicable to other Muslims, unless otherwise clearly indicated. Al-Ghazālī notes that these two types of assessment are unanimously upheld by all jurists including those who deny the authority of legal analogy. The third type is the extrapolation of an *ʿilla*, which stands for the identification of the proper *ʿilla* of a text-based rule for a given issue, which can then be extrapolated to another unstated one. The classic example in these discussions is the prohibition of wine, which is presumed on the basis of the extracted *ʿilla* that it has an intoxicating effect. This extracted *ʿilla* is then used, through legal analogy, to extrapolate the same ruling for any substance that has a similar intoxicating effect.[24]

Juristic discussions concerning legal construction, particularly with regard to new and novel cases (*nawāzil*), are usually located under the theme of *ijtihād*. For example, the prominent Mālikī jurist Abū Isḥāq al-Shāṭibī (d. 790/1388) distinguishes two main types of *ijtihād* on the basis of the foregoing discussion concerning *ʿilla*. The first type revolves around the actualization of the underlying *ʿilla* for legal rules. This type of *ijtihād* involves the process of implementing legal rules for individual cases. The other type of *ijtihād*, is not limited to mere implementation of legal rules but it also includes the process of deducing new rules.[25] In the pre-modern period, *ijtihād* was pursued mostly as an individual enterprise, undertaken by qualified and competent jurists. In the modern period, however, with the growing realization of the increased complexity of technical questions, a new form of collective *ijtihād* started to take shape. This new form of *ijtihād* relies on the combined efforts of religious scholars, as well as on the contributions from technical subject-matter experts.[26]

---

[23] Qur'an 2:144 and 2:149 (*al-Baqara*).

[24] Al-Ghazālī (n.d.), 2:230.

[25] Al-Shāṭibī notes that the first type is ongoing until the day of resurrection. The second type, on the other hand, may be interrupted before the day of resurrection. The second type is furthered divided into three main types, similar to the ones mentioned by al-Ghazālī: actualization (*taḥqīq*), verification (*tanqīḥ*), and extrapolation (*takhrīj*) of the underlying *ʿilla* of legal rules (*manāṭ*). Actualization under the second type, however, is distinguished from actualization under the first type in terms of degree and scope. While actualization under the first type is considered essential for all legal rules and it covers the process of identifying relevant species or genres (*anwāʿ*), actualization under the second type pertains to the process of implementing legal rules in light of the particular conditions and circumstances of individuals (*ashkhāṣ*). See al-Shāṭibī (2003), 4:73–87.

[26] Al-Khālid (2009), 70.

## 12.4 Interface Between Islamic Law and Science

One of the main features of modern culture has been the increased appreciation of specialized scientific knowledge (as organized, developed, transmitted, and implemented by trained professionals within specific academic disciplines and communities of practice).[27] Outsiders, including religious scholars, can only choose to ignore verified scientific information within established disciplines and fields at the risk of ridiculing themselves. Since scientific knowledge is constantly evolving, jurists need to consult with technical experts on the current state of scientific knowledge in a given field. A quick survey of modern Islamic legal discourses would reveal greater sensitivity to the role of modern science, particularly in the case of technical questions that require expert knowledge. The process of legal construction is predicated on two main elements: knowledge of scriptural sources (*maṣādir*, sing. *maṣdar*); and knowledge of the lived reality (*wāqiʿ*) within which constructed rulings are to be implemented.[28]

In the legal tradition Muslim jurists discuss the extent to which factual information, especially in the case of specialized knowledge within certain professions, can be incorporated in the process of legal construction. These discussions usually fall under the general theme of expertise (*khibra*). Classical jurists used terms such as *maʿrifa* (knowledge), *tajriba* (experience), and *baṣar* (practical insight) to denote specialized knowledge or technical expertise. They also discussed several examples of the issues that require the involvement of experts, particularly within judicial proceedings. Because the judge is not expected to have detailed technical knowledge of certain issues or certain professions, he may resort to experts such as translators, distributors, physiognomers, evaluators, physicians, and veterinarians.[29] Juristic discussions on the issue of expertise include the qualifications for a specific expert and also whether it would be sufficient to rely on one expert only. These discussions often involve the distinction between an expert, a witness, and a judge.[30]

[27] Max Weber (d. 1920) describes modern scientific progress as the culmination of a centuries-old intellectualization process, through which the world has been disenchanted. By this he means: 'there are no mysterious incalculable forces that come into play, but rather that one can, in principle, master all things by calculation. This means that the world is disenchanted. One need no longer have recourse to magical means in order to master or implore the spirits, as did the savage, for whom each mysterious power existed. Technical means and calculations perform the service. This above all is what intellectualization means.' Weber (2009), 138–9.

[28] Dār al-Iftāʾ al-Miṣriyya (1434/2013), 34. The term for Islamic substantive law, *fiqh*, literally means understanding, as it seeks to construct legal rulings on the basis of an accurate understanding of reality. The technical definition of *fiqh* as a legal science is 'knowledge of the practical rulings of Sharīʿa, which are derived from their detailed textual foundations' (*al-ʿilm bi-al-aḥkām al-sharʿiyya al-ʿamaliyya al-muktasab min adillatihā al-tafṣīliyya*), see, for example, *al-Mawsūʿa al-fiqhiyya* (1982-), 32:193; al-Zarkashī (2010), 1:19–21.

[29] *Al-Mawsūʿa al-fiqhiyya* (1982-), 19:18.

[30] Ibrāhīm (2003), 723–4; Wāṣil (2002b), 161–4; Shanyūr (2005), 62. In the modern period Muslim jurists draw on similar discussions in modern (secular) legal studies concerning the issue of expertise (*khibra*). Three different types (or rather contexts within which expertise is sought and imple-

In general, modern Muslim jurists are acutely aware of the tremendous changes that transformed the world over the past two or three centuries, mainly due to impressive leaps in scientific knowledge and technological advances. For example, in his discussion on the need for the renewal of Islamic law, the Mufti of Egypt (2003–2013), ʿAlī Jumʿa, notes that one of the main tasks that Muslim jurists must undertake in the modern period is developing an accurate understanding of reality (*al-wāqiʿ*). The term *fiqh al-wāqiʿ* is often invoked to highlight the importance of recognizing differences emanating not from text-based rulings in themselves but rather from social-historical circumstances that may have an impact on how such rulings should be implemented.[31] As jurists reiterate, such differences may be attributed to changes in time, place, surrounding circumstances, or customs.[32] The true challenge lies not only in the proper understanding of textual sources in a theoretical, abstract or detached manner but rather in light of informed understanding of the context within which the jurist operates. Linking these two elements (foundational texts and contextual circumstances) to each other takes place in the mind of the jurist through actual and practical construction (*taṣwīr*).[33] This line of reasoning often aims to illustrate that classical legal methodology was developed in the past to address contemporary needs, as reflected in pre-modern legal corpuses. Here, ʿAlī Jumʿa is encouraging jurists in the modern period to follow the example of their forebears and develop rules that respond to modern needs. According to him, one of the main tools to get an accurate understanding of reality is scientific knowledge, which should be pursued in a manner that does not conflict with fundamental Islamic principles. *Ijtihād*, therefore, should be undertaken but it should be well-regulated within the boundaries of the definitive indications and moral vision of the scriptural sources. What is interesting to observe in this discussion is how he emphasizes the importance of scientific knowledge as one of the tools for the renewal of Islamic law. He notes that reality involves five 'worlds' (*ʿawālim*, sing. *ʿālam*): things (*ashyāʾ*); persons; (*ashkhāṣ*); events (*aḥdāth*); ideas (*afkār*); and systems

mented) are distinguished. The first is official judicial expertise, which is solicited by a judge with regard to a question involving specialized knowledge that the judge cannot ascertain on his own. Different legal systems regulate how and when this process is undertaken. The second is unofficial consultative expertise, which may be solicited at the initiative of private individuals or entities for verification or assessment purposes. The third type is also unofficial expertise, which is solicited on the basis of consensual agreement among disputing parties that they would acknowledge and uphold the opinion of a particular expert, which may be the case in arbitration procedures. See Shanyūr (2005), 42. On the issue of expert testimony, see Shaham (2010).

[31] See Jumʿa (2006), 258 (referring to the changes that occurred over the past three centuries and their unprecedented impact on changing the human understanding of the world). See also, Ibn Bayyah (2007), 149 (emphasizing the importance of developing a comprehensive understanding of the lived reality in the work of modern *fatwā* institutions).

[32] Dār al-Iftāʾ al-Miṣriyya (1434/2013), 35–46. On this, see also Ibn Qayyim al-Jawziyya (2002), 4:337.

[33] Jumʿa (2006), 261. For an examination of how the notion of *wāqiʿ* was invoked by the leaders of al-Jamāʿa al-Islāmiyya in Egypt in the revisions they undertook in the 1990s while serving prison terms, see Jackson (2009): 59, 63.

(*nuẓum*). Proper understanding of each of these worlds requires the employment of its own respective methods, deemed relevant to its subject matter. In the modern period, empirical science is considered indispensable for the understanding of the 'world of things.' Although he points out the distinction between the more general concept of knowledge in the Islamic tradition and the more specific concept of modern empirical science, his discussion does not imply total rejection of the latter. This discussion by ʿAlī Jumʿa reveals that modern science is understood as a form of sustained and systematic investigation of the natural world through the employment of empirical and experimental methods. In this sense, science, as a framework of discovery and problem solving, is deemed essential in allowing the legal tradition, any legal tradition, to accommodate emerging needs and changing circumstances. The practice of this scientific investigation, however, should be guided by and evaluated in light of Islam's normative principles and ethical objectives.

In the modern *fatwā* literature Islamic religious scholars often show deference to technical expertise, which may give the impression of a major transformation in the institution of *iftāʾ* by means of which the Mufti is turned into a 'concerned *mustaftī* who will evaluate the answer from the point of view of Islamic law and ethics.'[34] In other words, the Mufti is no longer viewed as the sole figure vested with the authority to provide normative guidance but must now rely on technical expertise to ensure the accuracy of the assessment. For example, in addressing complex economic questions, Muftis increasingly consult with lay economists and financial experts.[35] Similarly, Muftis do also often rely on lay technical experts in their deliberations on medical and healthcare issues.[36] For the purpose of the present study, one important question to explore is the extent to which such reliance on technical expertise constitutes a development or transformation in the juristic process, particularly in light of pre-modern discussions on expert testimony. The working thesis that I advance here is that the increasing reliance of modern jurists on technical expertise in the juristic process may signal a change in degree but not necessarily in nature.

As noted above, the acknowledged complexity of modern technical questions provided the impetus for the emergence of collective *ijtihād* institutions, which aim to combine the efforts of traditionally-trained jurists on the one hand and technical

---

[34] See Skovgaard-Petersen (2004), 94 (discussing the institution of *iftāʾ* in Syria, Lebanon, and Egypt against the background of *iftāʾ* practice during the Ottoman era).

[35] On the inclusion of secular expertise in the process of *fatwā*-issuing with reference to economic issues, see Skovgaard-Petersen (1997), 295–318; and Mallat (1996), 286–96 (arguing that in the case of modern technical questions Muftis increasingly realize the limitation of reliance on religious knowledge alone and seek to incorporate secular knowledge by technical experts).

[36] For example, while discussing the notion of brain death and its implications, the Mufti of Egypt (1986–1996) and Shaykh al-Azhar (1996–2010), Muḥammad Sayyid Ṭanṭāwī (d. 1431/2010), relegated the authority to determine when death takes place to physicians: 'Death is the separation from life, and those who can judge a separation from life are the physicians, not the religious scholars. So, if the doctor believes that the [patient], whose heart is beating although his brain has died, this is a matter of the physician ['s professional expertise]. [If] the heart of a patient continues to beat because he is hooked up to a machine, and his brain is dead, there is no fault in the family requesting the removal of the machine ... they are accepting God's decree.' Brockopp (2003), 178–8.

experts on the other.[37] But, the authority to issue *fatwās* has consistently been considered the prerogative of traditionally-trained scholars (*ʿulamāʾ*) to the extent that the issuing of *fatwās* by intellectuals outside the ranks of *ʿulamāʾ* or even their participation in the process is considered a departure from the standard practice or an 'aberration from the tradition of *iftāʾ*.'[38] Ultimately, juristic authority is defined by certain parameters such as having extensive knowledge of the scriptural sources, command of the legal tradition (including its technical language and normative precedents), as well as commitment to a particular methodology. The incorporation of secular knowledge (through technical experts) is meant to ensure the accuracy of the factual dimension of a *fatwā* rather than mark a transformation, by means of which a technical expert becomes an equal partner in the *fatwā*-issuing process.[39] On the other hand, ethical insights by Muslim technical experts are often coupled with the disclaimer that they should not be perceived as normative pronouncements.[40] As noted above, jurists often argue for the accommodation of modern

[37] In a recent study on some of the main institutions that facilitate this new form of collective *ijtihād*, Mohammed Ghaly observes that contributions by Muslim technical experts in bioethical deliberations occasionally include both technical and normative aspects and that it is not always easy to separate these two from each other. He argues that the increasing role of medical experts in normative bioethical deliberations reveals their growing influence on the *fatwā*-issuing process, and consequently allows them to assume the role of 'co-Muftis.' See Ghaly (2015). The term 'co-Mufti' suggests participation in the process of *fatwā*-issuing and one may argue that technical experts may qualify as co-Muftis since they participate at least in the factual dimension of a *fatwā*. If the term is meant to denote the ability or willingness of Muslim technical experts to formulate a normative argument, they would then be assuming the role of a full-fledged Mufti, provided that they meet the qualifications associated with juristic authority as mentioned above. In other words, technical experts may qualify as co-Muftis in light of their role in elucidating and clarifying the technical dimensions of a *fatwā*. In this case, however, one would need to explain how such role differs from that of the technical expert or expert witness in pre-modern juristic discussions. What is contested, however, is the claim that they can act as Muftis, by extending the scope of their contribution to the normative dimension of the *fatwā*. The jurists might rightly refuse to concede this role to technical experts in case they lack proper juristic credentials.

[38] See Nafi (2004) (discussing a *fatwā* issued jointly by Yūsuf al-Qaraḍāwī along with four other intellectuals: the Egyptian judge Ṭāriq al-Bishrī, the Egyptian lawyer Muḥammad Salīm al-ʿAwwā, the Syrian medical doctor Haytham al-Khayyāṭ, and the Egyptian journalist Fahmī Huwaydī. Although these four intellectuals are acclaimed thinkers and authors of numerous publications on Islamic issues, they are not considered *ʿulamāʾ* in the traditional sense and therefore their authority to issue *fatwās* is questioned.)

[39] For example, Mallat notes 'The modest tone of a religious expert who himself seeks the advice of experts in other fields can only strengthen the moral authority of the Mufti,' Mallat (1996), 296.

[40] For example, The Ethics Committee of the Islamic Medical Association of North America (2005) clearly indicates that the statement should not be perceived as a religious *fatwā*. For a comparative discussion on this statement and its position on brain death, see Padela, Shanawani, and Arozullah (2011): 64. Ghaly also notes that jurists do not generally show willingness to allow technical experts to engage in purely normative deliberations. See Ghaly (2015): 309. In his discussion on the work of *fatwā* institutions, the Mauritanian jurist ʿAbd Allāh Ibn Bayyah cautions against exaggerating the role of technical experts in issuing Sharīʿa-based rulings. See Ibn Bayyah (2007), 149.

scientific knowledge in the process of legal construction along the lines of traditional discussions on technical expertise or expert testimony.[41]

From a broader historical perspective, these discussions concerning the relationship between the jurists and technical experts as well as the proper scope of their respective contributions in the *fatwā*-issuing process should be traced to the larger social and cultural transformations that Muslim societies have undergone since the introduction of modern Western science, which resulted, among other things, in sharp bifurcation between religious sciences on the one hand and natural and applied sciences on the other.[42] With the increased secularization of technical knowledge and the consecration of the separation between religion and science, following the creation of dual (secular and religious) educational systems, the gap between religious scholars and modern science has steadily grown. Moreover, with the introduction of Western technologies, not only in biomedicine, but also in other modern scientific fields, Muftis have become dependent on technical experts for proper explanation of related scientific and technical information.

## 12.5 Interplay of Science, Law, and Ethics

Many of the concerns associated with modern biomedical applications touch on core ethical issues such as dignity of the human person and inviolability of the human body. It is generally assumed that science is not interested in purely moral or metaphysical questions, whose answers have to be located elsewhere.[43] This positivist view of science, however, is often challenged within the context of experimental research, particularly in biomedicine. For example, in her book on organ transplantation, Lesley A. Sharp notes:

> In contexts framed by highly experimental work – whether in transplant medicine or elsewhere – moral thinking figures prominently in scientific domains, where personal values, training, and experimentation determine scientists' commitments to certain projects over

[41] In fact, some researchers criticize the conceptualization of collective *ijtihād* as the combination of the efforts by religious scholars and technical experts (or scholars of text and context). Accordingly, this combination of efforts should be seen as a temporary and transitional stage. Ideally, the gap between religious and secular knowledge should be filled (at one point in the future) by a *mujtahid* who can combine these two bodies of knowledge within himself/herself. See al-Khālid (2009), 82.

[42] Seyyed Hussein Nasr notes that unlike Muslim reformers during the nineteenth century who embraced Western science, traditional scholars today have mostly kept a distance and isolated themselves from modern science. This, in turn, resulted in an increasing sense of 'cultural and social dislocation.' See Nasr (2010): 72.

[43] On this point Max Weber notes: 'Whether life is worthwhile living and when – this question is not asked by medicine. Natural science gives us an answer to the question of what we must do if we wish to master life technically. It leaves quite aside, or assumes for its purposes, whether we should and do wish to master life technically and whether it ultimately makes sense to do so.' See Weber (2009), 144.

> others. Should, for instance, one harness nuclear power for weaponry or for civilian energy needs? Are insects best understood as pests we must eliminate, or should we harvest them as viable protein sources? Are certain research funds, though hefty or lucrative, off-limits because their origins are morally suspect? How should one evaluate the economic, clinical, and social expense of employing various animal species in laboratories? Whose needs should be targeted in one's research – those of infants or the elderly, the wounded or the young and able-bodied, or destitute or paying clients? Is it morally responsible or reprehensible to attempt radically new procedures on or implant experimental devices within terminally ill patients if knowledge garnered from their end-of-life experiences could save others later? And what if these patient-subjects are children? Though muted or undervalued elsewhere, these sorts of questions shape scientists' convictions about the relevance, legitimacy, and social worth of their thoughts, beliefs, and actions when they forge ahead with highly experimental projects.[44]

In response to these moral questions and concerns, researchers point out the importance of devising regulatory frameworks to address the multifaceted effects of the modern biomedical revolution. Proposed regulatory frameworks range from private efforts on the basis of individual responsibility and control, professional efforts through institutions and organizations, communal efforts through oversight committees, as well as legal and legislative efforts.[45] In general, legal and legislative approaches to accommodate scientific knowledge as well as technical applications (through legislation, policies, and judicial procedures or decisions) may be the most effective and lasting in light of their connection with the power of the state and its law-enforcement prerogative. Different legal systems develop their own methods to govern the process through which scientific knowledge and applications are incorporated through legislative or judicial procedures. In most cases, the legal system provides a gatekeeping function that ensures its responsiveness to emerging social needs by integrating and incorporating verified scientific knowledge as well as validated technical developments.[46] Within the Muslim context, the Sharīʿa has always been a major source for moral reasoning, even after modern legal reform movements ended up either curtailing or eliminating its role in various legal and legislative areas. The growing and influential *fatwā* literature (covering not only issues of religious doctrine or rituals but also most aspects of private and public life) demonstrates the continuing role of the Sharīʿa as the main source of moral decision-making in the Muslim world. This unique role of the institution of *iftāʾ* within the Muslim context suggests that it participates in a significant way in the process of accommodating modern scientific knowledge and technical applications. The non-binding unofficial 'ethical gatekeeping' role that it plays often precedes and supplements the 'official' gatekeeping function of the state and its various regulatory bodies.

[44] Sharp (2013), 4–5.

[45] Morgan and Ford (2006), 271–2.

[46] For example, in the United States this gatekeeping function of the legal system is undertaken by the courts, although different states may use different standards. See Bernstein and Jackson (2004).

## 12.6 Islamic Law and Ethical Gatekeeping of Science Within the Context of Genetic and Reproductive Technologies: Different Modes of Interaction

Islamic bioethical discourses comprise different types of religious-normative literature such as treatises, monographs, journal articles (in regular journals of newly established journals dedicated to medical ethics or jurisprudence)[47] conference proceedings, recommendations, and statements. Considering the role of the *fatwā* as a 'mechanism of religious legitimization,'[48] the *fatwā* literature – whether in the form of individual *fatwās*, especially the ones issued by prominent scholars, or collective institutional *fatwās* – is particularly significant. The legitimizing power of the *fatwā* is usually highlighted in the area of politics but it is hardly limited to that domain. In many ways the dominance of the *fatwā* literature in modern bioethical discourses reflects the increasing demand for ethico-legal rulings on the various bioethical issues and consolidates the authority of the *ʿulamāʾ* not only as guardians of a static and fixed ethical-legal tradition but also as active agents who are called upon to monitor and guide social and cultural transformations.[49] Within this diverse body of literature, responses to bioethical issues are often presented as forms of *ijtihād* in light of the novel nature of the issues and also the lack of exact historical precedents in the classical legal corpus.[50]

In general, Muslim jurists are mainly interested in maintaining the continuity of the tradition, which they pursue through a number of strategies such as investigating the range of interpretive possibilities of scriptural sources, searching for relevant precedents, or selective appropriation of opinions from different legal schools within the vast and extended legal tradition of Islam. In the process they utilize the various tools of classical legal methodology such as juristic analogy (*qiyās*), appeal to relevant legal maxims (*qawāʿid*), or invoke the ultimate objectives of Sharīʿa (*maqāṣid*). The fluidity that marks these juristic efforts to address modern questions are sometimes criticized as unsystematic or instrumentalist.[51] This may partly be

[47] For example, the first issue of *Majallat al-Dirāsāt al-Ṭibbiyya al-Fiqhiyya* (established by the Saudi Association for Jurisprudential Medical Studies at Imam Muḥammad Ibn Saʿūd Islamic University) was published in 1436/2015.

[48] Masud, Messick, and Powers (1996), 9.

[49] See, for example, Zaman (2001). Still, however, the prominent role of the *fatwā* as the main source of proper religious-legal knowledge does not necessarily mean that the various social and cultural dimensions of these bioethical issues are always properly addressed. On this point, see Iqbal (2007), 182–3.

[50] Some researchers refer to collective *fatwās* as a form of collective *ijtihād*. Others, however, make a distinction between *ijtihād* and *iftāʾ*. Accordingly, *ijtihād* is based on the conviction of a jurist after expending his or her utmost in analysing a particular question and must therefore be individual. *Iftāʾ*, on the other hand, may involve more than one Mufti and can therefore take a collective form. See Ibn Bayyah (2007), 149.

[51] See, for example, Moosa (2002), 344 (analysing different *fatwās* on both organ transplantation and brain death, and arguing that Islamic legal deliberations are often concerned with finding a link

due to the multiple pressures that modern jurists feel in dealing with these issues. First, they are called upon to justify the continued relevance and applicability of the Sharīʿa and its underlying moral vision. After all, legal construction is not perceived as divorced from the underlying moral vision of the foundational sources and that is why it is often emphasized that not each and every scientific procedure or technical application can be legally or ethically sanctioned. Second, they feel the pressure of the modern hegemonic scientific culture, which challenges the viability of the Islamic legal system. As much as classical Muslim jurists were able to accommodate and incorporate the scientific culture of their time, jurists in the modern period feel they have a similar duty and responsibility. Third, they also feel the pressure to compete with and even to outperform secular legal systems that have managed to unseat Sharīʿa as the dominant legal system in the Muslim world.

Following the aforementioned discussion by the Egyptian Mufti, ʿAli Jumʿa, on the role of science in the renewal of Islamic law, Islamic bioethical discourses reveal different forms of interaction between Islamic law on the one hand and modern scientific knowledge and technical applications on the other. At the factual level, scientific knowledge is utilized to ensure accurate comprehension of the technical details that require elucidation from specialists and subject matter experts. Employment of scientific knowledge for the verification of factual details is often acknowledged as a critical and indispensable step for proper ethical analysis. At the ethical level, on the other hand, technical applications and procedures are evaluated in light of Islamic ethical principles as well as Islamic moral objectives. Accordingly, within the realm of genetic and reproductive technologies, qualifications accorded to the various applications of these technologies range from full embracement to reserved acceptance and even outright proscription.

## 12.7 Scientific Applications Embraced

One of the clearest examples to show the extent to which modern scientific knowledge has been used to revisit classical legal rules is the juristic discussion concerning the average pregnancy duration. Due to lack of a clear textual indication to either the minimum or the maximum period of a viable pregnancy, pre-modern jurists differ on the determination of the exact gestation period. Various juristic opinions, however, sought to bolster their arguments with references to, or rather inferences from, the Qur'an or the Prophetic tradition. In general, the determination of the minimum period of pregnancy was less controversial than the maximum period. Most jurists estimate the minimum period of pregnancy to be six months and some even cite consensus on this point. This estimate is based on deduction from two verses in the Qur'an. The first stipulates the proper breastfeeding period to be

with the tradition while overlooking modern ethical concerns. Moosa refers to the moral dimensions of Islamic law, which al-Ghazālī emphasized beyond mere formalistic constructions of legal rules. He describes this as the ritual function of the law (ibid., 353–4)).

two years.[52] The second stipulates the period from pregnancy to weaning to be thirty months.[53] Subtracting twenty-four months out of thirty leaves six months, which is taken to be the minimum duration of a viable pregnancy. Unlike the minimum period of pregnancy, the maximum period was subject to a great deal of juristic disagreement. In the pre-modern juristic tradition, several opinions were expressed ranging from nine month to an open-ended range.

In the modern period, most jurists, basing themselves on modern medical and scientific knowledge, choose a minimum pregnancy period of six months and a maximum of nine months.[54] They explain the disagreement among pre-modern jurists and their accommodation of extended maximum periods of pregnancy by the unavailability of accurate medical information and also by reliance on reported claims of these extended periods. Modern medical and scientific research now considers these reports of extended pregnancy periods as cases of false pregnancy or pseudocyesis, which has been confirmed by modern clinical studies. For example, according to the recommendations of the Islamic Organization for Medical Sciences on this issue, the average pregnancy period is 280 days or 40 weeks starting from the beginning of the last menstruation cycle preceding pregnancy. In some cases, this period may extend for one or two weeks at most.[55] Most personal status laws in Muslim majority countries have adopted the minimum of six months and the maximum of one full year to allow for the accommodation of extremely rare cases, in which pregnancy can last for more than nine months.[56]

Several other examples illustrate how modern scientific knowledge and technical applications have been accommodated, which include the use of DNA testing for paternity or forensic verification as well as the use of medical-genetic testing to determine suitability for marriage. The juristic debate on the legal status of DNA fingerprinting revolves around the possibility of integrating this new tool within the classical evidentiary structure. This issue has been addressed in a number of institutional resolutions that were issued after extensive deliberations among Muslim jurists and technical experts. During these deliberations, the scientific value of this tool was never questioned. The main reservations that the jurists made in the area of paternity had to do with the primacy of the licit sex principle in the definition of the parental connection between children and their fathers. In the area of criminal law, the main reservations had to do with the limited area of retaliation (*qiṣāṣ*) and stipulated punishments (*ḥudūd*).[57] Apart from these two main exceptions, DNA fingerprinting is considered a very useful tool, which can be utilized in order to serve the ultimate goals of the Islamic legal system by settling disputes and serving justice.

---

[52] Qur'an 2:233 (*al-Baqara*).

[53] Qur'an 46:15 (*al-Aḥqāf*).

[54] Al-Ashqar (1988).

[55] Al-Bārr (1984), 452; al-Ashqar (1988), 179.

[56] Al-Nūr (2007).

[57] This is mainly due to the understanding that *ḥudūd* and *qiṣāṣ* should be warded off if an accusation cannot be proven beyond doubt. DNA evidence is generally categorized as a type of circumstantial evidence, which cannot be used to categorically establish guilt in these cases.

The juristic discussions concentrate on the ethical guidelines that should govern the employment of this method, particularly in cases involving claims of unknown or contested paternity or identity. What is interesting to note in these discussions is that the process of integrating this new tool is pursued through comparison with the pre-Islamic Arabian practice of physiognomy (*qiyāfa*) to the extent that it is often described as its modern counterpart, although it is also often admitted that DNA fingerprinting is far more accurate than the primitive method of physiognomy.[58]

Similarly, the use of modern medical-genetic testing to determine suitability for marriage is predicated on the juristic discussions concerning defects that may justify annulment of the marital contract. In general, while a few jurists argued that prospective couples should not investigate each other's medical conditions prior to marriage,[59] most jurists argued that prospective couples should utilize these tests not only to ensure their own benefits (by precluding potential problems that may endanger the marital relationship), but also to achieve wider societal benefits (by ensuring the health and wellness of the prospective offspring). The main disagreement, however, was on whether such tests should be made compulsory or whether they should be left optional. In fact, some jurists have suggested that the state may intervene by developing legislation to prevent marriage when tests confirm that the children of a prospective couple will be at significant risk of having a serious illness.[60] These diverse opinions were also reflected in the various resolutions and collective *fatwās* that were issued on this topic. Three main examples are: the recommendations of the Islamic Organization for Medical Sciences in 1998; the resolution of the Islamic Fiqh Council (Muslim World League) in 2003; and the resolution of the International Islamic Fiqh Academy (Organisation of Islamic Cooperation) in 2013. While they all emphasize the importance of educating prospective couples and raising public awareness about the importance of medical-genetic pre-marital tests, the first two emphasize the importance of keeping these tests optional. The third, however, added the possibility that authorities may enforce premarital medical tests in case such a measure constitutes a considerable public interest.[61]

[58] For the congress hosted by the Islamic Organization for Medical Sciences, see al-ʿAwaḍī and al-Jindī (2005), 461–5. One of the main resolutions on this topic was issued by the Islamic Fiqh Council of the Muslim World League, see *Majallat al-Majmaʿ al-Fiqhī al-Islāmī* (2002): 478–81. For more on these discussions, see: Shabana (2014), and Shabana (2013).

[59] This opinion is attributed to the Mufti of Saudi Arabia (1993–1999), ʿAbd al-ʿAzīz ibn Bāz (d. 1420/1999). See al-Shuwayrakh (2007), 128–9.

[60] For the congress that the Islamic Organization for Medical Sciences hosted on this issue, see al-ʿAwaḍī and al-Jindī (2000). For a commentary on these discussions, see Shabana (2019).

[61] Shabana (2019), 92.

## 12.8 Scientific Applications Contested

One of the main examples that illustrates how modern scientific applications in the area of genetic and reproductive technologies have been contested has to do with the ban on third-party involvement in the reproductive process. As shown above in the case of DNA paternity testing, which has largely been approved as long as this new tool does not violate the licit sex principle, assisted reproductive technologies are also considered legitimate as long as they are pursued by married couples. This means that procedures involving any form of gamete donation or surrogacy arrangements are generally deemed impermissible. Although some jurists, mainly within the Shīʿī context, do allow these procedures on the grounds that they cannot be equated with illicit sexual relationship between unmarried couples, the majority view, mainly within the Sunnī context, do not distinguish these procedures from the physical act of adultery.[62] One of the earliest discussions on these issues dates back to the early 1980s, soon after the emergence and development of assisted reproductive technologies. The very first congress hosted by the Islamic Organization for Medical Sciences in 1983 brought together several prominent jurists and technical experts (physicians and scientists). It was during this congress that the main lines of the debate concerning the ethical reservations surrounding modern reproductive technologies from an Islamic perspective have been drawn.[63] While the concluding statement indicated that any form of third-party involvement would be impermissible, the collective deliberations among the participants show that the scientists and jurists engaged in an open and candid dialogue on the possibility of revisiting classical legal rules and doctrines. For example, while discussing the notion of 'womb renting,' the Egyptian Professor of Zoology at Ain Shams University in Cairo ʿAbd al-Ḥāfiẓ Ḥilmī (d. 1433/2012) raised a question about the importance of looking at this issue in light of two main considerations. The first is the changing reality, mainly under the influence of modern scientific knowledge and technical applications. The way we approach scriptural passages, according to him, should not ignore this fact. For example, the famous *ḥadīth* recounting foetal development describes the process inside the mother's womb. With assisted reproductive technologies, however, the process is now undertaken within the lab in a Petri dish. The second is the principle of necessity (*ḍarūra*) and the extent to which the need of infertile couples may serve as sufficient grounds to justify invocation of this principle in order to allow the involvement of a third party. He urged his interlocutors to examine the issue not only from an ideal normative perspective, but also to keep in mind the fact that some couples travel abroad to pursue infertility treatment, which may include some forms of third-party involvement. Ultimately, according to Dr Ḥilmī, since science can circumvent the main ethical reservation (confusion of lineages) by easily allowing the identification of the genetic contributors, referred to here as the real parents, ethical evaluation should transcend formal details and concentrate on

[62] Inhorn and Tremayne (2012).

[63] Al- ʿAwaḍī and al-Jindī (1983).

the essential ethical objectives. Dr Ḥilmī was extremely careful in explaining what he meant by emphasizing that he merely wanted to clarify the issue from the scientific perspective, but ultimate judgment would have to be made by the jurists: 'I am merely a witness and I present my testimony to the designated court. I am not speaking about permissibility or impermissibility. I realize that I am not qualified to pass such a judgment.'[64] The exchange between Dr Ḥilmī and the other participants, particularly the jurists, shows that the participating scientists saw themselves as expert witnesses in a court, within which the jurists assume the role of the judge who is invested with the authority to make the ultimate ethical assessment. Moreover, it also shows that scientists view the scope of their participation as limited to the factual/scientific dimension. Although he also invoked scriptural passages and made suggestions to see them in a new light that may inspire a new interpretation, he was careful to offer these suggestions in the form of queries rather than statements or conclusions. More broadly, this exchange shows the boundaries of the epistemic authority of the scientists and their scientific contributions in these Islamic moral-juristic deliberations. As Dr Ḥilmī put it, they serve as expert witnesses, rather than equal partners in the process of ethico-legal analysis. Subsequent resolutions on these issues along with accompanying collective discussions reveal the establishment of this division of labour between the jurists and technical experts. Moreover, they also reveal the confirmation of certain ethical assessments concerning some procedures, as is the case with the Sunnī ban on any form of third-party involvement in the procreative process.[65]

## 12.9 Conclusion

Islamic bioethical discourses on genetic and reproductive technologies reveal different forms of interaction between Islamic law and ethics and modern scientific knowledge and applications. Within these discourses, modern scientific knowledge is utilized mainly in clarifying the technical dimensions of the issue at hand. Consequently, technical applications and procedures are either accepted and embraced or contested and proscribed. Throughout, normative juristic discussions revolve around efforts to determine the scope of application, guidelines on proper integration within the Islamic juristic structure, and specification of relevant conditions and stipulations governing such integration. It is suggested here that these different patterns of interaction demonstrate the role of Islamic normative pronouncements in providing an unofficial ethical gatekeeping function, which, depending on the social-political context, would supplement, compete with, or work in parallel with other official gatekeeping functions associated with state-affiliated regulatory bodies. The question of Islam and science, however, cannot be isolated

[64] Ibid., 223.

[65] See Shabana (2015).

from the larger historical transformations that shaped Muslim-majority countries in the modern period. In addition to the relationship between religion and science, these transformations have also raised important questions about the relationship between religion and law, on the one hand, and between science and ethics, on the other.

**Acknowledgements** Earlier drafts of this chapter were presented at two meetings hosted by the 'Islam and the Human Sciences' Templeton project. The first was held at the Oxford Centre for Islamic Studies on November 22, 2017, and the second was held at the University of Chicago on September 9, 2018. I would like to thank Dr Afifi al-Akiti and Dr Aasim Padela, the principal investigators of this project and the conveners of these meetings, for inviting me to participate and for all the hard work they put in over the years. Research for my own chapter was supported by a Faculty Research Grant from Georgetown University in Qatar during the academic year of 2017–2018. It was also made possible by NPRP grant # NPRP8-1478-6-053 from the Qatar National Research Fund (a member of the Qatar Foundation). The results and statements made herein are solely the responsibility of the author.

## References

'Abd al-Bāqī, Muḥammad Fu'ād. 2001. *al-Muʿjam al-mufahras li-alfāẓ al-Qurʾān al-Karīm.* Cairo: Dār al-Ḥadīth.

al-Ashqar, ʿUmar Sulaymān. 1988. 'al-Ḥayḍ wa-al-ḥaml wa-al-nifās bayna al-fiqh wa al-ṭibb.' *Majallat al-Sharīʿa wa-al-Dirāsāt al-Islāmiyya* 11.

al-ʿAwaḍī, ʿAbd al-Raḥmān ʿAbd Allāh, and Aḥmad Rajāʾī al-Jindī, eds. 1983. *al-Islām wa-al-mushkilāt al-ṭibbiyya al-muʿāṣira: Awwalan, al-injāb fī ḍawʾ al-Islām: Thabt kāmil li-aʿmāl Nadwat al-Injāb fī Ḍawʾ al-Islām al-munʿaqida bi-tārīkh 11 Shaʿbān 1403 H, al-muwāfiq 24 Māyū 1983 M.* Kuwait: al-Munaẓẓama al-Islāmiyya li-al-ʿUlūm al-Ṭibbiyya.

———. 2000. *Ruʾya Islāmiyya li-baʿḍ al-mushkilāt al-ṭibbiyya al-muʿāṣira: Thabt kāmil li-aʿmāl nadwat: al-Wirātha wa-al-handasa al-wirāthiyya wa-al-jīnūm al-basharī wa-al-ʿilāj al-jīnī - ruʾya Islāmiyya al-munʿaqida fī al-Kuwayt fī al-fatra min 23-25 Jumādá al-ākhira 1419 H. - al-muwāfiq 13-15 Uktūbar 1998 M. 2 vols.* Kuwait: al-Munaẓẓama al-Islāmiyya li-al-ʿUlūm al-Ṭibbiyya.

———. 2002. *Ruʾya Islāmiyya li-baʿḍ al-mushkilāt al-ṭibbiyya al-muʿāṣira: Thabt kāmil li-aʿmāl nadwat: al-ʿUlūm fī al-Islām fī al-fatra min 28 Shawwāl - 1 Dhū al-Qaʿda 1421 H. - al-muwāfiq 23-25 Yanāyir 2001 M.* Kuwait: al-Munaẓẓama al-Islāmiyya li-al-ʿUlūm al-Ṭibbiyya.

———. 2005. *al-Mīthāq al-Islāmī al-ʿālamī lil-akhlāqiyyāt al-ṭibbīya wa-al-ṣiḥḥīya fī al-fatra min 29 Shawwāl - 2 Dhū al-Qaʿda 1425 H. al-muwāfiq 11-14 Dīsambir 2004 M.: al-Qāhira.* Kuwait: al-Munaẓẓama al-Islāmiyya li-al-ʿUlūm al-Ṭibbiyya.

al-Bārr, Muḥammad ʿAlī. 1984. *Khalq al-insān bayna al-ṭibb wa-al-Qurʾān.* Jeddah: al-Dār al-Saʿūdiyya.

Bāshā, Aḥmad Fu'ād. 2002. 'Naẓariyyat al-ʿilm al-Islāmiyya: Naḥwa ḥaḍāra Islāmiyya mustaqbaliyya: Asāsuhā al-dīn wa-al-ʿilm.' In *Ruʾya Islāmiyya li-baʿḍ al-mushkilāt al-ṭibbiyya al-muʿāṣira: Thabt kāmil li-aʿmāl nadwat: al-ʿUlūm fī al-Islām fī al-fatra min 28 Shawwāl - 1 Dhū al-Qaʿda 1421 H. - al-muwāfiq 23-25 Yanāyir 2001 M.*, eds. ʿAbd al-Raḥmān ʿAbd Allāh al-ʿAwaḍī and Aḥmad Rajāʾī al-Jindī. Kuwait: al-Munaẓẓama al-Islāmiyya li-al-ʿUlūm al-Ṭibbiyya.

Bernstein, David E., and Jeffrey D. Jackson. 2004. 'The Daubert Trilogy in the States.' *Jurimetrics* 44 (3): 351–366.

Brockopp, Jonathan E. 2003. 'The Good Death in Islamic Theology and Law.' In *Islamic Ethics of Life: Abortion, War, and Euthanasia*, ed. Jonathan E. Brockopp. Columbia, SC: University of South Carolina Press.

al-Būṭī, Muḥammad Saʿīd Ramaḍān. 2002. 'al-ʿUlūm fī al-Islām.' In *Ruʾya Islāmiyya li-baʿḍ al-mushkilāt al-ṭibbiyya al-muʿāṣira: Thabt kāmil li-aʿmāl nadwat: al-ʿUlūm fī al-Islām fī al-fatra min 28 Shawwāl - 1 Dhū al-Qaʿda 1421 H. - al-muwāfiq 23-25 Yanāyir 2001 M.*, eds. ʿAbd al-Raḥmān ʿAbd Allāh al-ʿAwaḍī and Aḥmad Rajāʾī al-Jindī. Kuwait: al-Munaẓẓama al-Islāmiyya li-al-ʿUlūm al-Ṭibbiyya.

Dār al-Iftāʾ al-Miṣriyya. 1434/2013. *Ḍawābiṭ al-ikhtiyār al-fiqhī ʿinda al-nawāzil*. Cairo: Maṭbaʿat Dār al-Kutub wa-al-Wathāʾiq al-Qawmiyya.

Ghaly, Mohammed. 2015. 'Biomedical Scientists as Co-Muftis: Their Contribution to Contemporary Islamic Bioethics.' *Die Welt Des Islams* 55 (3–4): 286–311.

al-Ghazālī. 2010. *Iḥyāʾ ʿulūm al-dīn*, ed. ʿAbd al-Muʿṭī Amīn Qalʿajī. 5 vols. Beirut: Dār Ṣādir.

———. n.d. *al-Mustaṣfā min ʿilm al-uṣūl*. 2 vols. Beirut: Dār al-Fikr.

Ḥatḥūt, Ḥassān. 2002. 'al-Ḥubb al-mafqūd bayna al-ʿilm wa al-dīn.' In *Ruʾya Islāmiyya li-baʿḍ al-mushkilāt al-ṭibbiyya al-muʿāṣira: Thabt kāmil li-aʿmāl nadwat: al-ʿUlūm fī al-Islām fī al-fatra min 28 Shawwāl - 1 Dhū al-Qaʿda 1421 H. - al-muwāfiq 23-25 Yanāyir 2001 M.*, eds. ʿAbd al-Raḥmān ʿAbd Allāh al-ʿAwaḍī and Aḥmad Rajāʾī al-Jindī. Kuwait: al-Munaẓẓama al-Islāmiyya li-al-ʿUlūm al-Ṭibbiyya.

Ibn Bayyah, ʿAbd Allāh. 2007. *Ṣināʿat al-fatwā wa-fiqh al-aqalliyyāt*. Jeddah: Dār al-Minhāj.

Ibn Ḥajar al-ʿAsqalānī. n.d. *Fatḥ al-Bārī bi-Sharḥ Ṣaḥīḥ al-Bukhārī*, eds. ʿAbd al-ʿAzīz ibn ʿAbd Allāh ibn Bāz, ʿAlī ibn ʿAbd al-ʿAzīz al-Shibl, and Muḥammad Fuʾād ʿAbd al-Bāqī. 13 vols. Beirut: Dār al-Maʿrifa.

Ibn Qayyim al-Jawziyya. 2002. *Iʿlām al-muwaqqiʿīn ʿan Rabb al-ʿālamīn*, ed. Abū ʿUbayda Mashhūr Āl Salmān. 7 vols. Riyadh: Dār Ibn al-Jawzī.

Ibrāhīm, Aḥmad. 2003. *Ṭuruq al-ithbāt al-Sharʿiyya*. Cairo: Dār al-Jumhūriyya.

al-Ījī.1997. *Kitāb al-Mawāqif*, ed. ʿAbd al-Raḥmān ʿUmayra. 3 vols. Beirut: Dār al-Jīl.

Inhorn, Marcia C., and Soraya Tremayne, eds. 2012. *Islam and Assisted Reproductive Technologies: Sunni and Shia Perspectives*. New York, NY: Berghahn Books.

Iqbal, Muzaffar. 2007. *Science and Islam*. London: Greenwood Press.

Islamic Medical Association of North America (IMANA) Ethics Committee. 2005. 'Islamic Medical Ethics: The IMANA Perspective.' *JIMA* 37: 33–42. Available at http://jima.imana.org/article/view/5528/37_1-33.

Jackson, Sherman A. 2009. 'Beyond Jihad: The new thought of the Gamāʿa Islāmiyya.' *Journal of Islamic Law and Culture* 11 (1): 52–69.

Jumʿa, ʿAlī. 2006. 'Tajdīd al-fiqh al-Islāmī.' In *Mawsūʿat al-tashrīʿ al-Islāmī*, ed. Maḥmūd Ḥamdī Zaqzūq. Cairo: al-Majlis al-Aʿlā li-al-Shuʾūn al-Islāmiyya.

al-Jurjānī. 2009. *al-Taʿrīfāt*, ed. Muḥammad Bāsil ʿUyūn al-Sūd. Beirut: Dār al-Kutub al-ʿIlmiyya.

al-Khālid, Khālid Ḥusayn. 2009. *al-Ijtihād al-jamāʿī fī al-fiqh al-Islāmī*. Dubai: Markaz Jumʿa al-Mājid li-al-Thaqāfa wa-al-Turāth.

al-Khayyāṭ, Muḥammad Haytham. 2002. 'al-Islām wa-al-ʿIlm.' In *Ruʾya Islāmiyya li-baʿḍ al-mushkilāt al-ṭibbiyya al-muʿāṣira: Thabt kāmil li-aʿmāl nadwat: al-ʿUlūm fī al-Islām fī al-fatra min 28 Shawwāl - 1 Dhū al-Qaʿda 1421 H. - al-muwāfiq 23-25 Yanāyir 2001 M.*, eds. ʿAbd al-Raḥmān ʿAbd Allāh al-ʿAwaḍī and Aḥmad Rajāʾī al-Jindī. Kuwait: al-Munaẓẓama al-Islāmiyya li-al-ʿUlūm al-Ṭibbiyya.

*Majallat al-Majmaʿ al-Fiqhī al-Islāmī* 2002. 13 (15): 478–81.

Mallat, Chibli. 1996. 'Tantawi on Banking Operations in Egypt.' In *Islamic Legal Interpretation: Muftis and Their Fatwas*, eds. Muhammad Khalid Masud, Brinkley Messick, and David S. Powers. Cambridge, MA: Harvard University Press.

Masud, Muhammad Khalid, Brinkley Messick, and David S. Powers. 1996. 'Muftis, Fatwas, and Islamic Legal Interpretation.' In *Islamic Legal Interpretation: Muftis and Their Fatwas*, eds. Muhammad Khalid Masud, Brinkley Messick, and David S. Powers. Cambridge, MA: Harvard University Press.

*al-Mawsūʿa al-fiqhiyya*. 1982-. 45 vols. Kuwait: Wizārat al-Awqāf wa al-Shuʾūn al-Islāmiyya.

Moosa, Ebrahim. 2002. 'Interface of Science and Jurisprudence: Dissonant Gazes at the Body in Modern Muslim Ethics.' In *God, Life, and Cosmos: Christian and Islamic Perspectives*, eds. Ted Peters, Muzaffar Iqbal, and Syed Nomanul Haq. Burlington: Ashgate.

Morgan, Derek, and Mary Ford. 2006. 'In Vitro Fertilization: Regulation.' In *Living with the Genome: Ethical and Social Aspects of Human Genetics*, eds. Angus Clarke and Flo Ticehurst. New York: Palgrave.

Nafi, Basheer M. 2004. '*Fatwā* and War: On the Allegiance of the American Muslim Soldiers in the Aftermath of September 11.' *Islamic Law and Society* 11 (1): 78–116.

Nasr, Seyyed Hussein. 2010. 'Islam and the Problem of Modern Science.' *Islam and Science* 8 (1): 63–74.

al-Nūr, Muḥammad Sulaymān. 2007. 'Muddat al-ḥaml bayna al-fiqh wa-al-ṭibb wa-baʿḍ qawānīn al-aḥwāl al-shakhṣiyya al-muʿāṣira.' *Majallat al-Sharīʿa wa-al-Dirāsāt al-Islāmiyya* 70.

Padela, Aasim I., Hasan Shanawani, and Ahsan Arozullah. 2011. 'Medical Experts and Islamic Scholars Deliberating over Brain Death: Gaps in the Applied Islamic Bioethics Discourse.' *Muslim World* 101 (1): 53–72.

al-Qaraḍāwī, Yūsuf. 2002. 'Mafhūm al-ʿilm wa-takwīn al-ʿaqliyya al-ʿilmiyya fī al-Qurʾān al-Karīm.' In *Ruʾya Islāmiyya li-baʿḍ al-mushkilāt al-ṭibbiyya al-muʿāṣira: Thabt kāmil li-aʿmāl nadwat: al-ʿUlūm fī al-Islām fī al-fatra min 28 Shawwāl - 1 Dhū al-Qaʿda 1421 H. - al-muwāfiq 23-25 Yanāyir 2001 M.*, eds. ʿAbd al-Raḥmān ʿAbd Allāh al-ʿAwaḍī and Aḥmad Rajāʾī al-Jindī. Kuwait: al-Munaẓẓama al-Islāmiyya li-al-ʿUlūm al-Ṭibbiyya.

al-Qārī, ʿAlī. 2001. *Mirqāt al-mafātīḥ Sharḥ Mishkāt al-maṣābīḥ*, ed. Jamāl ʿItānī. 12 vols. Beirut: Dār al-Kutub al-ʿIlmiyya.

Rāghib al-Iṣfahānī. 2010. *al-Mufradāt fī gharīb al-Qurʾān*, ed. Muḥammad Khalil ʿItānī. Beirut: Dār al-Maʿrifa.

al-Sallāmī, Muḥammad al-Mukhtār. 2002. 'Mafhūm al-ʿulūm fī al-Islām.' In *Ruʾya Islāmiyya li-baʿḍ al-mushkilāt al-ṭibbiyya al-muʿāṣira: Thabt kāmil li-aʿmāl nadwat: al-ʿUlūm fī al-Islām fī al-fatra min 28 Shawwāl - 1 Dhū al-Qaʿda 1421 H. - al-muwāfiq 23-25 Yanāyir 2001 M.*, eds. ʿAbd al-Raḥmān ʿAbd Allāh al-ʿAwaḍī and Aḥmad Rajāʾī al-Jindī. Kuwait: al-Munaẓẓama al-Islāmiyya li-al-ʿUlūm al-Ṭibbiyya.

Shabana, Ayman. 2013. 'Negation of Paternity in Islamic Law between *Liʿān* and DNA Fingerprinting.' *Islamic Law and Society* 20 (3): 157–201.

———. 2014. 'Islamic Law of Paternity between Classical Legal Texts and Modern Contexts: From Physiognomy to DNA Analysis.' *Journal of Islamic Studies* 25 (1): 1–32.

———. 2015. 'Foundations of the Consensus against Surrogacy Arrangements in Islamic Law.' *Islamic Law and Society* 22 (1–2): 82–113.

———. 2019. 'Transformation of the Concept of the Family in the Wake of Genomic Sequencing: An Islamic Perspective.' In *Islamic Ethics and the Genome Question*, ed. Mohammed Ghaly. Leiden: Brill.

Shaham, Ron. 2010. *The Expert Witness in Islamic Courts: Medicine and Crafts in the Service of Law*. Chicago, IL: University of Chicago Press.

al-Shakʿa, Muṣṭafā. 2002. 'Makānat al-ʿulūm wa-al-ʿulamāʾ fī al-Islām.' In *Ruʾya Islāmiyya li-baʿḍ al-mushkilāt al-ṭibbiyya al-muʿāṣira: Thabt kāmil li-aʿmāl nadwat: al-ʿUlūm fī al-Islām fī al-fatra min 28 Shawwāl - 1 Dhū al-Qaʿda 1421 H. - al-muwāfiq 23-25 Yanāyir 2001 M.*, eds. ʿAbd al-Raḥmān ʿAbd Allāh al-ʿAwaḍī and Aḥmad Rajāʾī al-Jindī. Kuwait: al-Munaẓẓama al-Islāmiyya li-al-ʿUlūm al-Ṭibbiyya.

Shanyūr, ʿAbd al-Nāṣir Muḥammad. 2005. *al-Ithbāt bi-al-khibra bayna al-qaḍāʾ al-Islāmī wa-al-qānūn al-dawlī wa-taṭbīqātuhā al-muʿāṣira: Dirāsa muqārana*. Amman: Dār al-Nafāʾis.

Sharp, Lesley A. 2013. *The Transplant Imaginary: Mechanical Hearts, Animal Parts, and Moral Thinking in Highly Experimental Science*. Berkley: University of California Press.

al-Shāṭibī. 2003. *al-Muwāfaqāt fī uṣūl al-sharīʿa*, ed. ʿAbd Allāh Darrāz. 4 vols. Cairo: al-Maktaba al-Tawfīqiyya.

al-Shuwayrakh, Saʿd ibn ʿAbd al-ʿAzīz ibn ʿAbd Allāh. 2007. *Aḥkām al-handasa al-wirāthiyya*. Riyadh: Dār Kunūz Ishbīliyā.

Skovgaard-Petersen, Jakob. 2004. 'A Typology of State Muftis.' In *Islamic Law and the Challenge of Modernity*, eds. Yvonne Yazbeck Haddad and Barbara Freyer Stowasser. Walnut Creek, CA: Alta Mira Press.

———. 1997. *Defining Islam for the Egyptian State: Muftis and Fatwas of the Dār al-Iftā.* Leiden: Brill.

Stearns, Justin. 2011. 'The Legal Status of Science in the Muslim World in the Early Modern Period: An Initial Consideration of *Fatwās* from Three Maghribī Sources.' In *The Islamic Scholarly Tradition, Studies in History, Law, and Thought in Honor of Professor Michael Allan Cook*, eds. Asad Q. Ahmed, Behnam Sadeghi, and Michael Bonner. Leiden: Brill.

al-Tamīmī, ʿAbd al-Jalīl. 2002. 'Dawr al-ʿulamāʾ wa-al-bāḥithīn al-ʿArab fī al-taʾthīr al-maʿrifī al-mustaqbalī li-al-ummah al-ʿArabiyya.' In *Ruʾya Islāmiyya li-baʿḍ al-mushkilāt al-ṭibbiyya al-muʿāṣira: Thabt kāmil li-aʿmāl nadwat: al-ʿUlūm fī al-Islām fī al-fatra min 28 Shawwāl - 1 Dhū al-Qaʿda 1421 H. - al-muwāfiq 23-25 Yanāyir 2001 M.*, eds. ʿAbd al-Raḥmān ʿAbd Allāh al-ʿAwaḍī and Aḥmad Rajāʾī al-Jindī. Kuwait: al-Munaẓẓama al-Islāmiyya li-al-ʿUlūm al-Ṭibbiyya.

al-Taskhīrī, Muḥammad ʿAlī. 2002. 'Mafhūm al-ʿilm min minẓār al-Islām.' In *Ruʾya Islāmiyya li-baʿḍ al-mushkilāt al-ṭibbiyya al-muʿāṣira: Thabt kāmil li-aʿmāl nadwat: al-ʿUlūm fī al-Islām fī al-fatra min 28 Shawwāl - 1 Dhū al-Qaʿda 1421 H. - al-muwāfiq 23-25 Yanāyir 2001 M.*, eds. ʿAbd al-Raḥmān ʿAbd Allāh al-ʿAwaḍī and Aḥmad Rajāʾī al-Jindī. Kuwait: al-Munaẓẓama al-Islāmiyya li-al-ʿUlūm al-Ṭibbiyya.

Wāṣil, Naṣr Farīd. 2002a. 'Makānat al-ʿilm wa-al-ʿulamāʾ fī al-Islām.' In *Ruʾya Islāmiyya li-baʿḍ al-mushkilāt al-ṭibbiyya al-muʿāṣira: Thabt kāmil li-aʿmāl nadwat: al-ʿUlūm fī al-Islām fī al-fatra min 28 Shawwāl - 1 Dhū al-Qaʿda 1421 H. - al-muwāfiq 23-25 Yanāyir 2001 M.*, eds. ʿAbd al-Raḥmān ʿAbd Allāh al-ʿAwaḍī and Aḥmad Rajāʾī al-Jindī. Kuwait: al-Munaẓẓama al-Islāmiyya li-al-ʿUlūm al-Ṭibbiyya.

———. 2002b. *Naẓariyyat al-daʿwa wa-al-ithbāt fī al-fiqh al-Islāmī.* Cairo: Dār al-Shurūq.

Weber, Max. 2009. 'Science as a Vocation.' In *From Max Weber: Essays in Sociology*, eds. Hans Heinrich Gerth and C. Wright Mills. New York, NY: Routledge.

Zaman, Muhammad Qasim. 2001. *The Ulama in Contemporary Islam: Custodian of Change.* Princeton, NJ: Princeton University Press.

al-Zarkashī. 2010. *al-Baḥr al-muḥīṭ fī uṣūl al-fiqh*, eds. ʿAbd al-Qādir ʿAbd Allāh al-ʿĀnī and ʿUmar Sulaymān al-Ashqar. 6 vols. Kuwait: Wizārat al-Awqāf wa-al-Shuʾūn al-Islāmiyya.

**Dr Ayman Shabana** is Associate Research Professor and Director of the Islamic Bioethics Project at Georgetown University in Qatar. His teaching and research interests include Islamic legal history, Islamic law and ethics, human rights, and bioethics. He is the author of *Custom in Islamic Law and Legal Theory*, in addition to several book chapters and academic journal articles, which appeared in *Islamic Law and Society*, *Journal of Islamic Studies*, *Journal of Qur'anic Studies*, *Zygon*, *Hawwa*, *Journal of Islamic Ethics*, *Religion Compass*, *Sociology of Islam*, and *Medicine Health Care and Philosophy*. He has also contributed to several reference works such as *Encyclopedia of Islam III*, *Encyclopedia of Islam and the Muslim World*, *Oxford Encyclopedia of Islam and Law*, *Oxford Handbook of Islamic Law*, *Routledge Handbook of Islamic Law*, *Oxford Handbook of Religious Perspectives on Reproductive Ethics*. He is also Chief Editor of the upcoming *Oxford Encyclopedia of Islamic Bioethics*.

# Chapter 13
# Integrating Science and Scripture to Produce Moral Knowledge: Assessing *Maṣlaḥa* and *Ḍarūra* in Islamic Bioethics and the Case of Organ Donation

**Aasim I. Padela**

## 13.1 Introduction

Every day appears to bring forth new discoveries about ourselves and the world around us. From gravitational waves to mitochondrial DNA, each discovery not only provides humankind greater knowledge about how things work but also, importantly, sets the stage for being able to manipulate the world and fashion a desired future. Arguably, mobilization of this knowledge is most rapid, and most significant, in the field of biomedicine. Only decades after uncovering mitochondrial DNA, for example, we not only know which diseases arise from specific DNA malfunctions,[1] we also have developed technologies to eradicate such diseases.[2] Since new data must be understood within its proper context, and newfound powers must be wielded ethically and responsibly, religious traditions are often called upon to address the nature and application of biomedical science.

Indeed, in Sunday school classrooms and mosque seminars congregants ask religious leaders to align scriptural teachings with biomedical knowledge, and in court houses and political forums religious authorities are asked to weigh in on the ethical implications of bio-law and healthcare policy. These tasks are not easy as they require religious scholars not only to be well-versed in theology and doctrine, but also to be scientifically literate and politically-savvy. In other words, in order to generate a religious perspective on biomedicine, religious experts must understand not only what the science communicates, but also how that squares with religious

[1] Zeviani and Di Donato (2004): 2153–72.

[2] Pfeffer et al. (2012): 2–40; and Fogleman et al. (2016): 39–52.

A. I. Padela (✉)
Department of Emergency Medicine & Institute for Health and Equity, Medical College of Wisconsin, Milwaukee, WI, USA
e-mail: apadela@mcw.edu



A. al-Akiti, A. I. Padela (eds.), *Islam and Biomedicine*, Philosophy and Medicine 137, https://doi.org/10.1007/978-3-030-53801-9_13

beliefs. And in order to speak on the 'rightness' of healthcare laws and policies, religious experts need to understand both the policy and legal question at hand as well as the socio-political context that circumscribes their role at the proverbial table. Consequently, religious authorities need to become multidisciplinary so that they can address the pressing questions arising from biomedicine; they either need to acquire expertise in the relevant fields of religion and science themselves, or to bring experts from the relevant disciplines together so as to avail themselves of their insights.[3]

This chapter seeks to further such multidisciplinary engagement at the intersection of religion and biomedicine. Religious experts need conceptual frameworks and process models to help them structure natural and social scientific data, and also to evaluate and integrate this information with scriptural knowledge so as to produce moral guidance. The chapter seeks to deliver such a framework and model by drawing upon the ideas of Thomas F. Torrance (d. 2009) about the relational nature and social coefficient of knowledge as well as the schema devised by al-Ghazālī (d. 505/1111) for *ḥuḍūrī* (presential) and *ḥuṣūlī* (attained) knowledge. I contend that scientific knowledge must be integrated with scriptural insights in order to meet the ultimate end-goal of Islamic morality – 'forestalling harms and procuring benefits' (*darʾ al-mafāsid wa-jalb al-maṣāliḥ*). Accordingly, I will demonstrate how the ethico-legal constructs of *maṣlaḥa* (human interest/public good) and *ḍarūra* (dire necessity) must bridge scriptural values with social reality. In closing I will illustrate the model's utility by turning to the 'Islamic bioethics' of organ donation. I will delineate specific questions that must be addressed on the basis of biomedical and social scientific data in order to proffer Islamic ethical perspectives on the act of donation and related policy questions.

## 13.2 Knowledge: Epistemic Concepts and Relational Schematics

Before building up a framework and model for acquiring and producing knowledge, be it scientific, moral, or some other category, we must define what we mean by knowledge. Herein knowledge (*al-ʿilm*) is defined according to how it is referred to within the Islamic moral sciences, as 'the perception of a thing or concept that is in correspondence to the thing itself.'[4] Important here is that knowledge resides in the subject, the one who wants to know, and that it stands at a distance from the object of that knowing. Although the knower desires information about the object of knowing that fully corresponds to the reality of that object, such information varies in its

[3] For a discussion on the role of technical experts and their changing relationship with Muslim religious authorities, see Chap. 12, 'Interface Between Islamic Law and Science: Ethico-Legal Construction of Science in Light of Islamic Bioethical Discourses on Genetic and Reproductive Technologies,' by Ayman Shabana in this book. Other works discussing the challenges and promise of such interaction include Ghaly (2015) and Padela, Shanawani, and Arozullah (2011).

[4] Al-Maydānī (1998).

accuracy and consequently so does the knower's conviction in it. So, for example, one can be fully certain that the sky is blue, believe that it is more likely or more doubtful that the sky is blue, or be certain that the sky is not blue. One's degree of conviction about their knowledge of the sky being blue can vary based on the evidence one has about the proposition, and, critically, this perception and accompanying conviction stands apart from the Ultimate Reality of the colour of the sky.

## 13.3 Thomas F. Torrance's Framework

With this foundational definition in hand, several aspects of Thomas F. Torrance's theological and epistemic frameworks are particularly useful for engaging the multidisciplinarity inherent to moral knowledge. Torrance was a Scottish Protestant theologian of the twentieth century who carried on the task of developing Reformed theology in the lineage of scholars such as John Calvin (d. 1564), Robert Bruce (d. 1631), and Karl Barth (d. 1968). Torrance held the post of Professor of Christian Dogmatics at the University of Edinburgh for nearly three decades and during that time made wide-ranging contributions to systematic theology, as well as methodologies for studying the intersection of science and theology.[5] While Torrance's principal interests were in advancing Christian thinking about the world, his work is relevant to non-Christian and non-theologian audiences as well. Indeed, his thoughts on the subjective and objective poles of knowledge, the relationship between these two, and about the social coefficient of knowledge are portable across traditions and disciplines. To be sure, the belief in a triune God, and as part of that the incarnate yet contingent nature of Christ, was incredibly important to Torrance's theological activities and such notions would be ardently contested in Muslim circles. However, the basic structure of his theory of relational knowledge does not depend on these beliefs and is useful for our discussion of moral knowledge.

To begin with he holds God to be the supreme Truth, ontologically beyond the grasp of human knowledge,[5] yet made somewhat discernible by His unveiling Himself in scripture and through His acts. Moving from God to the creation, he adopts a critical realist outlook in holding the external world to have a reality independent of human perceptions (i.e., knowledge) of that reality.[6] For him it is critical that there is a space between human knowledge and reality, or, said another way, between the truth of a statement about an object and the truth of that object's being. Such realist positions seek to strike a middle position where knowledge about an object is neither purely representational of the true nature of the object, nor is it purely constructionist and wholly decoupled from this nature. Further in his schema, the human being and the world around her reside in the same plane of existence, equidistant from, and in relationship with, the Creator. Since the subjective pole of

---

[5] Palma (1984): 2–46. See also, McGrath (1999).

[6] Miller (2013), esp. chap. 2.

knowledge (the human seeking information) and the objective pole (the thing that knowledge is sought about) are on the same ontological plane, they are both rightly-ordered when the reference point beyond them (the Creator) is properly acknowledged as the originator and the ultimate source of knowledge.

In the words of Kris A. Miller, Torrance's theological framework is unique in that it maintains a distinction between human knowledge and reality while at the same time emphasizing the ontological connection between the knower and the known.[7] It thus moves beyond ontological reductionism where 'reality is reduced to human thought, speech, experience and interpretation as if it can be explained solely in terms of subjective dimensions,' and epistemological reductionism where knowledge is 'reduced to an objective mirror of the mind-independent (or language-independent) reality.'[8] Knowledge instead emerges in the context of a relationship between the subject and the object, where the subject uses the full range of his capacities of discernment including the cognitive, affective, practical, ethical and spiritual to probe the object, and the object undergoes corresponding unveilings of its reality. This 'whole person' view of knowing is a key aspect of Torrance's schema because he views human knowing to be an emergent capacity that cannot be cut off, or function separately, from other aspects of our being. Rather the knowing being is the whole person, and knowledge involves all of the ontological dimensions/capacities of the human being. When we consider once again the connection between knowledge and reality, we need to remember first of all that reality and human knowledge neither correspond fully to each other nor are reducible to one another. Since human knowledge and the reality we are able to grasp are both at some distance from God, who is ultimate truth and reality, our knowledge about any matter can never be fully complete or fully certain. Epistemic humility is therefore required in all knowledge-seeking activities.

Another valuable concept Torrance develops is the 'social coefficient' of knowledge. For Torrance, human knowledge is generated through communities. Reflecting initially on knowledge about God he states that 'we are unable to know God in any onto-relationship way without knowing him in the togetherness of our personal relations with one another.'[9] Although knowing God is a personal (a whole-person) experience as God reveals himself to individuals, individuals can share their experiences and knowledge within a community, and in the Christian view the Holy Spirit continues God's self-revelation through the church community. As such the Church provides the social coefficient for knowledge of God. The idea of their being communities is integral to the process of knowing, that there is a social component to knowledge, is not unique to Torrance. Alasdair MacIntyre holds a similar view arguing that nothing is learned or known without the medium of a knowing community (or tradition),[10] and Eric G. Flett builds upon Torrance's ideas to note that knowl-

[7] Ibid., 102, 146 and Conclusion.

[8] Ibid., 176 and 167.

[9] Torrance (2003), 46.

[10] Lutz (2021).

edge is embodied in communities where community rituals, practices, and actions represent the practical aspect of theoretical knowledge.[11] For our purposes the idea that understanding a certain piece of knowledge about an object – or if the correspondence between reality and knowledge is high, a certain aspect of the object's true nature – requires the medium of community is key because it introduces space for distinct disciplinary experts. While one's knowledge of God might be better understood through the knowing community of theologians, one's knowledge about cars might be made more accurate and better understood through the mediation of the community of mechanics.

Save for notions about the Holy Spirit and Christ, the parts of Torrance's framework I have laid out above would resonate with Islamic teachings. Indeed, in the Muslim tradition one of God's names is *al-Ḥaqq* (the Truth) and revelation represents the primary, and most certain, means of knowledge about Him. All of our reality is but a shadow of God's Ultimate Reality, and our knowledge is but perception and limited in scope and accuracy. Rather than laying out a lot of schemata, it suffices to say that critical realist theories also abound within the Islamic intellectual tradition, and the ontological and epistemic division between creation and the Creator is doctrinal.

## 13.4 Al-Ghazālī's Division of Knowledge into *Ḥuḍūrī* (Presential) and *Ḥuṣūlī* (Attained)

Adding in a Ghazālian classification rubric for knowledge, and orienting the framework towards 'Islamic' moral ends will help to furnish a more complete multidisciplinary Islamic model for moral knowledge acquisition and production. Among the various divisions for the intellectual sciences and knowledge al-Ghazālī sets up, the division of knowledge into *ḥuḍūrī* (presential) and *ḥuṣūlī* (attained) is most fundamental.[12] These two categories are distinguished by their content and the means of acquisition. Presential knowledge covers primarily religious knowledge, knowledge that is oriented towards God and the afterlife, though its content may relate to the worldly or spiritual realm. This type of knowledge is knowledge from on high (*ʿilm ladunī*) and thus it is supra-rational or intuitive and is acquired immediately via a grant from God or through focused contemplation and spiritual reflection. It includes the knowledge the Prophets receive via revelation from God (*waḥy*), and knowledge saints and pious individuals gain from inspiration (*ilhām*) or similar spiritual modes (*inkishāf*).[13]

Attained knowledge, on the other hand, primarily concerns affairs of this world though such knowledge can also be instrumental for the hereafter, and is

[11] Flett (2012).

[12] Bakar (1998), 204.

[13] Ibid., 204 and 218–22.

rationally-derived or discursively-gained. It is important to note that the categories of *ḥuḍūrī* (presential) and *ḥuṣūlī* (attained) are porous in so far as they concern moral knowledge. This is so because al-Ghazālī sought to counter narratives of a dichotomy between faith and reason, as well as between religious disciplines and worldly ones. Rather he aimed to build bridges across these divides in the formation of moral knowledge, while simultaneously proclaiming a hierarchy of certitude where revelation and spiritual modes of knowing were at the top. This division of knowledge and modes of knowing lays the foundation for a division of labour among scholars as well. Scholars of religion who study revelation (*waḥy*), the Prophetic tradition (Sunna), and undertake spiritual exercises can glean moral insights about an object or into a certain matter and thereby contribute to moral knowledge. At the same time, scholars of the *ḥuṣūlī* ilk apply rational tools, and use empirical, social scientific, and other research methods to disclose morally-relevant information about the object of study.

## 13.5 *Maṣāliḥ* (Human Interests), *Mafāsid* (Harms) and the *Maqāṣid al-Sharīʿa* (Higher Objectives of Islamic Law)

The final pieces to consider in building up a conceptual framework and process model for moral assessment and knowledge production are end-goals. The types of knowledge to be acquired by the subject and the corresponding information that needs to be gleaned about the object (or issue) depend on the aims of the enterprise. At the level of theology, the ultimate aim of the Islamic message is humankind's salvation, and accordingly all human actions should strive for Divine pleasure. This theological objective implicates legal theory as scripture and Prophetic statements come to be the primary sources for gleaning which actions and corresponding societal conditions align with Divine approval or disapproval. While it is beyond the scope of this chapter to show how theology informs legal theory and to describe the sources and methods of Islamic law, it is necessary for the reader to realize that the principal aim of Islamic ethics and law is 'to forestall harm and procure benefits' (*darʾ al-mafāsid wa-jalb al-maṣāliḥ*), whereas 'forestalling harms takes precedence over procuring benefits' (*darʾ al-mafāsid muqaddam ʿalā jalb al-maṣāliḥ*). The ultimate harm is represented by Divine punishment meted out in hell as the execution of His justice, and the highest of benefits is seeing God in paradise through His grace. Human actions are assessed using the tools and devices of Islamic law with respect to whether they produce Divine pleasure and thus benefits in the afterlife or Divine disapproval and thus punishment.[14] However, the notions of benefit and harm in Islamic law relate to the life of this world as well. These ideas are most

[14] Jackson (2009), 99–125; Reinhart (1983): 195; and Reinhart (1995), 161–74.

closely tied together in the framework of the higher objectives of Islamic law (*maqāṣid al-sharīʿa*).

The *maqāṣid* (sing. *maqṣid*) refer to the overarching purposes/goals of Islamic law and 'the underlying reasons which the Lawgiver has placed within each of its rulings.'[15] After inductively surveying all of the ordinances of the Sharīʿa, pre-eminent Islamic ethico-legal theorists identified five goods that the Sharīʿa aims to protect and preserve: religion (*dīn*), life (*nafs*), intellect (*ʿaql*), progeny (*nasab*) or lineage (*nasal*), and wealth (*māl*).[16] These five goods together constitute complete human welfare and reflect human beneficial interests (*maṣāliḥ al-ʿibād*). According to al-Shāṭibī (d. 790/1388), a famous legal theorist and Malikī jurist who is arguably the 'father' of the *maqāṣid* frameworks, these five goods are the necessary (*ḍarūrī*) *maqāṣid* which 'establish interests of the *dīn* [literally 'religion' but connotes the hereafter in this usage], and the *dunyā* [this world] … their absence leads to corruption and trials as well as loss of life,' and consequently leads to 'loss of success and blessings' in the hereafter.[17] On top of these most fundamental *maqāṣid* is the category of the needful (*ḥājī*) *maqāṣid* which are required to attain facility and remove obstacles such that without them humans face difficulty and hardship prevails; while the enhancing (*taḥsīnī*) *maqāṣid* represent acquiring the 'good things' and avoiding the 'deceptive' things, such that the actions and practices are ornamented and perfected, and are thus optional.[18] The relationship between the three categories is that the *ḥājī* supplement the *ḍarūrī*, while the *taḥsīnī* complement the *ḥājī*. Although the necessary (*ḍarūrī*) *maqāṣid* were gleaned from an inductive reading of revelation, al-Shāṭibī states that the needful and enhancing objectives of Islamic law can be founded upon rational deliberation about actions and means that support and complement the necessary objectives. To put it another way, scientific data can help identify how best to service the goals of the necessary *maqāṣid*.[19]

Harkening back to the idea that Islamic ethics and law seeks 'to forestall harms and procure benefits' (*darʾ al-mafāsid wa-jalb al-maṣāliḥ*), a good or benefit (*maṣlaḥa*) is anything that promotes the obtainment of these five higher goods; whereas a harm (*mafsada*) is that which harms these goods or promotes what is contrary to the five higher goods. As the prominent Shāfiʿī legal theorist ʿIzz al-Dīn Ibn ʿAbd al-Salām (d. 660/1262) summarizes: 'The Sharīʿa in its entirety is comprised of securing all types of goods (*maṣāliḥ*) … and warding off all types of detriments (*mafāsid*).'[20] Similarly, al-Ghazālī offers 'what we mean by interests (*maṣāliḥ*) are those interests that conform specifically to the objectives of Islamic law (*maqāṣid*),' and harms are likewise detriments to these interests.[21] Additionally

[15] Al-Raysūnī (2005), xxiii.

[16] Al-Shāṭibī (2011), 2:10; Auda (2008), 3. al-Raysūnī (2005), 136–144; Nyazee (2005), 243

[17] Al-Shāṭibī (2011), 2:9. al-Raysūnī (2005), xxiii

[18] Al-Shāṭibī, 2:10.

[19] Al-Raysūnī (2005), 270–285.

[20] Ibn ʿAbd al-Salām (2000), 1:39.

[21] Abdur-Rashid, Furber, and Abdul-Basser (2013): 89.

when the necessary (*ḍarūrī*) *maqāṣid* are at risk at the collective or the individual level, e.g., when humankind may cease to exist or an individual's life is threatened, the state of affairs becomes a dire necessity or *ḍarūra.* Removing this state of affairs becomes a priority and the high level of probable harm may grant exemptions from normative prohibitions as long as the condition endures, and no alternative recourse is available. The paradigmatic example for this idea is found in the Qur'an which allows for a person dying of thirst to partake of wine, for instance, when no other nourishment is available, only in enough quantity to forestall death.[22] In this scenario the probability of death represents the dire condition where it becomes necessary to drink wine, which is normally prohibited. Certifying when a dire necessity, traditionally considered to be reflected in a credible life-threatening situation or a similarly extreme difficulty, exists requires detailed contextual knowledge. In summary, advancing human interests represented by the higher objectives of Islamic law, as well as removing threats to these, is our purpose in seeking knowledge about an object and thereby offering moral guidance.

Notably, the schema of *maṣāliḥ* and *mafāsid* is further classified into those *maṣāliḥ* and *mafāsid* that relate to human existence in this world as well as the hereafter (*al-ākhira*), i.e., life after death. As the renowned ethico-legal theorist of the modern era Muḥammad Saʿīd Ramaḍān al-Būṭī (d. 1434/2013) states, Islamic law 'actualize(s) both categories of human goods: those that relate to this world and the hereafter.'[23] Since Sharīʿa ordinances relate to the worldly and the hereafter dimensions of human existence, the question of whether the *maṣāliḥ* and *mafāsid* can be accurately known arises. Ibn ʿAbd al-Salām contends that 'the majority of the goods of this world and its detriments are discernible by the intellect as are the goods and detriments of the Sharīʿa.'[24] An example, provided by Ibn ʿAbd al-Salām, of a good and of a detriment that relates to the worldly existence of human beings is health and sickness because these states occur in a person's life in this world. Relatedly, the science of medicine, which aims to preserve health and remove the harm of sickness, is a worldly good that is primarily discerned by the intellect. However, goods that relate to human existence in the hereafter cannot be rationally-derived. He states, 'the goods of the hereafter and its harms are only known by virtue of transmitted knowledge [from Prophets].'[25] These ideas align with al-Ghazālī's category of *ḥuḍūrī* (presential) knowledge as information about the hereafter and religious ends is gained from revelation, and is inspired. At the same time, *ḥuṣūlī* knowledge is rationally-derived and principally concerns matters of this world and includes harms and benefits to human interests in this life. In these respects, these epistemic categories align with Torrance's framework for knowledge.

[22] Qur'an 5:3 (al-Māʾida).

[23] Al-Būṭī (2000), 79.

[24] Ibn ʿAbd al-Salām (2000), 1:39.

[25] Ibid., 1:11.

## 13.6 The Conceptual Framework and Process Model Synthesized

Bringing together the aforementioned concepts and schema furnishes a conceptual framework and process model that is multidisciplinary, incorporates schema for knowledge and ways of knowing from within the Islamic tradition, and serves the moral purposes of Islamic ethics and law. (See Fig. 13.1 below).

On one end we have a person (or a group of individuals) who seeks information to evaluate the moral status of an object or a state of affairs. In order to make a moral assessment the information seeker (the subjective pole of knowledge) needs to do two things. First, she requires information about the object/issue as it is in present reality. If the objective pole of knowledge is a piece of technology, then the subject needs information about its nature, its purposes, its social implications, its limits, and the like. On the other hand, if the objective pole is a state of affairs, then the knower needs information about why the affairs are as they are, the ethical concerns that are driving the present conditions, what the cultural, legal, and social dimensions the issue at hand are, and similar data. This first aspect of knowing wholly relates to matters of this life: information about the present reality and the world. Secondly, she needs to evaluate whether present conditions or a future proposed

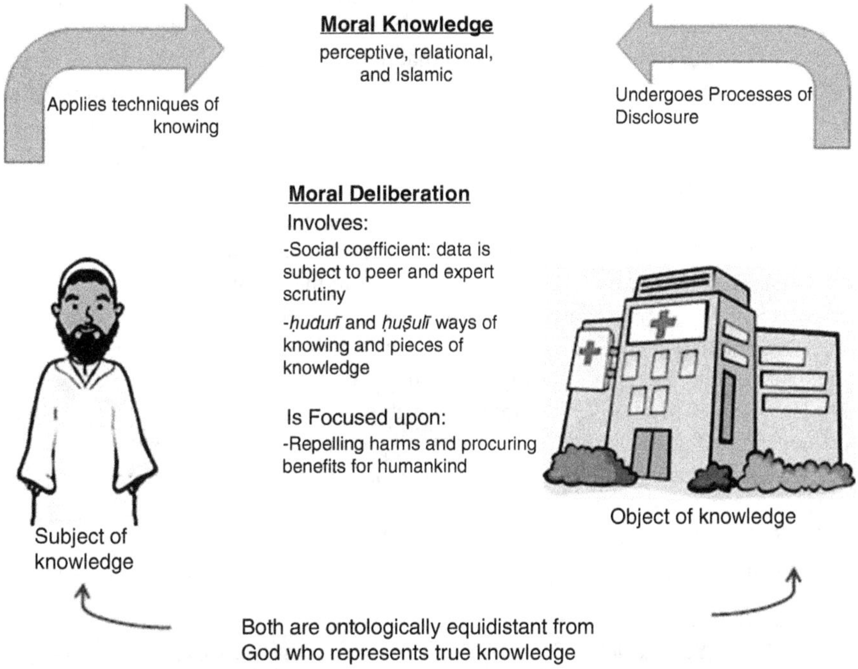


**Fig. 13.1** A schema of ways of knowing for the production of moral knowledge in the Islamic tradition

state, based on the data gleaned about the object/issue, furthers the end-goals of Islam. In other words, this second aspect of moral evaluation focuses upon the forestalling of harms from, and procuring of benefits for, humankind in this life and the next. In this way the moral evaluation can be said to be 'Islamic,' and the information being sought – perceptive moral knowledge. Since the benefits and harms are related to both this world and the next, this second aspect of knowing incorporates data about this world, yet it also requires obtaining knowledge about the world to come. Having gleaned these items of knowledge, i.e., the present realities of the object/issue and how it relates to the moral end-goals of Islam, the subject can then issue an edict about the moral status of the object and/or issue[26] and thus produce moral knowledge.

Having identified the end-goals of, and types of information needed for, Islamic moral assessment, the model also specifies how to obtain the requisite knowledge. Both the object and the subject of knowledge are located in the same plane of existence, and the former undergoes processes of disclosure as the latter probes its reality using rational and supra-rational faculties. The ontological connection between the subject and the object produces knowledge that is relational in nature, in so far as it relates to matters on the same plane of existence, i.e., not about God or the afterlife. Thus, when the subject desires to glean the 'this world' reality of the technology or state of affairs, i.e., whether these are harmful or beneficial to humankind from the perspective of this life, she must recognize her own multidimensionality and that of the object of knowledge. She must utilize the full range of her capacities of discernment including the cognitive, affective, practical, ethical and spiritual to probe the object, and account for the fact that the object has social, biological, legal, cultural, historical dimensions and implications. The necessity of a full and holistic knowing about the object/state of affairs' benefits and harms mandates multidisciplinary analysis, as does the requirement that all of the human being's tools of knowing be employed. The subject must either themselves possess the skill-sets needed for such investigation, or draw in the relevant disciplinary experts to provide the requisite information. Accordingly, this world-oriented knowledge is rationally-derived and scientific, and classified as *ḥuṣūlī* (attained). Moreover, each type of knowledge, be it social, scientific, biological or otherwise, must be articulated and verified through a community of scholars learned in that field. This social coefficient provides the locus of meaning to the information and transforms it into actionable knowledge. Much like the probative value of a statement of the Prophet that was never acted upon by the Companions is ambiguous, so is a piece of data that is dismissed by the community of scholars who are expert in that area.

The second part of moral discernment seeks information about the afterlife benefits and harms (God's approval or disapproval) of the deployment of a certain technology or the occurrence of a state of affairs. This knowledge can only be gleaned

---

[26] In this chapter the 'Islamic' moral status of an action refers to its Islamic legal (or ethico-legal) status. In other words, whether the action is evaluated to be obligatory, meritorious, permitted, reprehensible, or forbidden by Islamic law. This judgement of moral status takes into account the benefits procured and harms avoided in both this life and the afterlife.

from revelatory sources, be inspired, or result from spiritual reflection, and as such is *ḥuḍūrī* (presential). Theologians and jurists are most learned in the scriptural texts and ways of deriving moral values from them, versed in these modes of esoteric knowing, and possess the spiritual insights (*baṣīra*), to opine on the correspondence of a said state of affairs with God's approbation and afterlife benefits and harms. At times the afterlife harms and benefits are not linked to harms and benefits of this world. An example of this is the prohibition of wine and gambling where the Qur'an recognizes that there are human benefits in this world to both but that the sin in them, i.e., the afterlife harm, outweighs benefit in this world.[27] However, in many issues the afterlife's harms and benefits coincide with, or are predicted based on, harms and benefits of this world. In these latter cases the theologian-jurist must properly account for the testimony of disciplinary experts as they enumerate the worldly benefits and harms of a technology or state of affairs. This idea is encapsulated by the ethico-legal construct of *maṣlaḥa* which can include rationally-derived human benefits and interests beyond those vocalized by scripture. These *maṣāliḥ* are by themselves, according to certain schools of law and in certain circumstances, sufficient grounds for an Islamic moral judgement.[28]

As applied to Islamic bioethical rulings, this framework and model resists allocating all moral knowledge, and thereby all moral authority, to religious scholars. Rather it demands an interaction between knowledge of the texts and contexts to discern Islamic moral perspectives. While the traditionally-trained religious scholar has greater insight into scriptural values and where Divine pleasure resides, assessing whether present conditions and applications of technology or proposed future ones cohere with those values and Divine sanction requires data from multiple sources. These data then assist with fully mapping out the technology/state of affairs and the human benefits and harms that accompany it. The necessity of there being an active interplay between religious scholars and natural and social scientists in order to generate Islamic ethico-legal rulings is not a novel idea. Indeed, it is captured by the following legal maxim of Islamic law: *al-ḥukm ʿalā shayʾ farʿan taṣawwurihi* (the ethico-legal assessment of a matter comes after its accurate conceptualization). This maxim cautions jurists against haste and misgiven conceptualizations, in other words, giving a wrong diagnosis. Rather, in so far as possible, the subject at hand must be investigated to the fullest extent, the context and ramifications of the matter at hand must be completely understood, and all dimensions of the issue comprehensively probed. Moreover, the idea that religious scholars are primarily responsible for deriving moral values and theory from scripture, and that experts of the field from which the ethical issue arises must certify whether or not scriptural values are furthered or threatened by a present state of affairs, is part and parcel of Islamic jurisprudential theory. Indeed al-Shāṭibī and al-Ghazālī both divide the process of rendering an ethico-legal judgement on a matter not univocally addressed by revelation into three possible moves: *tanqīḥ al-manāṭ*, *takhrīj al-manāṭ*,

[27] Qur'an 2:219 (*al-Baqara*).

[28] Kamali (2005), 235–247; Nyazee (2005), 216–244.

and *taḥqīq al-manāṭ*. *Tanqīḥ al-manāṭ* involves isolating a possible effective cause (moral grounds) for a ruling mentioned in the Qur'an or Sunna when multiple possibilities are indicated by the texts. *Takhrīj* refers to deducing such grounds when they are not mentioned, while *taḥqīq* refers to ascertaining whether the moral grounds delineated by *takhrīj* and *tanqīḥ* are present in the case at hand.[29] While *takhrīj* and *tanqīḥ* are in the purview of religious scholars, *taḥqīq* is best done by those in the field. The model presented herein builds upon these complementary roles by describing how knowledge of moral import should be received, and how moral knowledge should be generated in a holistic and multidisciplinary way.

## 13.7 *Maṣlaḥa*, *Ḍarūra*, and the 'Islamic' Bioethics of Organ Donation

Islamic legists have been deliberating over the moral status of organ donation for decades.[30] As the science and technology of organ transplantation has improved, the once-experimental therapy has become a mainstay for treating certain types of organ failure. Indeed, organ transplantation is the optimal option for heart, lung, liver, and pancreas failure when patient factors allow for it. At the same time, kidney transplantation is the preferred option for treating kidney failure as it portends improved quality, and at times increased duration, of life over dialysis. More recently uterus, face, and limb transplants are being introduced as therapeutic options. The focus on transplantation as therapy is motivated by the fact that the number of individuals suffering from organ failure continues to rise.[31] The global prevalence of diseases such as hypertension and diabetes are increasing, and with it rates of kidney failure.[32] As Muslim countries struggle to provide healthcare to their citizenry and are beset with patients with organ failure, social contexts and healthcare needs have forced Islamic scholars to consider the ethics and legality of organ donation. Indeed health policy makers and transnational healthcare stakeholders routinely convene scientists and jurists in high-profile meetings to mete out Islamic stances on organ donation and transplantation with the hope of informing state polices and laws, as well as garnering public support for these practices.[33]

Although a definitive and durable Islamic verdict on organ donation is unattainable because the matter is not univocally addressed by the Qur'an and Sunna, Islamic ethico-legal perspectives on the matter can be grouped into three broad

---

[29] Al-Ghazālī (1993), 4:98–104.

[30] Al-Bar and Chamsi-Pasha (2015), 209–223; Yacoub (2001), 254–275.

[31] Health Resources and Services Administration (USA): https://optn.transplant.hrsa.gov/data/view-data-reports/national-data/.

[32] World Health Organization (2011).

[33] Rasheed and Padela (2013): 635–54; Ali and Maravia (2020); Al Barwani and Tithecott (2018).

positions.[34] The first view is that organ donation is categorically impermissible. This position is based on the idea that the processes of procuring an organ from a living or deceased donor is a direct threat to the inviolability (*ḥurma*) of the body and also detracts from human sanctity (*karāma*). These violations are particularly unjustified because they do harm to the donor without the prospect of any personal benefit. The second perspective also holds organ donation to be impermissible in principle, but overturns this prohibition and allows for contingent permissibility on the basis of dire necessity (*ḍarūra*). The many lives at-risk due to organ failure and organ donation (and thereby subsequent transplant) being the best (and in some cases only) option for treatment are judged to meet the threshold conditions for invoking the maxim of 'dire necessity rendering the prohibited permissible' (*al-ḍarūra tubīḥu al-maḥẓūrāt*), at an individual and/or societal level. The third position argues that organ donation falls within the domain of permitted actions, and it can gain the status of a merit-gaining act based on the donor's intention. This view is based on the idea that organ donation serves a general human interest, improving health and/or quality and quantity of life, and thus the ethico-legal construct of *maṣlaḥa* serves as its grounding.[35] Each of these moral judgements is nuanced, especially through various conditions that are attached to them. Some scholars draw moral distinctions between living donation and donation after neurological criteria for death are met, some between whether the organ donation is life-saving or life-enhancing, others change their views if there are alternatives to organ transplant, e.g., dialysis, and still others amend their judgement based on whether a Muslim or a non-Muslim is involved.

Despite this diversity, each camp invokes notions of harm and benefit in their rulings. In other words, in order to morally evaluate the practice, Islamic scholars seek to identify the harms and benefits that accompany organ donation, and they seek to determine whether the harms or benefits predominate. To be sure, scriptural evidence and ethico-legal concepts derived from scriptural sources certainly frame juridical decisions, and they inform what sorts of things are to be considered a benefit and a harm. However, because the scriptural sources are not univocal, scholars can draw upon a variety of evidence to buttress their views. For example, the camp that judges organ donation to be prohibited supports their position with a Prophetic *ḥadīth* that declares breaking the bone of a dead body to be akin to breaking the bone of a living person.[36] After learning that organ procurement involves surgical incisions and disruption of the vascular, tissue, and at times skeletal structures of the body, some Islamic jurists marshalled the aforementioned *ḥadīth* as evidence against the practice. Obviously, they had to learn that organ procurement involves such procedures which appear harmful from the vantage-point of this world. The *ḥadīth* allowed them to claim that organ donation is harmful from an

---

[34] Padela and Duivenbode (2018): 1–12;

[35] Moosa (1993): 385–86; and Moosa (1998): 292–317.

[36] Rasheed (2011), 10. Hussaini (2007), 10–15.

afterlife perspective as well because similar activities met with the Prophet's condemnation.[37]

The other two camps use constructs that more heavily privilege the this-world register of harms and benefits. The contingent permissibility camp invokes *ḍarūra,* while the categorical permissibility group cites *maṣlaḥa*. As indicated above, *ḍarūra* refers to a condition of dire necessity where there is a credible threat to the life of an individual and/or when societal conditions are so extreme that humankind is at risk. In this way one of the necessary higher objectives of Islamic law, the preservation of life (*ḥifẓ al-nafs*), is threatened. Determining the likelihood that a patient will die because a specific organ is failing, and assessing whether humankind will perish on account of the lack of organ donation, is beyond the pale of scriptural authorities. Rather, biomedical and societal data are needed in order to establish the threshold conditions to invoke that it is now a dire necessity. Arguably, *ḍarūra* is a 'fuzzy' concept as jurists differ on how credible a life threat needs to be in order for prohibitions to be overturned, and they also disagree over what other types of significant harms, be they societal or individual, can be classified as *ḍarūra.* Nonetheless, conditions in this world must be accounted for when the construct is invoked to ground a moral assessment, and, as such, expertise beyond the juridical is needed.

*Maṣlaḥa* works in a similar way and represents the opposite spectrum of considerations. Saving the life of an individual is an interest/benefit sourced within the Qur'an, yet when the construct of *maṣlaḥa* is used to ground Islamic rulings the convention is that the benefit should be societal (*al-maṣlaḥa al-ʿamma*). This general, societal notion of benefit as the foundation for rulings based on *maṣlaḥa* is easily recognizable in the *maqāṣid al-sharīʿa* which provide additional scaffolding for *maṣlaḥa*-based rulings. Using *maṣlaḥa* as grounds for a ruling therefore requires assessing societal conditions and benefits, and demands that jurists engage with social scientific knowledge and expertise.

The extent to which Islamic jurists incorporate scientific data in making moral pronouncements about biomedicine varies. While many transnational juridical academies incorporate expert testimony from clinicians when deliberating over bioethics, they often do not critically examine the clinical insights these experts offer. Moreover, critical analyses of the ethical deliberations reveal that all sorts of other information are missing. Elsewhere, I have pointed out that social scientific, epidemiologic, and health policy data is not appropriately incorporated into these moral assessment activities.[38] Other scholars decry that some jurists still operate under the premise that the majority of medical practice aims at curing disease, and do not recognize that much of clinical care is devoted to chronic disease management

---

[37] Some may argue that in the case of deceased organ donation, i.e., donation made after the declaration of death by cardiac or neurologic criteria (i.e., 'brain death'), there is no harm to the donor. However, based on many scriptural texts, many Muslim jurists note that the human body is judged to be dignified and inviolable whether or not it contains a soul. Thus the process of procuring organs from a body, irrespective of whether it is considered alive or dead, is still considered a harm.

[38] Padela (2013): 655–70; Padela et al. (2014): 59–66; Padela, Shanawani, and Arozullah (2011): 53–72.

today.[39] With respect to morally evaluating the practice of organ donation, the aforementioned views capture some aspects of social reality and biomedical data, but appear to miss others.

## 13.8 An Enhanced Approach to Judging the Moral Status of Organ Donation from an Islamic Perspective

The general ethico-legal verdicts on organ donation all involve conceptions of worldly conditions. The moral judgements invoke constructs that translate social conditions into the edifice of Islamic law; a certain state of affairs represents dire need, while another general public benefit, and yet another view sees harms to donors outweighing any benefits that may be accrued. This is necessarily so because the jurists are attempting to issue rulings that cohere with the ethos of 'forestalling harms and procuring benefits' (*dar' al-mafāsid wa jalb al-maṣāliḥ*). Consequently, they are charged with identifying and measuring the harms and benefits of organ donation and to see if these harms and benefits align with scriptural analogues of harm and benefit. Although plurality can be accommodated in Islamic law, and different perspectives on the same evidence can be justified, I would suggest that the conceptual framework and process model we have developed would allow for a more complete, and more specific, assessment of the moral status of organ donation.

Recall that knowledge is viewed as perceptive and relational within our model. Knowledge neither fully reflects the reality of the object of knowing, nor is it fully reduced to the perceptions the knower has about the object. Taking this perspective in receiving information about the state of affairs, jurists would have to inquire about the certitude with which experts make claims based on data, and also evaluate how likely it is that the data corresponds with reality. The 'fact' that organ donation is life-saving or that organ failure is a death sentence, for example, needs to be interrogated (Is it for one specific person or for humanity is general? Is there a 30% chance of death or is it 51%?). Clinicians would need to back up such truth claims by vocalizing how sure they are about this 'fact' and by providing the evidentiary basis for the claim. While jurists may not be able to interrogate these data, other scientists may look at the same data and interpret it differently. Hence the data-point and truth claim must be interpreted in light of a community of disciplinary experts (more on this point later). Certainly, the assertion that someone will die based on a single empirical study is different than making such a statement based on hundreds of studies. Similarly, a claim made with 20% conviction in its accuracy is different from one made with 80% conviction. These differences are important to recognize and must be accounted for when making moral claims on the behalf of a tradition.

Other pieces of data would require similar inspection. With respect to organ donation, there are many tools and research data that provide greater detail into its

[39] Ghaly (2015): 286–311.

life-saving and enhancing nature, and similar resources exists to estimate mortality risk. Today, we can estimate, for example, a patient's life-expectancy with kidney failure based on their own physiological profile and historical data. We can also estimate the likelihood a certain organ transplant will not be rejected along with its subsequent contribution to an anticipated increase in quantity as well as quality of life. These research data and prognostic tools have different kinds of limitations, and variable coefficients of error, both of which must be accounted for when making predictions about the case at hand. Nonetheless, such data are morally-relevant as they assist with measuring harms and benefits, and also to the specification of general moral values to concrete cases.[40] As such, a critical realist approach, such as that of Torrance's, opens up the space for bringing in epidemiological data and a community of experts into the fold, and offers much needed nuance to claims about the lives saved or lives lost in the context of organ donation.

At the same time, when rendering their final moral verdict, jurists need to couch their own claims by noting how certain they are that their derived ruling accords with Divine pleasure or displeasure. The conventional way juridical authorities reflect the possibility that their view is incomplete or may be inaccurate is by appending the statement '*wa-Llāhu aʿlam*' (only God knows best!) at the end of their pronouncements. While such a statement communicates epistemic humility and a modicum of uncertainty, it does not provide insight to how 'shaky' the foundations for the moral evaluation are. Islamic law contains schema for grading and prioritizing different types of evidence, and for evaluating the probative value of scriptural and scientific reports.[41] When rending moral opinions about 'new' matters not univocally treated by the Qur'an and Sunna, and especially when diverse views about an issue exist, jurists would be better served by designating the level of certainty they attach to their position based on the quality of the evidence they marshal, and the logic they have utilized.

Accounting for the relational aspect, and social coefficient, of knowledge also affects the reception of expert testimony. Beginning with the latter, as religious scholars sift through the evidence presented by technical experts about the harms related to organ donation, the dire need it represents, and the benefits it procures, they also need to evaluate how a community of experts views such data. Every expert carries their own biases into data interpretation and a communal perspective serves to limit the effect of such biases. For example, if a clinician notes that a certain type of donation carries no risk and provides data to support such a claim, the claim and the evidence must be subject to peer/community scrutiny. Procedurally this means that juridical authorities may need to reach out to professional societies and/or disciplinary experts to certify that the assumption is accurate, or to grade the quality of the evidence presented. This task is made easier, at least with respect to clinical research and epidemiological data, by the fact that grading schema for such

[40] Richardson (1990): 279–310.

[41] On this point, see Chap. 11, 'Science in the Framework of Islamic Legal Epistemology: An Exploratory Essay,' by Kamaluddin Ahmed in this book.

data already exist, and a hierarchy among the various data sources is already well-agreed upon by biomedical scientists.[42] When judging evidence coming from social, scientific, legal, or other domains, a similar assessment must be made. Again, such a process is not novel to Islamic law as it coheres with the practice of certifying the authenticity of Prophetic reports, and to treating a Prophetic statement that is not acted upon by the Companions as lower grade evidence than one that is acted upon. Some legists go so far in privileging the 'community of experts' perspective that they afford greater weight to the practice of the early Muslim community (*ʿamal ahl al-Madīna*) than a statement from the Prophet to its contrary, even if the communal practice is not backed up by scriptural evidence or by another Prophetic report.[43] Accounting for the social coefficient of knowledge in the process of disclosing the reality of the issue at hand requires undertaking peer and/or professional review of the data presented by the disciplinary experts at the table of dialogue. This added scrutiny will help generate a more precise understanding of the context at hand, and thereby inform a more appropriate Islamic moral evaluation.

Moral knowledge is received and produced within a relationship between those who are desiring to know and the issue they wish to understand. Both the subject and the object exist in the same ontological plane, one that is distant from the source and master of all knowledge, God. Just as the critical realist perspective motivates epistemic humility, so too does this relational notion. The knower's probity is limited and cannot compare to God's knowledge about the object's true nature and its moral significance. Accordingly, any moral judgment made by the knower should be accompanied by one or more caveats. At the same time, the relational aspect of knowledge highlights the link between social reality and scriptural values for generating Islamic morality. This idea sets up the ethico-legal constructs of *ḍarūra*, *maṣlaḥa* and the like, as ones that bridge to social reality. These constructs, though sourced in scripture, are not invested with their full moral content until the social realities they refer to are made known.

More to the point, the necessity of taking a multidisciplinary and multidimensional approach to the ethics of organ donation is also tied to the idea of relational knowledge. The knower is a multidimensional being equipped with several different techniques of knowing, and the object/issue similarly has multiple different facets to its nature. Building bridges of knowledge between the knower and the object/issue requires that the knower apply all of the different techniques of knowing in order to disclose all of the relevant aspects of the object/issue at hand. As one tool is applied, one aspect is disclosed, and thus the relationship between the knower and the to-be-known generates knowledge. Making an Islamic moral assessment about organ donation, for instance, necessitates disclosure of the social, clinical, legal, biological, emotional, and other dimensions relating to organ donation. Consequently, in making a moral assessment, juridical authorities need to bring in experts who can present information about these dimensions of the issue, and they need to reflect

[42] Straus et al. (2005).

[43] Dutton (1999), 41–2.

upon using rational, intuitive, spiritual and other modes of knowing intrinsic to our nature as human beings. In this way those seeking moral knowledge incorporate both *ḥuḍūrī* (presential) and *ḥuṣūlī* (attained) knowledge into their decision-making process.

With respect to the extant rulings regarding organ donation, it is clear that certain types of evidence were not discussed and certain types of moral knowing not incorporated into the deliberative process. For example, many juridical academies have not probed the affective dimension of organ donation by seeking out the voices of organ donors, recipients and their families. These experts are important because they provide experiential and emotional insights that are morally-relevant, and the evidence they present requires that the affective facilities of knowing are employed by juridical authorities during the moral deliberation. A similar case could be made for social anthropological expertise which remains largely marginalized in *fiqh* academies.

The end-point of moral deliberation occurs when the juridical authorities come to a conclusion, to a reasonable degree of certainty, about whether the benefits, or the harms, of organ donation are preponderant. Given that the issue is subject to *ijtihād*, i.e., its moral status is not univocally addressed within the Qur'an and Sunna, the benefit/harm calculation focuses on the knowable effects in this life. Only after proceeding down the multidisciplinary path of inquiry we have outlined above, and cogitating over the morality of organ donation using all of the different faculties of moral knowing, can the *maqāṣid al-sharīʿa* frameworks provide a final 'rational' check. Although these frameworks are subject to revision, and can be a source of debate, some scholars find the *maqāṣid* to be a valuable cognitive tool for moral decision-making.[44] In the process of *ijtihād,* the *maqāṣid* can serve as principles, or an axiology, by which the accuracy of a moral assessment can be examined. If a particular judgement contravenes multiple *maqāṣid* considerations, it is by definition threatening human interests, and thus requires revision. The same would be the case when a ruling lowers a *maqāṣid* at the risk of violating a higher-order *maqāṣid.* In this way the *maqāṣid* are not merely principles by which new rulings are generated, but can also serve as safeguards in Islamic moral evaluation. With respect to the moral status of organ donation, the *maqāṣid*, at least as formulated by al-Shāṭibī, do not provide a clear-cut answer. Certainly, the act of donation, in so far as it is life-saving or life-enhancing, promotes the preservation of life. Yet in the context of a deceased's donation, where organs are procured from individuals meeting neurological criteria for death, the 'Dead Donor Rule' is arguably violated. This violation is more serious for jurists who see the 'brain dead' state as a living one.[45] Despite this ambiguity, Islamic ethics and law 'prioritize the repelling of harms over the procuring of benefits' (*darʾ al-mafāsid awlā/muqaddam min jalb al-maṣāliḥ*). Thus, if organ donation threatens any of the *maqāṣid* more clearly than it advances

---

[44] Auda (2008), 22–25; See, for example: Nassery (2018), 75–88; Larsen (2018), 260–274; and Kamali (2012).

[45] Padela and Abdul-Basser (2012): 433–50; Padela, Arozullah and Moosa (2011): 132–139.

them, its permissibility comes into question or becomes bounded by specific contingencies. In any case, considering how organ donation relates to the higher objectives of Islamic law would help juridical authorities in making a more nuanced moral assessment of the issue.

In summary, our conceptual framework and process model allows for a multidisciplinary engagement and delineates the types of expertise and knowledge needed for a holistic Islamic moral evaluation. It emphasizes generating moral knowledge both from scriptural insights as well as scientific facts, yet in a humble way. And it also accounts for the end-goals of Islamic morality, namely, the removal of harms and procuring of benefits for humankind.

In deploying this model to address the moral status of organ donation, some may decry that our discussion generates more questions than it answers. In response, we would note that such critiques are somewhat off-base in that a topic is considered to be in the realm of *ijtihād* precisely because a definitive and singular moral judgement cannot be derived solely on the basis of the scriptural source-texts. If anything, the biomedical case discussed in this chapter suggests that the extant rulings are incomplete as they miss critical perspectives and overlook certain pieces of data. It also suggests that the moral status of organ donation might need to be evaluated on a case-by-case basis. All organs are not equal in the benefits they may procure; all patients are not equally harmed by the failure of different organs; and the legal frameworks, social culture, and medical capabilities of healthcare systems also differ. A universal ruling, in our view, does not properly recognize these different considerations, and undermines the inherent plurality of the Islamic ethico-legal tradition. As such it may be even appropriate for us to say that the moral status of organ donation is something indeterminate in Islam, and that it can become either *ḥarām* (prohibited), *mubāḥ* (permissible), or *mandūb* (meritorious) depending on its context, or on a case by case basis. Regardless, our model provides the foundation for a more informed discourse about the Islamic bioethics of organ donation.

## 13.9 Conclusion

The growing complexity of biomedical science in society can be bewildering to the religiously-minded public as well as to their scholars. Both seek to find their moral compass from their tradition and struggle to see how their scriptural values speak to the issues of the day. This chapter showcased the building of a bridge between 'the religious' and 'the scientific' by describing the ways in which these categories overlap in the production of moral knowledge. By drawing upon ideas and concepts giving weight to social dimensions of knowledge, correspondence theory, and moral ends, it presents us with a conceptual framework and process model for Islamic moral evaluation that incorporates natural, social, and other 'scientific' and worldly data. This framework and model also service the essential goals of Islamic morality by facilitating the identification of harms and benefits associated with the matter at hand. Our reflection closes by illustrating how that model could be used to address the morality of organ donation from an Islamic perspective that can definitely be described as ambivalent.

**Acknowledgements** Part of this research was supported by a grant from the Templeton Religion Trust (Conversations on Islam and the Human Sciences; TRT0214) and the Health Resources and Services Administration (Informing American Muslims about Living Donation; R39OT40203-01-00).

## References

Abdur-Rashid, Khalil, Steven Woodward Furber, and Taha Abdul-Basser. 2013. 'Lifting the Veil: A Typological Survey of the Methodological Features of Islamic Ethical Reasoning on Biomedical Issues.' *Theoretical Medicine and Bioethics* 34 (2): 81–93.

Al Barwani, Ahmed, and Andrea Tithecott. 2018. 'Oman: New Human Organ & Tissue Donation & Transplantation Regulations.' Law Update: Latest Legal News and Developments from the MENA Region 312. Available at https://www.tamimi.com/law-update-articles/oman-new-human-organ-tissue-donation-transplantation-regulations/.

Ali, Mansur, and Usman Maravia. 2020. 'Seven Faces of A Fatwa: Organ Transplantation and Islam.' *Religions* 11 (2): 1–22.

Auda, Jasser. 2008. *Maqasid al-Shariah as Philosophy of Islamic Law: A Systems Approach*. London: International Institute of Islamic Thought.

Bakar, Osaman. 1998. *Classification of Knowledge in Islam: A Study in Islamic Philosophies of Science*. Cambridge: Islamic Texts Society.

al-Bar, Mohammed Ali, and Hassan Chamsi-Pasha. 2015. *Contemporary Bioethics: Islamic Perspective*. New York, NY: Springer.

al-Būṭī, Muḥammad Saʿīd Ramaḍān. 2000. *Ḍawābiṭ al-maṣlaḥa fī al-sharīʿa al-Islāmiyya*. Beirut: Muʾassasat al-Risāla.

Dutton, Yasin. 1999. *The Origins of Islamic Law: The Qur'an, the Muwatta'and Madinan Amal*. Surrey: Curzon.

Flett, Eric G. 2012. *Persons, Powers, and Pluralities: Toward a Trinitarian Theology of Culture*. Cambridge: James Clarke.

Fogleman, Sarah, Casey Santana, Casey Bishop, Alyssa Miller, and David G. Capco. 2016. 'CRISPR/Cas9 and Mitochondrial Gene Replacement Therapy: Promising Techniques and Ethical Considerations.' *American Journal of Stem Cells* 5 (2): 39–52.

Ghaly, Mohammed. 2015. 'Biomedical Scientists as Co-Muftis: Their Contribution to Contemporary Islamic Bioethics.' *Die Welt Des Islams* 55 (3–4): 286–311.

al-Ghazālī. 1993. *al-Mustaṣfá min ʿilm al-uṣūl*, ed. Ḥamzah ibn Zuhayr Ḥāfiẓ. 4 vols. Medina: Dār al-Nashr.

Health Resources and Services Administration (USA). 'Organ Procurement and Transplantation Network: National Data.' Available at https://optn.transplant.hrsa.gov/data/view-data-reports/national-data/.

Hussaini, Mohammad Omar. 2007. 'Organ Transplantation: Classical Hanafite Perspectives.' Working paper, Pureway Non-Profit Organisation, Tampa, Florida. Available at https://pureway.org/Writings/organ_transplant.pdf.

Ibn ʿAbd al-Salām, ʿIzz al-Dīn. 2000. *al-Qawāʿid al-kubrā al-mawsūm bi-qawāʿid al-aḥkām fī iṣlāḥ al-anām*, eds. Nazīh Kamāl Ḥammād and ʿUthmān Jumʿa Ḍumayriyya. 2 vols. Damascus: Dār al-Qalam.

Jackson, Sherman A. 2009. *Islam and the Problem of Black Suffering*. Oxford: Oxford University Press.

Kamali, Mohammad Hashim. 2005. *Principles of Islamic Jurisprudence*. 3rd ed. Cambridge: Islamic Texts Society.

———. 2012. *Maqāṣid al-Sharīʿah, Ijtihad and Civilisational Renewal*. Occasional Papers Series, no. 20. London: International Institute of Islamic Thought.

Larsen, Lena. 2018. How Muftis Think: Islamic Legal Thought and Muslim Women in Western Europe. Leiden: Brill.
Lutz, Christopher Stephen. 2021. 'Alasdair Chalmers MacIntyre.' In *The Internet Encyclopedia of Philosophy*. Available at https://www.iep.utm.edu/.
al-Maydānī, 'Abd al-Raḥmān Ḥasan Ḥabannaka. 1998. *Ḍawābiṭ al-ma'rifa wa-uṣūl al-istidlāl wa-al munāẓara: Ṣiyāgha li-al-manṭiq wa-uṣūl al-baḥth mutamashshiya ma'a al-fikr al-Islāmī*. Damascus: Dār al-Qalam.
McGrath, Alister E. 1999. *Thomas F. Torrance: An Intellectual Biography*. London: T&T Clark.
Miller, Kris A. 2013. 'Participating in the Knowledge of God: An Engagement with the Trinitarian Epistemology of T. F. Torrance.' PhD diss., Durham University.
Moosa, E. 1993. 'Brain Death and Organ Transplantation: An Islamic Opinion.' *South African Medical Journal* 83 (6): 385–6.
———. 1998. 'Transacting the Body in the Law: Reading Fatawa on Organ Transplantation.' *Afrika Zamani: Annual Journal of African History* 6: 292–317.
Nassery, Idris. 2018. 'The Inviolability of Human Dignity.' In *The Objectives of Islamic Law: The Promises and Challenges of the Maqasid al-Shari'a*, 75–88. Lanham, MD: Lexington Books.
Nyazee, Imran Ahsan Khan. 2005. *Theories of Islamic Law: The Methodology of Ijtihād*. Islamabad: Islamic Research Institute.
Padela, Aasim I. 2013. 'Islamic Verdicts in Health Policy Discourse: Porcine-based Vaccines as a Case Study.' *Zygon* 48 (3): 655–670.
Padela, Aasim I., and Taha A. Basser. 2012. 'Brain Death: The Challenges of Translating Medical Science into Islamic Bioethical Discourse.' *Medicine and Law* 31 (3): 433–50.
Padela, Aasim I. and Rosie Duivenbode. 2018. 'The Ethics of Organ Donation, Donation after Circulatory Determination of Death, and Xenotransplantation from an Islamic Perspective.' *Xenotransplantation* 25 (3): 1–12.
Padela, Aasim I., Ahsan Arozullah, and Ebrahim Moosa. 2011. 'Brain Death in Islamic Ethico-Legal Deliberation: Challenges for Applied Islamic Bioethics.' *Bioethics* 27 (3): 132–139.
Padela, Aasim I., Hasan Shanawani, and Ahsan Arozullah. 2011. 'Medical Experts and Islamic Scholars Deliberating over Brain Death: Gaps in the Applied Islamic Bioethics Discourse.' *The Muslim World* 101 (1): 53–72.
Padela, A.I., Aasim I., Steven W. Furber, Mohammad A. Kholwadia, and Ebrahim Moosa. 2014. 'Dire Necessity and Transformation: Entry-points for Modern Science in Islamic Bioethical Assessment of Porcine Products in Vaccines.' *Bioethics* 28 (2): 59–66.
Palma, Robert J. 1984. 'Thomas F. Torrance's Reformed Theology.' *Reformed Review* 38 (1): 2–46.
Pfeffer, Gerald, Kari Majamaa, Douglass M. Turnbull, David Thorburn, and Patrick F. Chinnery. 2012. 'Treatment for Mitochondrial Disorders.' *Cochrane Database of Systematic Reviews* 4 (CD004426): 1–37.
Rasheed, Shoaib [A.]. 2011. 'Organ Donation among Muslims: An Examination of Medical Researchers' Efforts to Encourage Donation in the Muslim Community.' BA Hons. diss., University of Michigan.
Rasheed, Shoaib A., and Aasim I. Padela. 2013. 'The Interplay between Religious Leaders and Organ Donation among Muslims.' *Zygon* 48 (3): 635–654.
al-Raysūnī, Aḥmad. 2005. *Imām al-Shāṭibī's Theory of the Higher Objectives and Intents of Islamic Law*, trans. Nancy Roberts. Herndon, VA: International Institute of Islamic Thought.
Reinhart, A. Kevin. 1983. 'Islamic Law as Islamic Ethics.' *Journal of Religious Ethics* 11 (2): 186–203.
———. 1995. *Before Revelation: The Boundaries of Muslim Moral Thought*. New York, NY: State University of New York Press.
Richardson, Henry S. 1990. 'Specifying Norms as a Way to Resolve Concrete Ethical Problems.' *Philosophy and Public Affairs* 19 (4): 279–310.
al-Shāṭibī. 2011. *The Reconciliation of the Fundamentals of Islamic Law: Al-Muwāfaqāt fī Uṣūl al-Sharī'a*, trans. Imran Ahsan Khan Nyazee and Raji M. Rammuny, 2 vols. Reading: Garnet Publishing.

Straus, Sharon E., Paul Glasziou, W. Scott Richardson, and R. Brian Haynes. 2005. *Evidence-based Medicine: How to Practice and Teach It*. 3rd ed. Edinburgh: Churchill Livingstone.
Torrance, Thomas F. 2003. *Reality and Evangelical Theology: The Realism of Christian Revelation*. Eugene, OR: Wipf and Stock Publishers.
World Health Organization (WHO). 2011. *'Global Status Report on Noncommunicable Diseases 2010'*. Geneva: World Health Organization.
Yacoub, Ahmed Abdel Aziz. 2001. *The Fiqh of Medicine: Responses in Islamic Jurisprudence to Developments in Medical Science*. London: Ta-Ha Publishers.
Zeviani, Massimo, and Stefano Di Donato. 2004. 'Mitochondrial Disorders.' *Brain* 127 (10): 2153–72.

**Dr Aasim I. Padela** is a clinician, health researcher, and bioethicist at the Medical College of Wisconsin. He utilizes methodologies from health services research, religious studies, and comparative ethics to examine the encounter of Islam with contemporary biomedicine through the lives of Muslim patients and clinicians, and in the writings of Islamic scholars. His scholarship develops intellectual frameworks through which Islamic theology (both moral and scholastic) can engage with contemporary natural and social scientific data.

# Index




A. al-Akiti, A. I. Padela (eds.), *Islam and Biomedicine*, Philosophy and Medicine 137, https://doi.org/10.1007/978-3-030-53801-9

CPSIA information can be obtained
at www.ICGtesting.com
Printed in the USA
LVHW051541120323
741461LV00005B/501

9 783030 538002